THEORETICAL MODELS AND EXPERIMENTAL APPROACHES IN PHYSICAL CHEMISTRY

Research Methodology and Practical Methods

Innovations in Physical Chemistry: Monograph Series

THEORETICAL MODELS AND EXPERIMENTAL APPROACHES IN PHYSICAL CHEMISTRY

Research Methodology and Practical Methods

Edited by

A. K. Haghi, PhD
Sabu Thomas, PhD
Praveen K. M.
Avinash R. Pai

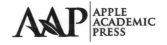

APPLE ACADEMIC PRESS

Apple Academic Press Inc.
3333 Mistwell Crescent
Oakville, ON L6L 0A2
Canada

Apple Academic Press Inc.
9 Spinnaker Way
Waretown, NJ 08758
USA

© 2019 by Apple Academic Press, Inc.

First issued in paperback 2021

Exclusive worldwide distribution by CRC Press, a member of Taylor & Francis Group
No claim to original U.S. Government works

ISBN 13: 978-1-77-463072-3 (pbk)
ISBN 13: 978-1-77-188632-1 (hbk)

Library and Archives Canada Cataloguing in Publication

Theoretical models and experimental approaches in physical chemistry : research methodology and practical methods / edited by A.K. Haghi, Sabu Thomas, Praveen K.M., Avinash R. Pai.

(Innovations in physical chemistry : monograph series)
Includes bibliographical references and index.
Issued in print and electronic formats.
ISBN 978-1-77188-632-1 (hardcover).--ISBN 978-1-315-10263-4 (PDF)

1. Chemistry, Physical and theoretical--Methodology.
I. Thomas, Sabu, editor II. Haghi, A. K., editor III. K. M., Praveen, editor IV. Pai, Avinash R., editor V. Series: Innovations in physical chemistry. Monograph series

QD453.3.T54 2018   541   C2018-904541-8   C2018-904542-6

CIP data on file with US Library of Congress

Apple Academic Press also publishes its books in a variety of electronic formats. Some content that appears in print may not be available in electronic format. For information about Apple Academic Press products, visit our website at **www.appleacademicpress.com** and the CRC Press website at **www.crcpress.com**

CONTENTS

ABOUT THE INNOVATIONS IN PHYSICAL CHEMISTRY: MONOGRAPH SERIES

This book series aims to offer a comprehensive collection of books on physical principles and mathematical techniques for majors, non-majors, and chemical engineers. Because there are many exciting new areas of research involving computational chemistry, nanomaterials, smart materials, high-performance materials, and applications of the recently discovered graphene, there can be no doubt that physical chemistry is a vitally important field. Physical chemistry is considered a daunting branch of chemistry—it is grounded in physics and mathematics and draws on quantum mechanics, thermodynamics, and statistical thermodynamics.

Editors-in-Chief

A. K. Haghi, PhD
Editor-in-Chief, International Journal of Chemoinformatics and Chemical Engineering and Polymers Research Journal; Member, Canadian Research and Development Center of Sciences and Cultures (CRDCSC), Montreal, Quebec, Canada Email: AKHaghi@Yahoo.com

Lionello Pogliani, PhD
University of Valencia-Burjassot, Spain
Email: lionello.pogliani@uv.es

Ana Cristina Faria Ribeiro, PhD
Researcher, Department of Chemistry, University of Coimbra, Portugal
Email: anacfrib@ci.uc.pt

Books in the Series

- **Applied Physical Chemistry with Multidisciplinary Approaches**
  Editors: A. K. Haghi, PhD, Devrim Balköse, PhD, and Sabu Thomas, PhD

- **Chemical Technology and Informatics in Chemistry with Applications**
  Editors: Alexander V. Vakhrushev, DSc, Omari V. Mukbaniani, DSc, and Heru Susanto, PhD

- **Engineering Technologies for Renewable and Recyclable Materials: Physical-Chemical Properties and Functional Aspects**
  Editors: Jithin Joy, Maciej Jaroszewski, PhD, Praveen K. M., Sabu Thomas, PhD, and Reza Haghi, PhD

- **Engineering Technology and Industrial Chemistry with Applications**
  Editors: Reza Haghi, PhD, and Francisco Torrens, PhD

- **High-Performance Materials and Engineered Chemistry**
  Editors: Francisco Torrens, PhD, Devrim Balköse, PhD, and Sabu Thomas, PhD

- **Methodologies and Applications for Analytical and Physical Chemistry**
  Editors: A. K. Haghi, PhD, Sabu Thomas, PhD, Sukanchan Palit, and Priyanka Main

- **Modern Physical Chemistry: Engineering Models, Materials, and Methods with Applications**
  Editors: Reza Haghi, PhD, Emili Besalú, PhD, Maciej Jaroszewski, PhD, Sabu Thomas, PhD, and Praveen K. M.

- **Physical Chemistry for Chemists and Chemical Engineers: Multidisciplinary Research Perspectives**
  Editors: Alexander V. Vakhrushev, DSc, Reza Haghi, PhD, and J. V. de Julián-Ortiz, PhD

- **Physical Chemistry for Engineering and Applied Sciences: Theoretical and Methodological Implication**
  Editors: A. K. Haghi, PhD, Cristóbal Noé Aguilar, PhD, Sabu Thomas, PhD, and Praveen K. M.

- **Theoretical Models and Experimental Approaches in Physical Chemistry: Research Methodology and Practical Methods**
  Editors: A. K. Haghi, PhD, Sabu Thomas, PhD, Praveen K. M., and Avinash R. Pai

ABOUT THE EDITORS

A. K. Haghi, PhD, is the author and editor of over 165 books, as well as 1000 published papers in various journals and conference proceedings. Dr. Haghi has received several grants, consulted for a number of major corporations, and is a frequent speaker to national and international audiences. Since 1983, he has served as professor at several universities. He is currently editor-in-chief of the *International Journal of Chemoinformatics and Chemical Engineering* and *Polymers Research Journal* and serves on the editorial boards of many international journals. He is also a member of the Canadian Research and Development Center of Sciences and Cultures (CRDCSC), Montreal, Quebec, Canada. He holds a BSc in urban and environmental engineering from the University of North Carolina (USA), an MSc in mechanical engineering from North Carolina A&T State University (USA), a DEA in applied mechanics, acoustics and materials from the Université de Technologie de Compiègne (France), and a PhD in engineering sciences from the Université de Franche-Comté (France).

Sabu Thomas, PhD, is Pro-Vice Chancellor of Mahatma Gandhi University and Founding Director of the International and Inter University Center for Nanoscience and Nanotechnology, Mahatma Gandhi University, Kottayam, Kerala, India. He is also a full professor of polymer science and engineering at the School of Chemical Sciences of the same university, and a fellow of many professional bodies. Professor Thomas's research group has specialized in many areas of polymers, which includes polymer blends, fiber-filled polymer composites, particulate-filled polymer composites and their morphological characterization, ageing and degradation, pervaporation phenomena, sorption and diffusion, interpenetrating polymer systems, recyclability and reuse of waste plastics and rubbers, elastomeric crosslinking, and dual porous nanocomposite scaffolds for tissue engineering, etc. Professor Thomas's research group has extensive exchange programs with different industries and research and academic institutions all over the world and is performing world-class collaborative research in various fields. Professor Thomas's center is equipped with various sophisticated instruments and has established state-of-the-art experimental facilities, which cater to the needs of researchers within the country and abroad.

Professor Thomas has published over 750 peer-reviewed research papers, reviews, and book chapters and has a citation count of 31,574. The H index of Prof. Thomas is 81, and he has six patents to his credit. He has delivered over 300 plenary, inaugural, and invited lectures at national/international meetings across 30 countries. He is a reviewer for many international journals. He has received MRSI, CRSI, nanotech medals for his outstanding work in nanotechnology. Recently Prof. Thomas has been conferred an Honoris Causa (DSc) by the University of South Brittany, France, and University of Lorraine, Nancy, France.

Praveen K. M. is Assistant Professor of mechanical engineering at SAINTGITS College of Engineering, India. He is currently pursuing a PhD in engineering sciences at the University of South Brittany—Laboratory IRDL PTR1, Research Center "Christiaan Huygens," in Lorient, France, in the area of coir-based polypropylene microcomposites and nanocomposites. He has published an international article in *Applied Surface Science* and has also presented posters and conference papers at national and international conferences. He has also worked with the Jozef Stefan Institute, Ljubljana, Slovenia; Mahatma Gandhi University, India; and the Technical University in Liberec, Czech Republic. His current research interests include plasma modification of polymers, polymer composites for neutron shielding applications, and nanocellulose.

Avinash R. Pai is a fulltime doctoral student at the International and Inter University Center for Nanoscience and Nanotechnology, Mahatma Gandhi University, under the guidance of Prof. Sabu Thomas. He received his bachelor's degree in polymer engineering from Mahatma Gandhi University and holds a master's degree in polymer engineering from the Institute of Chemical Technology, Mumbai, India. He is also a recipient of the Visvesvaraya PhD fellowship instituted by Media Lab Asia, MeitY, Government of India. His research interests include the development of flexible polymer nanocomposites for various technological applications.

LIST OF CONTRIBUTORS

Laxmi
Inorganic Materials Research Laboratory, Department of Chemistry, Jamia Millia Islamia, New Delhi 110025, India

Ann Rose Abraham
School of Pure and Applied Physics, International & Inter University Centre for Nanoscience and Nanotechnology, Mahatma Gandhi University, Kottayam, Kerala 686560, India

Cristobal N. Aguilar
Food Research Department, School of Chemistry, Universidad Autónoma de Coahuila, Blvd. V. Carranza and González Lobo s/n, ZIP 25280. Saltillo, Coahuila, México
E-mail: cristobal.aguilar@uadec.edu

Antonio F. Aguilera-Carbo
Department of Food Science and Technology, Universidad Autónoma Agraria Antonio Narro, Buenavista, Saltillo, Coahuila, México

Manoj B.
Material Sciences Research Laboratory, Department of Physics, Christ University, Bengaluru 560029, Karnataka, India

Tamal Banerjee
Department of Chemical Engineering, Indian Institute of Technology Guwahati, Guwahati 781039, Assam, India

Ruth E. Belmares
Food Research Department, School of Chemistry, Universidad Autónoma de Coahuila, Blvd. V. Carranza and González Lobo s/n, ZIP 25280. Saltillo, Coahuila, México

Gloria Castellano
Departamento de Ciencias Experimentales y Matemáticas, Facultad de Veterinaria y Ciencias Experimentales, Universidad Católica de Valencia San Vicente Mártir, Guillem de Castro-94, E-46001 València, Spain

Edith M. Colunga-Urbina
Analytical Chemistry Department, School of Chemistry, Universidad Autónoma de Coahuila, Blv. V. Carranza and González Lobo s/n, ZIP 25280, Saltillo, Coahuila, México

Juan C. Contreras-Esquivel
Food Research Department, School of Chemsitry, Universidad Autónoma de Coahuila, Saltillo, 25280, Coahuila, México

Soma Das
Department of Chemistry, CMR Institute of Technology, Bangalore 560037, India

Dulce A. Flores-Maltos
Food Research Department, School of Chemistry, Universidad Autónoma de Coahuila, Blvd. V. Carranza and González Lobo s/n, ZIP 25280, Saltillo, Coahuila, México

Pedro Furtado
Departamento de Engenharia Informatica, Faculdade de Ciências e tecnologia da Univrsidade de Coimbra, Coimbra, Portugal, E-mail: pnf@dei.uc.pt

Neelam Gautam
Botanical survey of India, Allahabad, India

Sushma P. Ijardar
Department of Chemistry, Veer Narmad South Gujarat University, Surat 395007, India;
Salt and Marine Chemicals Division, CSIR—Central Salt and Marine Chemicals Research Institute (CSIR-CSMCRI), Council of Scientific & Industrial Research (CSIR), Bhavnagar 364002, India
E-mail: sushmaijardar@yahoo.co.in

Rajesh A. Joshi
Department of Physics, Toshniwal Arts, Commerce and Science College, Sengaon 431542, Dist. Hingoli, Maharashtra, India, E-mail: urajoshi@gmail.com

Nandakumar Kalarikkal
School of Pure and Applied Physics, International & Inter University Centre for Nanoscience and Nanotechnology, Mahatma Gandhi University, Kottayam, Kerala 686560, India; International & Inter University Centre for Nanoscience and Nanotechnology, Mahatma Gandhi University, Kottayam, Kerala 686560, India, E-mail: nkkalarikkal@mgu.ac.in

Shabnam Khan
Inorganic Materials Research Laboratory, Department of Chemistry, Jamia Millia Islamia, New Delhi 110025, India

Arvind Kumar
Salt and Marine Chemicals Division, CSIR—Central Salt and Marine Chemicals Research Institute (CSIR-CSMCRI), Council of Scientific & Industrial Research (CSIR), Bhavnagar 364002, India

Debashis Kundu
Department of Chemical Engineering, Indian Institute of Technology Guwahati, Guwahati 781039, Assam, India

Jerald A. Lalman
Department of Civil and Environmental Engineering, University of Windsor, Windsor, ON N9B 3P4, Canada

Naved I. Malek
Applied Chemistry Department, S. V. National Institute of Technology, Surat 395007, India
E-mail: navedmalek@chem.svnit.ac.in, navedmalek@yahoo.co.in

Zubin R. Master
Applied Chemistry Department, S. V. National Institute of Technology, Surat 395007, India

Anu N. Mohan
Material Sciences Research Laboratory, Department of Physics, Christ University, Bengaluru 560029, Karnataka, India; Department of Physics, School of Graduate Studies, Jain University, J C Road, Bengaluru 560027, Karnataka, India, E-mail: anunmohan@gmail.com

C. O. Mohan
Senior Scientist, Fish Processing Division, ICAR-Central Institute of Fisheries Technology, CIFT Junction, Matsyapuri P.O., Willingdon Island, Kochi, Kerala 682029 India
E-mail: comohan@gmail.com

Nahid Nishat
Inorganic Materials Research Laboratory, Department of Chemistry, Jamia Millia Islamia,
New Delhi 110025, India, E-mail: nishat_nchem08@yahoo.com

Sukanchan Palit
Assistant Professor (Senior Scale), Department of Chemical Engineering, University of Petroleum
and Energy Studies, Post Office Bidholi via Premnagar, Dehradun 248007, Uttarakhand, India;
43, Judges Bagan, Post-Office Haridevpur, Kolkata 700082, India
Tel.: 0091-8958728093, E-mail: sukanchan68@gmail.com, sukanchan92@gmail.com

Arely Prado-Barragan
Department of Biotechnology, Universidad Autonoma Metropolitana Unidad Iztapalapa,
Mexico City, Mexico

C. N. Ravishankar
ICAR—Central Institute of Fisheries Technology, CIFT Junction, Matsyapuri P.O.,
Willingdon Island, Kochi, Kerala 682029, India

Srimanta Ray
Department of Chemical Engineering, National Institute of Technology, Agartala 799046,
Barjala, Jirania, West Tripura, Tripura, India
E-mail: rays.nita@gmail.com, srimanta.chemical@nita.ac.in

Armando Robledo
Food Research Department, School of Chemsitry, Universidad Autónoma de Coahuila,
Saltillo, 25280, Coahuila, México

Raúl Rodríguez
Food Research Department, School of Chemistry, Universidad Autónoma de Coahuila,
Blvd. V. Carranza and González Lobo s/n, ZIP 25280, Saltillo, Coahuila, México

L. V. Rodríguez-Duran
Food Research Department, School of Chemistry, Universidad Autónoma de Coahuila,
Blvd. V. Carranza and González Lobo s/n, ZIP 25280, Saltillo, Coahuila, México

Raul Rodríguez-Herrera
Food Research Department, School of Chemsitry, Universidad Autónoma de Coahuila,
Saltillo 25280, Coahuila, México

Mitali Saha
Department of Chemistry, National Institute of Technology, Agartala 799055, India

José Sandoval-Cortés
Analytical Chemistry Department, School of Chemistry, Universidad Autónoma de Coahuila,
Blv. V. Carranza and González Lobo s/n, ZIP 25280, Saltillo, Coahuila, México
E-mail: josesandoval@uadec.edu.mx

Leonardo Sepulveda-Torre
Food Research Department, School of Chemsitry, Universidad Autónoma de Coahuila,
Saltillo 25280, Coahuila, México

Eram Sharmin
Department of Pharmaceutical Chemistry, College of Pharmacy, Umm Al-Qura University,
PO Box 715, 21955 Makkah Al-Mukarramah, Saudi Arabia

Anamika Singh

Department of Botany, Maitreyi College, University of Delhi, Delhi, India
E-mail: arjumika@gmail.com

Rajeev Singh

Department of Environmental Studies, Satyawati College, University of Delhi, Delhi, India

P. Suresh

Department of ECE, Veltech Dr. RR, Dr. SR University, Avadi, Chennai 600062, Tamil Nadu, India

Heru Susanto

Department of Computer Science & Information Management, Tunghai University, Taichung, Taiwan; Computational Science, The Indonesian Institute of Sciences, Serpong, Indonesia

Sabu Thomas

International & Inter University Centre for Nanoscience and Nanotechnology, Mahatma Gandhi University, Kottayam, Kerala 686560, India

Francisco Torrens

Institut Universitari de Ciència Molecular, Universitat de València, Edifici d'Instituts de Paterna, P. O. Box 22085, E-46071 València, Spain

R. R. Usmanova

Ufa State Technical University of Aviation, Ufa 450000, Bashkortostan, Russia
E-mail: Usmanovarr@mail.ru

Zuber S. Vaid

Applied Chemistry Department, S. V. National Institute of Technology, Surat 395007, India

Fahmina Zafar

Inorganic Materials Research Laboratory, Department of Chemistry, Jamia Millia Islamia, New Delhi 110025, India, E-mail: fahmzafar@gmail.com

G. E. Zaikov

N. M. Emanuel Institute of Biochemical Physics, Russian Academy of Sciences, Moscow 119991, Russia, E-mail: chembio@chph.ras.ru

LIST OF ABBREVIATIONS

AA	ascorbic acid
AAD	average absolute deviation
ABTS	2,2′-azino-bis(3-ethylbenzthiazoline-6-sulphonic acid)
AFM	atomic force microscope
AIDS	Acquired immunodeficiency syndrome
AMHs	alkali metal halides
ANS	anisole
ATP	adenosine tri-phosphate
BET	Brunauer–Emmett–Teller
BTC	1,3,5 benzene tricarboxylic acid
CA	cluster analysis
CA4	combretastatin A 4
cAMP	cyclic adenosine monophosphate
CBD	chemical bath deposition
CCNT	carbon nanotube
CDs	carbon dots
CIA	collagen-induced arthritis
CMC	critical micellar concentration
CNDs	carbon nano-diamonds
CNN	convolution neural network
CNSL	cashew nut shell liquid
COL	colchicine
CT	computed tomography
CV	cyclic voltammetry
CVB	cylindrical vector beams
DEM	discrete element method
DES	drug eluting stent
DG	digol
DMSO	dimethyl sulfoxide
DNS	direct numerical simulation
DNT	2, 4 dinitrotoluene
DO	dissolve oxygen

DOE	diffractive optical element
DOTA	1, 4, 7, 10-tetraaza-1, 4, 7, 10-tetra kis (carboxymethyl) cyclododecane
DOX	doxorubicin
DPPH	2,2-diphenyl-1-picrylhydrazyl
DPV	differential-pulse voltammetry
DSCP	disuccinate cisplatin
EA	ellagic acid
EBI	European Bioinformatics Institute
EDX	energy dispersive X-ray spectrum
EFI	eye fundus image
EMI	electromagnetic interference
EPR	Einstein–Podolsky–Rosen
ETs	Ellagitannins
FACS	fluorescence-activated cell sorting
FCC	face-centered cubic
FCCU	fluid catalytic cracking unit
FESEM	field emission-gun scanning electron microscope
FRET	fluorescence resonance energy transfer
FTIR	Fourier-transform infrared spectroscopy
GA	gallic acid
GA	genetic algorithm
GC	gas chromatography
GNL	graphene nanolayers
GQDs	graphene quantum dots
GTR	general theory of relativity
H2	4,4′bipyrazole
H2Et4BPZ	3,3″5,5′ tetraethyl4,4′ bipyrazole
H2Me4BPZ	3,3″5,5′ tetramethyl4,4′ bipyrazole
H2Thz	2,5-thiazolo(5,4-d)thiazoledicarboxylic acid
H3BTC	trimesic acid 4,4′-bipy 4,4′-bipyridine
HBP	hydroxybutyl phthalate
HDI	hexa methylene diamine
HGB	hollow Gaussian beam
HHDP	hexahydroxydiphenic acid
HOG	histogram of oriented gradients
HPLC	High-performance liquid chromatography
HPP	mono (hydroxyl pentyl) phthalate

IAA	indole acetic acid
IBA	indole-3-butyric acid
IC50	concentration for 50% Inhibition
IPDI	isophorone diisocyanate
LBP	local binary patterns
LES	Large Eddy Simulation
LLE	liquid–liquid extraction
LO	longitudinal optical
LOD	limit of detection
LOQ	limit of quantification
LPG	liquefied petroleum gas
LSPR	localized surface plasmon resonance
LSV	linear sweep voltammetry
MB	methylene blue
MRI	magnetic resonance imaging
MSNPs	mesoporous silica nanoparticles
MTBE	tert-butyl methyl ether
MWCNT	multiwall carbon nanotube
NAA	naphthalene acetic acid
NCs	nanocrystals
NCPs	nanoscale coordination polymer particles
NEA	N-ethylaniline
NGS	next-generation sequencing
NMOFs	nanoscale metal organic frameworks
NRTL	non-random two-liquid
OI	optical imaging
OTF	optical transfer function
PBS	phosphate buffer solution
PC	principal component
PCA	principal components analysis
PCD	partial correlation diagram
PCL	polycaprolactone
PcMF	metallo-fluoro-phthalocyanines stack polymer
PDT	photodynamic therapy
PEG	polyethylene glycol
PGA	polyglycolic acid
PIC	2 phenylindole 3 carbaldehyde
PL	photoluminescence

PL	periodic law
PLA	polylactic acid
PLGA	lactide-co-glycolide copolymers
POE	polyortho ester
PSQN	polysilsesquioxane nanoparticles
PT	periodic table
PU	polyurethane
Pz	pyrazole
QC	quantum computer
QD	quantum decoherence
QM	quantum mechanics
QSAR	quantitative structure–activity relationship
RAM	radar-absorbing material
RANS	Reynolds Averaged Navier–Stokes
RMSD	root mean square deviation
SAR	specific absorption rate
SAR	structure–activity relationship
SARS	severe acquired respiratory syndrome
SBML	systems biology markup language
SG	splits graph
SIFT	scale-invariant feature transform
SILAR	successive ionic layer adsorption and reaction
SLIC	simple linear iterative clustering
SMHs	sodium metal halides
SOP	state of polarization
SPIONs	superparamagnetic iron oxide nanoparticles
SSF	solid-state fermentation
SVM	support vector machines
SWV	square wave voltammetry
TCA	trichloroacetic acid
TDI	toluene diisocyanate
TEA	triethanolamine
TEM	transmission electron microscopy
THF	tetrahydrofuran
THP	Total hydrolyzable phenols
TNT	2,4,6 trinitrotoluene
TO	transverse optical
TPA	dye-two photons absorbing

TPA	texture profile analysis
TPU	thermoplastic polyurethane
TTIP	titanium tetraisopropoxide
UNIQUAC	UNIversal QUAsi Chemical
UT	polyuria
WF	wave function
XRD	X-ray diffraction

LIST OF SYMBOLS

%	percent
Δn_D	deviation in refractive index
°C	degree Celsius
μ_g	dynamic viscosity of gas
CO_2	carbon dioxide
d_p	diameter of corpuscles
E_g	band gap energy
KBr	potassium bromide
KCl	potassium chloride
KI	potassium iodide
NaBr	sodium bromide
NaCl	sodium chloride
NaF	sodium fluoride
n_D	refractive index
q_S	specific substrate uptake rate
r	a geometry of the apparatus
R	Rao's molar sound function
TiO_2	titanium dioxide
X_M	maximal biomass level
$Y_{P/X}$	enzyme/biomass yield
ZnO	zinc oxide
α	hydrogen bond donating value
β	hydrogen bond accepting value
ε	dielectric constant
μ	specific growth rate
μ_M	maximal specific growth rate
ρ_p	corpuscle density
v_g	speed of radial
v_z	speed of axis
v_φ	speed of tangential
P	pressure

PREFACE

This book presents an up-to-date review of modern materials and physical chemistry concepts, issues, and recent advances in the field. Distinguished scientists and engineers from key institutions worldwide have contributed chapters that provide a deep analysis of their particular subjects.

It presents a modern theoretical and experimental approach in applied physical chemistry. The volume discusses the developments of advanced chemical products and respective tools to characterize and predict the chemical material properties and behavior.

This volume generates understanding through numerous examples and practical applications drawn from research and development chemistry. The authors allow a greater understanding of problems more quickly and easily than purely intuitive methods. It emphasizes the intersection of chemistry, mathematics, physics, and the resulting applications across many disciplines of science and explores applied physical chemistry principles in specific areas. At the same time, each topic is framed within the context of a broader more interdisciplinary approach, demonstrating its relationship and interconnectedness to other areas. The premise of this work, therefore, is to offer a comprehensive understanding of applied science and engineering as a whole as well as thorough knowledge of individual subjects. This approach appropriately conveys the basic fundamentals, state-of-the-art technology, and applications of the involved disciplines, and further encourages scientific collaboration among researchers.

The book is divided into following three parts:

PART 1—Experimental Innovations and Theoretical Methods
PART 2—Biophysical Chemistry from a Different Angle
PART 3—Multidisciplinary Perspectives

This new book fills the gap within modeling texts, focusing on applications across a broad range of disciplines, and presents information on many important problems of physical chemistry. These investigations are accompanied by real-life applications in practice. Some other highlights of this volume are:

1. It highlights some important areas of current interest in new products and chemical processes.
2. It focuses on topics with more advanced methods.
3. It emphasizes precise mathematical development and actual experimental details.
4. It analyzes theories to formulate and prove the physicochemical principles.
5. It provides an up-to-date and thorough exposition of the present state of the art of complex materials.

PART I

Experimental Innovations and Theoretical Methods

CHAPTER 1

COORDINATION POLYMERS: A BRIEF OVERVIEW FROM SYNTHESIS TO ADVANCED APPLICATIONS

LAXMI[1], SHABNAM KHAN[1], ERAM SHARMIN[2], FAHMINA ZAFAR[1,*] and NAHID NISHAT[1,*]

[1]*Inorganic Materials Research Laboratory, Department of Chemistry, Jamia Millia Islamia, New Delhi 110025, India*

[2]*Department of Pharmaceutical Chemistry, College of Pharmacy, Umm Al-Qura University, PO Box 715, 21955 Makkah Al-Mukarramah, Saudi Arabia*

Corresponding author. E-mails:fahmzafar@gmail.com; nishat_nchem08@yahoo.com

CONTENTS

ABSTRACT

This chapter deals with brief overview of coordination polymers (CPs), metal organic frameworks (MOFs), nano metal organic frameworks (NMOFs), classification, synthesis methods, strategies for incorporating the biomedically relevant agents within NMOFs with their advanced applications.

1.1   INTRODUCTION

Metal ion-incorporated polymers are area of keen interest due to alarming rise in the current field of chemical research. The idea of metal ions incorporation into monomeric or polymeric ligands in different arrays[1–6] has captured the great attention of researchers to develop new materials with desirable physical as well as chemical properties. These desirable properties can be achieved with the use of different metal ions and organic linkers. During the past two decades, enormous research efforts have been made to develop the metal-containing polymers or metal organic frameworks (MOFs) or coordination polymers (CPs) or coordination networks by self-assembling[7–9] simple and small ligands to large mesoporous frameworks,[10,11] which are frequently used in almost all fields of science because of their unique architectural motifs and topologies. They are used in material chemistry,[12] adsorption,[13] pollutant sequestration,[14] gas adsorption, separation, biomedical fields (antibacterial, antifungal, and anticancer agents), healthcare products, catalysis,[15] magnetism,[16] optics,[17–20] sensors,[21,22] biosensing,[23–26] medical diagnostics,[27,28] energy storage, batteries,[29,30] data storage,[31,32] and others.[33]

The chemical and physical properties along with advanced applications of these solid materials are mainly dependent on the shape and size of the microscopic entities.[34–36] This fact becomes more prominent when the size of the material falls in the nanoscale region. Facts and knowledge accumulated in the field of coordination chemistry during the past decade enable material scientists and chemists to engineer and synthesize different polymeric materials. A massive expansion has been recorded in the class of CPs along with the MOFs.

The chapter deals with brief overview of CPs, MOFs, nano metal organic frameworks (NMOFs), classification, synthesis methods, strategies for incorporating the biomedically relevant agents within NMOFs with their advanced applications.

1.2 COORDINATION POLYMERS (CPs)

CPs is a class of hybrid materials made up of metal nodes (having vacant sites to coordinate) and mono- or poly-dentate organic ligands (also called bridging linkers or ligand) (Fig. 1.1).[37] Thus, for self-assembling, selection of organic ligands (e.g., carboxylates, imidazolates, or phosphonates, porphyrin, cyclodextrin, adeninate, L-valine, serine derivative, peptides, polyurea, polyurethane (PU), N-heterocyclics, and others) seems to be important along with the metal ion clusters connected through the coordinate or other weak chemical bonds under mild conditions.[38–43] Since small change in organic ligands leads to considerable changes in coordination framework, thus physiochemical properties of CPs can be conveniently tuned for a particular application.

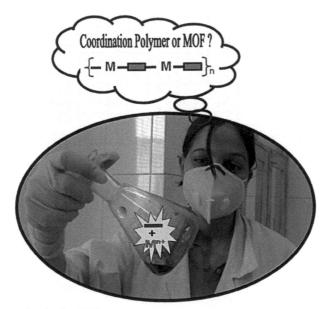

FIGURE 1.1   Synthesis of CP.

However, the synthesis of CPs has many limitations as it takes a very long completion time with the emission of toxic volatile organic solvents after proceeding through multistep processes. So, to design the CPs with desirable properties, field has to move in several different directions depending on their individual properties.

1.2.1   CLASSIFICATION OF CPs

On the basis of arrangement of metal ions and bridging ligands in space, CPs may be classified into one-, two-, or three-dimensional CPs.

Structure extending along the x-axis is called one-dimensional (Fig. 1.2).

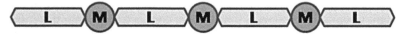

FIGURE 1.2   One-dimensional CP.

Structure extending along two directions, x- and y- axes is called two-dimensional (Fig. 1.3).

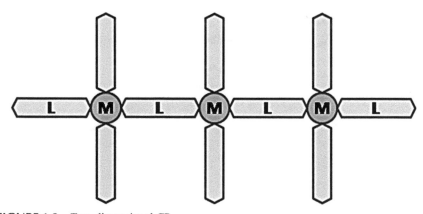

FIGURE 1.3   Two-dimensional CP.

Structure extending in all three directions, x-, y-, and z- axes is called three-dimensional[44] (Fig. 1.4).

CPs have been further classified into different groups by varying the position of metal.

   i)   **Metal as a pendant group:** Coordination complexes or CPs containing functionalized ligands and metals act as part of pendant substituents and undergo polymerization. On the basis of ligands

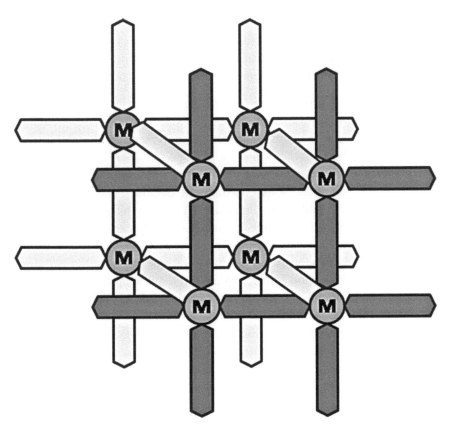

FIGURE 1.4   Three-dimensional CP.

having different chelating abilities, they are categorized as mono-dentate and poly-dentate.

- **Mono-dentate pendant CPs:** In the formation of mono-dentate pendant CPs, low molecular weight ligands mask the central metal ions leaving one unoccupied position. The mono-dentate type CPs can be synthesized by carrying out the reaction among polymeric ligand and excess amount of metal ions, which decrease the possibility of substitution of second labile ligand and leading to the synthesis of mono-dentate type CPs.[45]

- **Poly-dentate pendant CPs:** These polymers are bridged, stable metal complexes.[46] For example, 1, 1-disubstituted ferrocenes with radical or cationic initiation undergo cyclopolymerization and form poly-dentate pendant CPs.

ii) **Metal as a crosslinking agent:** Several substituted ferrocenes condense to form linear polymeric chain, which is cross-linked to the ferrocene moieties. Multidentate polymers yield metal cross-linked CPs.

iii) **Metal as an integral part of polymer backbone:** The nature of ligands and metal ions coordination decide the dimensionality (one-, two-, and three-dimensional) of the polymer. They are amorphous and insoluble in nature.[47] Polymers having metals as part of the backbone are coordinated to two different metal atoms simultaneously, which have the potential for the addition and polymerization connecting the monomeric units. For example, polymers containing halides or pseudohalide bridges form one-, two-, or three-dimensional polymers.

iv) **Parquet polymers:** These polymers are flat, net-like organic molecules where the metal is entangled in the net.[48] They are synthesized by the polymerization of organic net without disturbing the metal environments, thus increasing the coordination number of the metal with the retention of monomeric organic unit. Polyphthalocyanato, polyporphyrinato, and polyporphyrinato copper complexes are examples of such polymers. Polyporphyrinato copper complex is synthesized by reacting tetracyanoethylene with copper (II)-acetylacetonate under particular conditions (200°C and vacuum).[49]

v) **Stacked metal chain complexes:** A complex without macrocyclic ligands is called stacked metal chain complex. In such complexes, the ligands do not chelate the metal ion. For example, tetra-cyanoplatinate is a stacked complex. These materials act as one-dimensional conductor with conductivities greater than $1 \ \Omega^{-1}cm^{-1}$.[50,51]

vi) **Magnus green salt:** Magnus green salt is a class of compound with a linear chain of platinum atoms, developed from the columnar stacking of the constituent planar complex units. It is synthesized by mixing an aqueous solutions of $[Pt \ (NH_3)_4]^{2+}$ with $[PtCl_4]^{2-}$.[52]

vii) **Polymetallocenes:** These organometallic polymers possess transition metal ions in their main chain and slight change in their chemical structure leads to tuned properties of polymer. For example, Multidecker sandwich structure.[53]

viii) **Poly-ynes:** The transition metal poly-ynes polymer[54,55] is an unusual class of organometallic polymers in which transition metal is bound to the carbon atom of the main chain, which might be considered as CP. Platinum and palladium copolymers, having rod-like structure belong to this class.

ix) **Shish kebab CPs:** It is the class of stacked macrocyclic metal complexes based on CP in which bridging ligand connects the macrocyclic complexes through axial coordination.

- **O-bridged polymeric compounds:** Metallo-macrocycles like phthalocyanine (Pc) crystallize in stacks to have straight line pattern and conduct electricity through their metal ligand linkages along stack axis. Metal phthalocyanin gives M (Pc)(OH)$_2$, where (MO)$_n$ is repeating unit. It is made by the polycondensation yielding metallo-phthalocyanines co-facial arrays.

- **S-bridged polymeric compounds:** When sulfur replaced the oxygen in a polymeric compound to observe whether overlapping of d-orbital has any influence on the conductivity before and after doping they are called S-bridged polymeric compounds, for example, poly (thio-1,4-phenylene) polymer.[56]

- **F-bridged polymeric compound:** Kenney et al.[57] have reported bridging metallo fluoro-phthalocyanines stack polymer, (PcMF)$_n$ (where M=Al, Ga, Cr. PcAlOH, and PcGaOH). They have been synthesized by reacting PcAlCl and PcGaCl in NH$_4$OH or pyridine. The PcAlOH and PcGaOH thus formed are treated with concentrated aqueous (48%) HF to give (PcMF)$_n$.

- **Alkynyl-bridged polymers:** These polymers are achieved by the reaction of phthalocyaninato metal dichloride and the appropriate Grignard reagent.[58] These are usually transition metal complexes with flat π-conjugated ligands.[59,60]

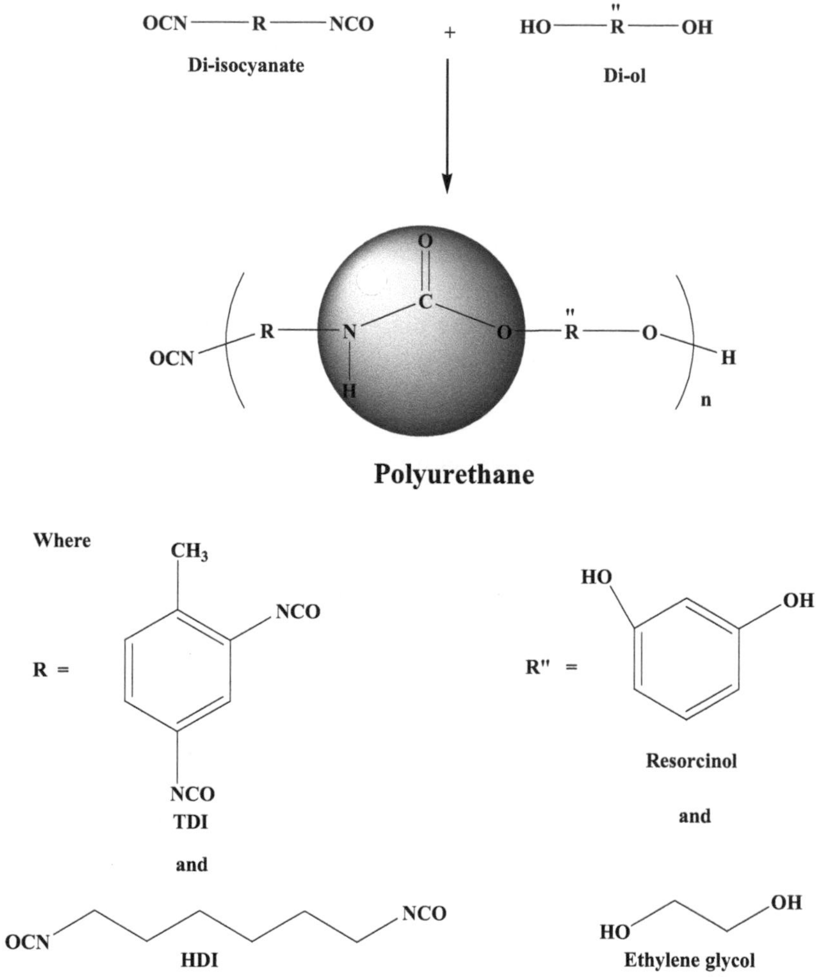

FIGURE 1.5   Polyurethanes synthesis.

1.2.2   CPs WITH DIFFERENT FUNCTIONAL LINKAGES

1.2.2.1   CPs WITH URETHANE LINKAGES (COORDINATED POLYURETHANES)

PU is basically a polymer composed of repeating organic units, joined by a urethane (carbamate) linkage Fig. 1.5. They are commonly synthesized by reacting diisocyanate with a polyol in presence of a catalyst or by activation by ultraviolet light. The diisocyanate used is either aliphatic (hexa methylene diisocyanate (HDI), isophorone diisocyanate (IPDI)), aromatic (Toluene diisocyanate (TDI)), or both and the polyol maybe a polyether polyol, that is, poly (oxy ethylene) glycol, and poly (oxy-propylene) glycol. They have versatile applications.

PU, irrespective of other synthetic polymers, has very poor thermal stability that can be improved by the presence of high cross-linking density. Hydrolytic stability of PUs also varies with the change in temperature, physical state, and degree of cross-linking of PU. The performance/prop-erties of PU (e.g., solubility, thermal stability, flexibility, fire retardancy) can be enhanced by incorporating metals in it.[61]

Coordinated PUs are formed by urethanation reaction of diol with diisocyanate, followed by metallation reaction (metal salts) of hydroxyl terminated monomers or prepolymers. R. Jaykumar et al. synthesized calcium-containing poly (urethane ether) by the reaction of calcium-salt of mono (hydroxypentyl) phthalate with TDI or HMDI, showing better coating properties.[62] R. Arun Prasath et al. synthesized metal-containing PU by reacting HMDI or TDI and mono (hydroxybutyl) phthalate metal salts and digol mixture leading to good thermal stability.[63]

1.2.2.2   CP WITH UREA LINKAGE (COORDINATED POLYUREAS)

Polyurea is a polymer that has recurring organic units joined by urea (–NH–CO–NH–) linkage. It is synthesized by the addition polymeriza-tion of isocyanate with an amine as shown in Fig. 1.6. It shows better properties like melting points, thermal stability, and chemical resistance to hydrolysis than polyesters, linear polyethylene PU, and polyamides.[64]

Metals can be incorporated in the polyurea chains through the donor groups such as C, O, –OH, –COOH, –NH$_2$ for improving their solubility-finding applications as resins, additives, catalysts, textile sizes, and in biomedical field.[65] Nahid Nishat et al. synthesized metal coordinated polyurea Fig. 1.7 by the condensation polymerization of polymeric ligands, that is, N (5 (formyl amino) 2 methylphenyl) dicarbonimidic diamide (synthesized by the addition polymerization of urea and TDI) with transi-tion metal ions. Since it showed elevated thermal stability and adsorption capacity, it can be used as an adsorbent for dyes.[66] Her research group synthesized metal-chelated polyurea by reacting TDI with chelated Schiff base diamine. The metal incorporation enhanced the thermal as well as antimicrobial activities, hence can be used as antifungal and antifouling coating purpose.[67]

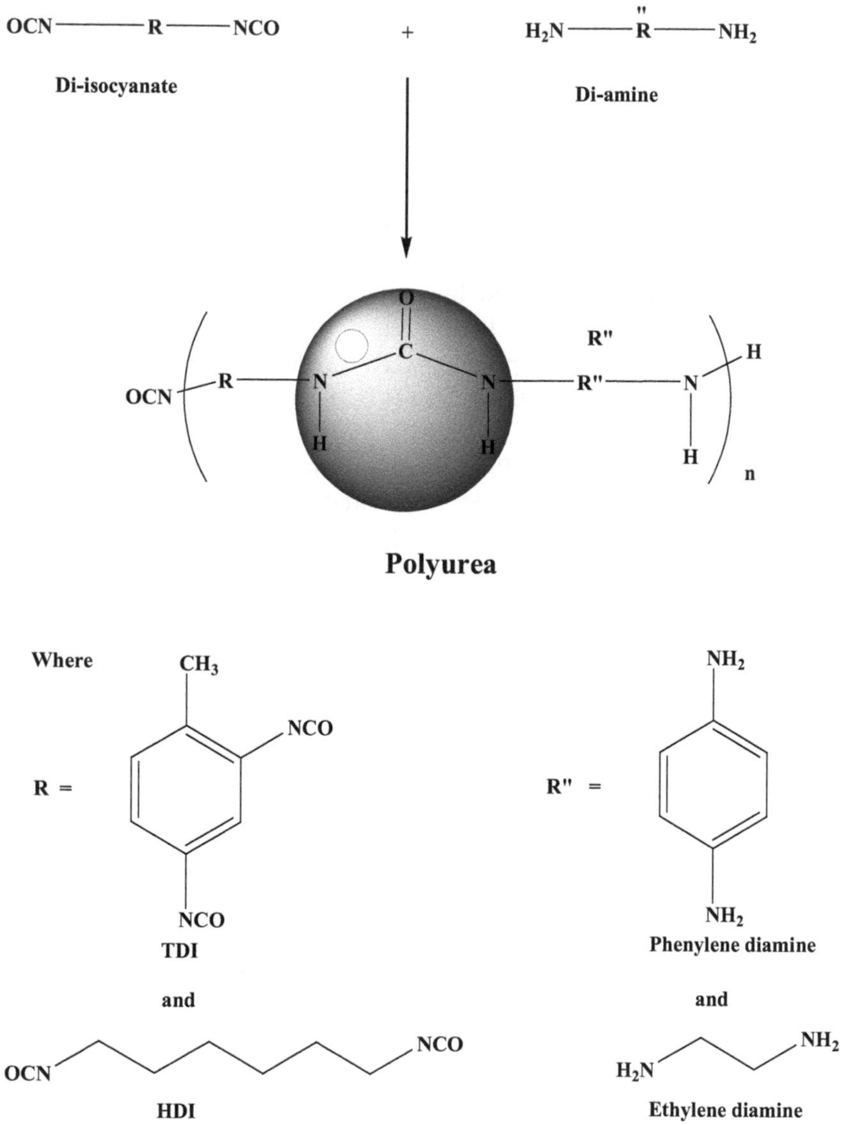

Polyurea

FIGURE 1.6   Polyureas synthesis.

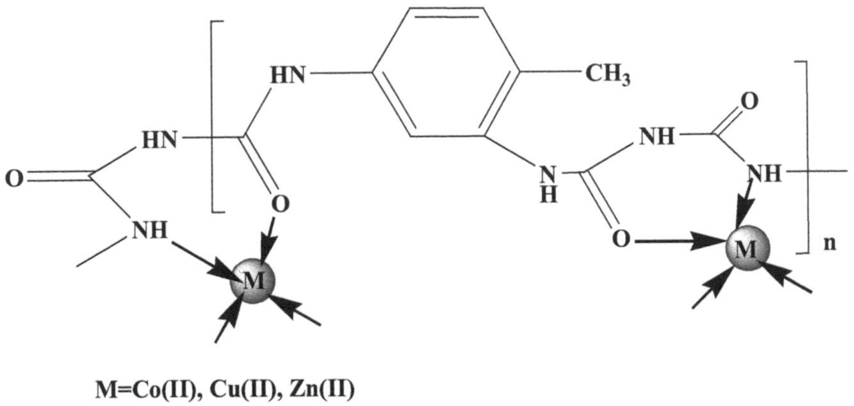

M=Co(II), Cu(II), Zn(II)

FIGURE 1.7 Synthesis of coordinated polyuria.

1.2.2.3   CPs WITH SCHIFF BASE

Metal-containing PU was synthesized (Fig. 1.8) by polymerizing the Schiff base complex incorporating N, N' bis (salicylidene) thiosemicarbazide (with transition metals) with TDI by Nahid Nishat group. It displayed high thermal stability and biocidal activities, which can be used in medical and biomaterial devices.[68] Her research group also synthesized number of metal-polychelates using polymeric Schiff as a ligand, showing excellent antibacterial and antifungal activity against *Escherichia coli, Aspergillus niger, Candida albicans*, and others.[69]

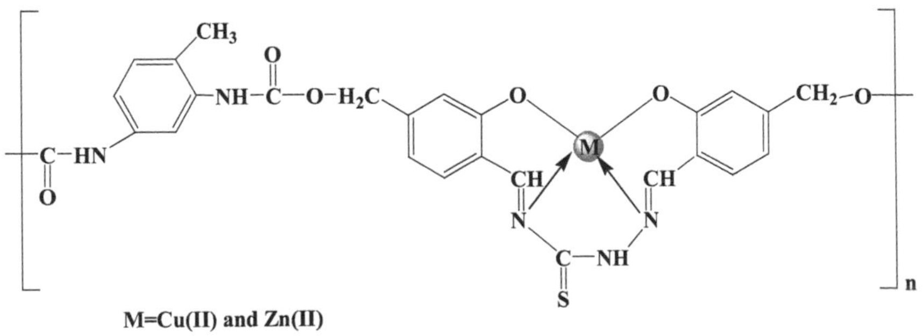

M=Cu(II) and Zn(II)

FIGURE 1.8 Synthesis of Schiff base containing coordinated PU.

TABLE 1.1 List of The CPs Reported in Literature.

S. No	Coordination polymer	Synthesis methods	Geometry	Characteristics	Applications	Ref.
1.	$Ca(HPP)_2–PEG–HMDI$	Precipitation method	–	Thermally stable, abrasion resistance	Coating	[62]
2.	$Ca(HBP)_2\text{-}HMDI\text{-}DG$	Precipitation method	–	Thermally stable	–	[63]
3.	UT–Mn (II)	Precipitation method	Octahedral	Thermally stable	Adsorption	[66]
4.	ColF-Mn-PU	Condensation followed by urethanation	Octahedral	Thermally stable	Adsorption	[85]
5.	$Tb_2(DSCP)_3(H_2O)_{12}$	Nano precipitation method	–	–	As anticancer drug	[106]
6	$Cu_2(OH)(BTC)(H_2O)$	Microwave assisted			Biomedical application	[118]
7.	$Co(H_2Me_4BPZ)_2(S_2O_6)$	Slow diffusion	Hexagonal	–	Adsorption	[218]
8.	$Co(H_2Me_4BPZ)Cl_2]\cdot2CH_3OH$	Slow diffusion	Octahedral	Thermally stable	Adsorption	[219]
9.	$Zn(H_2BPZ)_2(H_2O)_2](ClO_4)_2 \cdot 3.5\ CH_3OH$	Slow diffusion	Octahedral	Thermally stable	Adsorption	[219]
10.	$Zn(H_2BPZ)_2(H_2O)_2(NO_3)_2$	Slow diffusion	Octahedral		Adsorption	[219]
11.	$Co_4O(3,5\text{-}Me_2Pz)_6$	Microwave assisted	Cubic	Thermally stable	Adsorption	[220]
12.	Gd-benzene hexacarboxylic acid	Surfactant template solvothermal	–	–	Biological and biomedical applications	[108]
13.	$Gd(BDC)_{1.5}(H_2O)_2$	Reverse microemulsions		Crystalline	Biological and biomedical applications	[108]

TABLE 1.1 (Continued)

S. No	Coordination polymer	Synthesis methods	Geometry	Characteristics	Applications	Ref.
14.	Fe$_3$ (μ_3O)Cl(H$_2$O)(terephthalic acid)$_3$	Solvothermal method	Octahedral	Crystalline	Biomedical application	[107]
15.	Co$_2$ (H$_2$Me$_4$BPZ)$_4$ (SiF$_6$) (NCS)$_2$].3CHCl$_3$	Slow diffusion	Octahedral	–	Adsorption	[221]
16	Ni (BPZ).CH$_3$CN	Slow diffusion	Distorted octahedral	–	Adsorption	[222]
17	Cd (BPZ) (DMF)	Solvothermal method	Octahedral	Thermally stable	Adsorption	[222]
18	Cu$_2$ (H$_2$Me$_4$BPZ) Br.0.5H$_2$O	Solvothermal method	Hexagonal	Thermally stable	Use in UV-NIR region	[223]
19	Cu$_2$ (Et$_4$ BPZ)	Solvothermal method	Tetrahedral	Thermally stable	Selective adsorption and gate opening adsorption	
20	Co (H$_2$ BPZ) Cl]$_2$CH$_3$OH	Slow diffusion	Tetrahedral	Thermally stable	Adsorption	

1.3 NANOSTRUCTURED CP

If CP scaled down to nanosize range then they show many time improved overall performance of the final materials. Recently, our research group has synthesized nanostructured and nanoporous coordinated PUs. Here, the hydroxyl-terminated PU has been used as an organic linker and divalent metal ions such as Mn (II), Ni (II), and Zn (II) as metal ion nodes. The coordinated PU have been prepared through condensation polymerization of hydroxyl terminated PU with metal salts in presence of an acid catalyst Fig. 1.9). The synthesis has been carried out in very short time with minimal use of solvent. The synthesized material has been characterized by elemental analysis, conductivity, Fourier-transform infrared spectroscopy (FTIR), UV-Visible, X-ray diffraction (XRD), scanning electron microscopy–energy-dispersive X-ray spectroscopy (SEM-EDX), transmission electron microscopy (TEM), and thermogravimetric analysis (TGA).[70] In the synthesized coordinated PU, the divalent metal ions are pieced together with PU linker and arranged in octahedral (Mn (II), Ni (II)) and tetrahedral (Zn (II)) geometry, amorphous behavior, high thermal stability, layered structure having immense number of nanopores that are distributed all over the surface Fig. 1.10–1.14) and can be employed as a potent adsorbent for dye removal from waste.

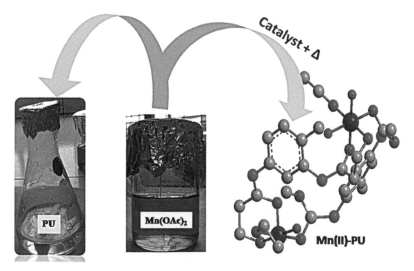

FIGURE 1.9 Synthesis of nanostructured coordination PU.

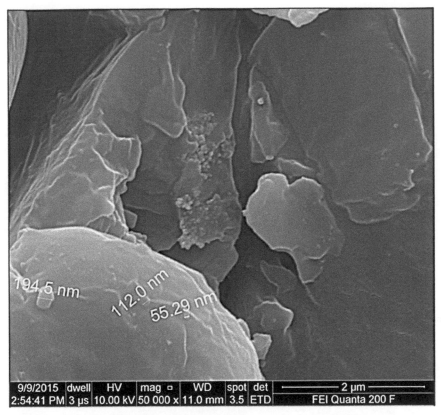

FIGURE 1.10   SEM image of nanostructured manganese coordinated PU.

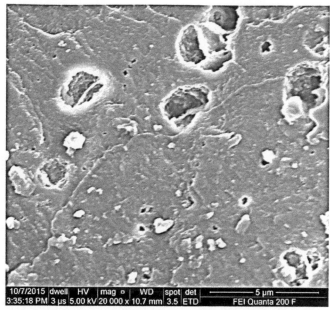

FIGURE 1.11   SEM image of nanostructured nickel coordinated PU.

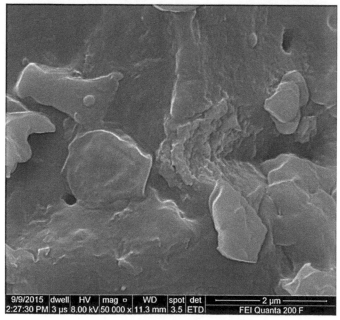

FIGURE 1.12   SEM image of nanostructured zinc coordinated PU.

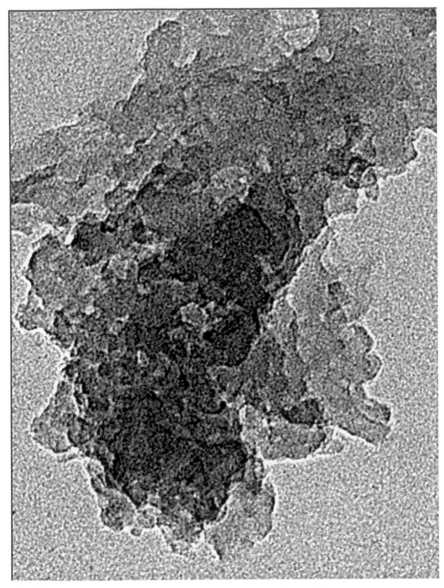

FIGURE 1.13   TEM image of nanostructure zinc coordinated PU.

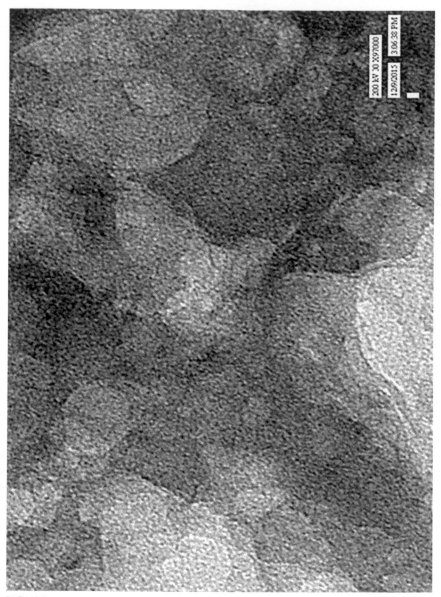

FIGURE 1.14   TEM image of nanostructured nickel coordinated PU.

As mentioned earlier, the properties and applications of CPs not only depend on metal ions but also on organic linker's geometry, length, ratio, functional group, and connectivity. In our recent work, our research group has developed nanostructured CPs from cashew nut shell liquid (CNSL)-derived ligands as organic linkers and transition metal ions via green chemistry route, which provides an alternative eco-friendly route for the scientists to develop CP with desirable properties (Fig. 1.15).[71–83]

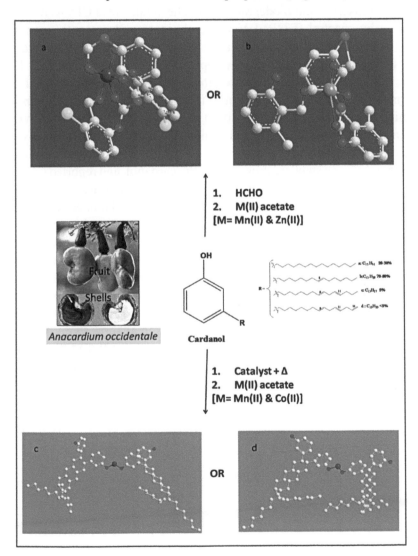

FIGURE 1.15 Synthesis of cardanol-based nanostructured CP (a) ColF-Mn-PU (b) ColF-Zn-PU (c) Col-Mn, and (d) Col-Co.

We have developed nanostructured CP (Figs. 1.16 and 1.17) self-standing transparent films from cardanol (CNSL constituent) as bridging ligand and Mn (II) and Co (II) as metal nodes via solid-state in situ method.[84] Cardanol is known for its unique characteristic features like low viscosity, phenolic hydroxyl group, high unsaturation, abundant availability, nontoxicity, and biodegradability. The synthesized CPs were characterized by spectral (FTIR, UV-Vis) techniques and magnetic moment measurements. The film curing was assessed by FTIR-ATR (attenuated total reflectance) spectral technique. Optical microscopy, SEM-EDX, HR TEM, and XRD techniques were used to investigate the morphology of the final material. TGA/DTA (differential thermal analysis) and (differential scanning calorimetry) DSC were used to analyze the thermal behavior. Antibacterial activity was assessed against *Staphylococcus aureus, Escherichia coli,* and *Pseudomonas aeruginosa* by agar disc diffusion methods and compared with standard drug ampicillin, cardanol, and reported CNSL-based CP. The synthesized CP films showed nanoporous morphology, amorphous behavior, thermal stability up to 300°C, and moderate antibacterial activity against *S. aureus, E. coli,* and *P. aeruginosa* and good antibiofilm activity. In another recent work,[85] we have developed nanostructured coordination PU free standing films from cardanol-formaldehyde[86] used as an organic linker and Mn (II) and Zn (II) divalent metal ions used as inorganic metal centers. The in situ synthesis of the aforementioned CPs involved formylation (with formaldehyde) of cardanol with formaldehyde in the presence of acid catalyst (citric acid), metallation (with divalent metal salts) of substituted methylol group (at ortho position) followed by urethanation with diisocyanate. The following reactions were confirmed by FTIR and UV-Vis spectral techniques.

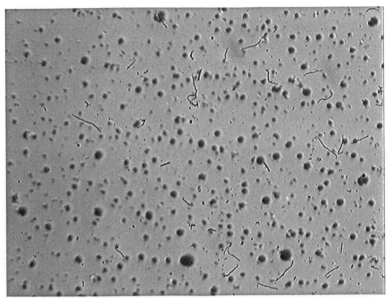

FIGURE 1.16   Optical micrographs of cardanol-based (a) Mn (II) nanostructured CP at 100×.

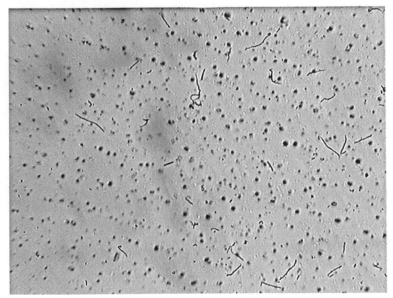

FIGURE 1.17   Optical micrographs of cardanol-based (b) Co (II) nanostructured CP at 100×.

The forenamed techniques (except antibacterial activity) along with preliminary adsorption properties for Congo red dye were used to characterize the coordination PU. They showed amorphous/semicrystalline and layered nanostructured and nanoporous patterns (Figs. 1.18 and 1.19) along with the optimum adsorption capacity (the amount of dye adsorbed per unit weight of absorbent) of 150 and 165 mg/g for Mn (II) and Zn (II) based coordination PU, respectively, at higher dye concentration.

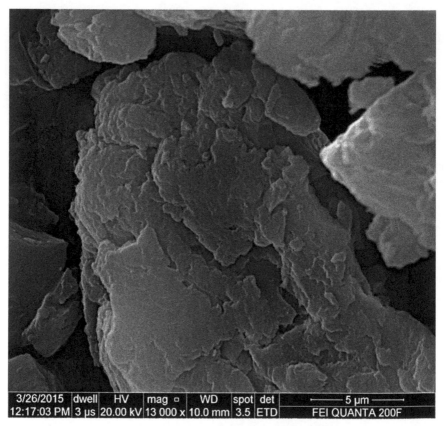

| 3/26/2015 | dwell | HV | mag □ | WD | spot | det | 5 μm |
| 12:17:03 PM | 3 μs | 20.00 kV | 13 000 x | 10.0 mm | 3.5 | ETD | FEI QUANTA 200F |

FIGURE 1.18   SEM image of cardanol-formaldehyde and Mn (II)-based nanostructured coordination PU.

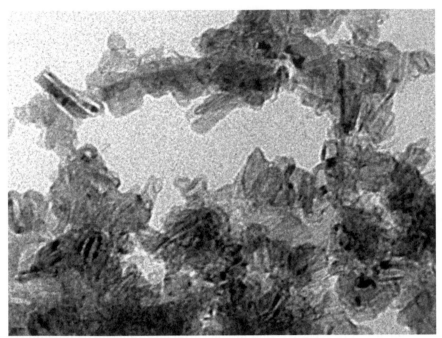

FIGURE 1.19 TEM image of cardanol-formaldehyde and Mn (II)-based nanostructured coordination PU.

1.4 METAL ORGANIC FRAMEWORKS (MOFs) AND NANO METAL ORGANIC FRAMEWORKS (NMOFs)

CPs having permanent porosity are referred as either porous CPs or MOFs. They show gas storage,[87,88] drug delivery, chromatographic separations,[89,90] gas sensing,[91] and biomedical applications[92] whereby metal nodes have served as magnetic resonance imaging (MRI), contrast agent,[93,94] and organic ligands have been used as therapeutic molecules,[95] in chemical sensing,[96–98] light harvesting,[99,100] thus raising interests at industrial level.[101]

NMOFs are the scale down of MOFs to the nanoscale region (1 nm = 10^{-9} m) and are designed as interesting nanomaterials for biological and biomedical applications. NMOFs contain metal ion in the center, linked by the polydentate bridging ligands having average diameter 1 nm to several microns. Synthesis and assembling of NMOFs in an organized array to make them operational and functional is very critical. Based on their structural regularity, NMOFs can be classified into two main groups.

- **Amorphous:** These are known as nanoscale CP particles (NCPs), can decrease the interfacial free energy present between the particle and solvent by adopting spherical morphology.
- **Crystalline:** These (known as NMOFs) have distinct morphology (non-spherical), which indicates that crystal lattice energy predominates over the particle. Its metal-ligand bond is labile, which is cleaved easily and degrades quickly, thus can be considered as essentially biodegradable.
- Since many of NMOFs materials tend to dissociate in aqueous medium they must be stabilized to enhance their utility in biological system. They have strong optical absorption, high electron density, magnetic moment, phosphorescence, or fluorescence and have great importance for the imaging and therapeutic use, for example, Au-nanoparticles and localized surface plasmon resonance (LSPR) arises by collectively oscillating the conducting electrons present in the metal nanoparticle and interact with electromagnetic radiations of appropriate frequency.[102] LSPR intensity, wavelength and shape do not change with nanoparticles composition but change only with the variation in dielectrial properties.[103] Gold nanoparticles after absorbing the light, get excited rapidly converting its excitation energy to heat that can be used in photothermal anticancer therapy.[104] Excluding Raman enhancement and Plasmon resonance, some gold nanoparticles have been publicized to exhibit strong photoluminescence,[105] which may be used in biosensing and bioimaging. The gold nanoparticle may be coated and functionalized with small molecules, polymers, and biomolecules.

1.4.1   METHODS FOR THE SYNTHESIS OF NMOFs

For NMOFs particles synthesis, various mechanistic methods have been in use, which can be useful in controlling their shape and size. There are four well-established methods commonly used to synthesize NMOFs.

1.4.1.1   NANOPRECIPITATION METHOD

To the mixture of ligand and metal cation, solvent is added, which leads to the precipitation of complex. This method produces nanoparticles because they are insoluble while the precursor remains dissolved in the same solvent. It is a surfactant free synthesis. For example, NMOFs synthesis containing anticancer drug c,c,t Pt(NH$_3$)Cl(Succinate)$_2$ (DSCP), and Tb^{3+}. Other nanocarriers have not been used to load cisplatin in high quantity[106] shown in Figure 1.20.

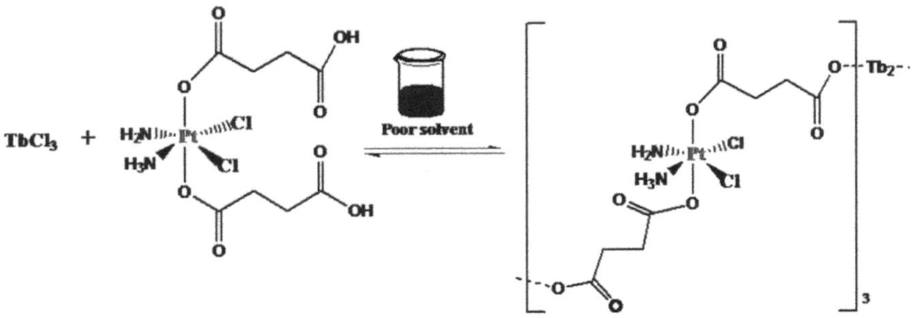

FIGURE 1.20   NMOFs particle synthesis.[106]

1.4.1.2   SOLVOTHERMAL METHOD

This method involves the high reaction temperature for the synthesis of NMOFs either by conventional heating or microwave. Since, the NMOFs building blocks are water soluble, they require high reaction temperature to complete the reaction. Temperature and heating provide additional parameters to control NMOFs growth and nucleation of the particles in crystalline forms and before the NMOFs nanoparticles formation, transformation of precursor takes place. Thus, by varying the reaction temperature, particle size can be controlled as high temperature favors the synthesis of large particles.[106] For example, Fe$_3$(μ_3O)Cl(H$_2$O)(terephthalic acid)$_3$.

In recent times, Jung and Oh demonstrated a method for NMOFs synthesis and that the change comes in particle's morphology during synthesis.[107] N, N-phenylene bis(salicylidene imine)dicarboxylic acid solution in dimethyl sulfoxide (DMSO) was added to the DMF solution having Zn (OAc)$_2$ (two equivalents). Out of two equivalents, one coordinates to a ligand salen pocket, whereas the other connects the resulting metallo ligands. The resulting solution was heated at 120°C for 60 min;

in this time, the nanowires transformed into nanocubes by the process of aggregation and intra-structural fusion and also demonstrated that by changing the reaction conditions, the nanocubes size could be tuned, as by decreasing the solubility of nanowires with the use of poor solvent mixture or with decrease of temperature.[107]

1.4.1.3   REVERSE MICROEMULSION

Reverse microemulsion was used for the synthesis of crystalline nanorods. In this method, surfactants were used for stabilizing the water droplets in nonpolar organic phase, for example, Gd (terephthalic acid)$_{1.5}$ (H$_2$O)$_2$.[108] In addition, by varying the ratio of water to the surfactant (water/surfactant) in microemulsion, nanoparticle size as well as morphology can be controlled.

1.4.1.4   SURFACTANT TEMPLATE SOLVOTHERMAL METHOD

In this method, the growing NMOFs particles can be coated under solvothermal conditions. The surfactant molecules can also be used for templating NMOFs synthesis and define the morphology of NMOFs significantly, for example, Gd-benzene hexacarboxylic acid NMOFs. Spontaneous precipitation of NMOFs has been studied by incorporating metal ions into the ligands by applying appropriate conditions. The NMOFs are then collected by centrifugation. Lin et al. synthesized the Ln$_2$ (1,4-benzenedicarboxylate)$_3$ (H$_2$O)$_4$ NMOFs (where Ln = Eu^{3+}, Gd^{3+}, or Tb^{3+}) by reacting LnCl$_3$ and di (methylammonium) benzene dicarboxylate in cationic system such as cetyltrimethyl ammonium bromide, isooctane, 1-hexanol, water microemulsion, and others.[108] The particle size (uniform) decreases with increasing concentration of reactants because they occupied more micelles to generate more nucleation site. The kinetics of nucleation and nanocrystal growth may be altered by elevating the temperature because it favors the synthesis of nanomaterials of uniform size under hydrothermal conditions.

In order to develop desirable industrial applications of MOFs, currents methods soon replaced by the microwave synthetic approach[109] with overcoming the described limitations of conventional synthesis such as complex, multistep synthesis,[110] requiring long reaction time (day to week), using bulky equipment with heavy energy consumption.[111] The reduction in reaction time[112] facilitates selectivity of phase[113] and control of crystal morphology as well.[114]

1.4.1.5   MICROWAVE ASSISTED SYNTHESIS

It has beneficial effects on material's properties and performances as compared to conventional method as it controls the optical and mechanical properties of the product perfectly,[115] for example, $[Mn[O_2Ph(C_6H_5)]_2(4,4'-bipy)]$,[116] $[Cu_2(OH)(BTC)(H_2O)]\cdot2nH_2O$, $Co_4O(3,5-Me_2Pz)_6]$.[117,118]

Wang et al. first reported non-cyano-metallate nano CPs synthesis in 2005.[119] They obtained spherical colloidal particles (submicrometer scale) simply by combining H_2PtCl_6 and p-phenylene diamine in aqueous medium.

Lin et al. have reported the NCPs synthesis of anticancer drug (disuccinatocisplatin and TbIII).[120] To reproduce it, the pH of $TbCl_3$ and dimethyl ammonium solution was adjusted to about 5.5 with sodium hydroxide solution, methanol addition induces the formation of NCPs of 58 ± 11.3 nm. Sweigart, Son, and coworkers have reported the formation of nanoparticles with an average diameter of 340 nm, by incorporating Al^{3+} metal ion $[Al (OiPr)_3]$ into organo-rhodium complex $[(\eta^6 - 1, 4$ hydroquinone) Rh (cod)]^+$.[121] It also showed that with increasing concentrations of the reagent, particle size increased which indicated that particle size has an influence on particle growth rate.

1.4.2   STRATEGIES FOR INCORPORATING THE BIOMEDICAL RELEVANT AGENTS WITHIN NMOFs

To incorporate therapeutic agents, for imaging and other applications, into the NMOFs, different methods have been developed. The strategies of agent loading generally fall into two categories:

1.4.2.1   DIRECT INCORPORATION DURING NMOFs SYNTHESIS

In this strategy, the biomedically relevant agents, either the metal connecting points[108,120,122,123] or the bridging ligands,[124] are used for assembling NMOFs. To form the NMOFs, paramagnetic metal ions such as Gd, Fe, and Mn are used, which not only connect the ligand but also function as MRI contrast agent. This plan has high agent loading tendency with distributing it uniformly. This strategy can be modified by taking a small amount of dopant with multifunctional NMOFs during the reaction process. This method encapsulates different agents with different properties such as optical dye, protein, chemotherapeutic, and smaller nanoparticles.[125–131] However, this method has some limitations, such as:

- Low drug loading
- The agent release kinetics may not be similar to framework decomposition rate

1.4.2.2   POST-SYNTHESIS LOADING

In this strategy, the NMOF pores are loaded by the biomedically active agents via covalent or non-covalent interactions.

- **Non covalent drug loading:** In this method, the drug can be loaded by the use of bulk phase MOFs that is means MOFs are arranged unprecedently in bulk, for example, 1 g MOFs can load 1.4 g of ibuprofen,[132] showing sustained release of the drug with minimal burst effect. To afford the high loading of agent, the size of NMOF pores must be larger than the encapsulated agents. Since the loading of the drug is reversible, the NMOF may lead to agent's premature release.
- **Covalent drug loading:** In this approach, the biomedically active agents are released only when NMOFs decompose. Therefore, the agents should be attached covalently through the functional groups present in the NMOFs.[133,134] But under specific biological conditions, the NMOFs–drug linkage can be cleaved. The loading of agents all over the NMOF particles may or may not be uniform.

Abovementioned methods allow the multimodal imaging agent or theranostic nanoparticle development by loading different types of agents in porous NMOFs.

1.5 APPLICATIONS

NMOFs with variety of composition and properties show interesting characteristics which have potential applications[135–150] in medicine, catalysis, adsorption, magnetism, optics, sensors, biological sensing, medical diagnostic, energy storage, spin crossover, templating, and drug delivery. NMOFs are expected to have broad impact in technological area of medicines.

1.5.1 ENCAPSULATION

The surface coating of the NMOFs can slow down the NMOF degradation and release of the encapsulated material under physiological conditions. Thus, to avoid intrinsic instabilities of many NMOFs, surface modification is particularly important. NMOFs surface can be modified by encapsulating the surface with silica and coating with organic polymers. The therapeutic agents are incorporated into NCPs in two ways, by encapsulating drug into the interstitial space of NCPs (Fig. 1.21) or by applying the pro-drug or drug as the building block for the polymer. Encapsulation of doxorubicin (DOX) in NCPs was successful and showed about 80% faster release at hours ascribed to the drug diffusion.[128] Drug degradation before reaching the target cells can be protected by encapsulating the drug inside the nanoparticles and thus helps in protecting the patient from adverse side effects. By attaching the peptides, antibodies, and aptamers to the particle surface, active targeting of cancer tissue can be achieved. [151] Horcajada et al. developed crystalline NCPs from Fe^{3+} and carboxylate ligands for encapsulating various anti-HIV drugs, anticancer drugs, showing its applications in theranostics, while performing drug delivery and MRI simultaneously.[152] Imaz et al. demonstrated NCPs capability, synthesized from Zn^{2+} and 1,4-bis (imidazole-1-ylmethyl) benzene, for encapsulating different types of functional moieties starting from iron oxide nanoparticles, quantum dots to florescent dyes. NCPs are not open framework structure so the encapsulation property of various functional moieties can be modified by tuning their compositions.[153] Microscale amorphous CP or NCP particles of diameter 300 ± 23 nm can encapsulate the drugs like DOX, SN-38, camptothecin, and daunomycin with 21% effectiveness.[154]

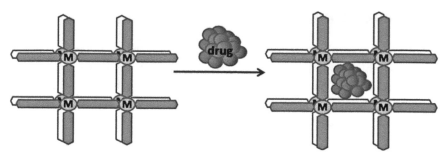

FIGURE 1.21   Loading of drug into NCPs via encapsulation, only one unit was shown for clarity.

Alternative encapsulation can be done by using biologically active metal ions (connecting building block) and organic drugs (bridging ligands). Pt based NCPs treated different types of cancer significantly.[155–158] Nitrogen containing bis-phosphonates (N-BPs) are constitutive building block drugs, which are effective antitumor agents and downregulate the integrins by inhibiting the activity of matrix metalloproteinase[159] because injected dose (N-BPs) is either quickly cleared by renal filtration or binds to bone. Liu et al. directly integrated two N-BPs, pamidronate (Pam) and zoledronate (Zol), into crystalline particles using Ca (II) ions as metal connecting nodes[160] to improve this.

A new concept in MOF nanocarrier's field is to protect the degradation of oligonucleotides (like DNA or RNA) and to facilitate their cellular uptakes by encapsulation. Mirkin and coworkers reported UiO-66-N$_3$ MOF-based nucleic acid-MOF nanoparticle conjugates.[161]

1.5.2   DRUG-ENCAPSULATED CARRIERS

For the specific release of therapeutic agents under desired conditions, chemists try to develop polymeric structures having desirable physical and chemical properties. There are various pharmaceutical formulations for drug encapsulation in the polymer, which are nano- and microparticles, nano- and microcapsules, capsosomes, and micelles.

1.5.2.1   NANO- AND MICROPARTICLES

In the formulation of these particles, drug is normally absorbed on to the polymer particles. The polymer protects transports and releases the drug through the polymer pores by diffusion under controlled conditions (Fig. 1.22). The drug carriers consist of the polymers of hydrophilic nature as gel and hydrogels. Hydrogels are nontoxic with three-dimensional structures, which help in controlled release of the drugs and therefore they are broadly used in drug encapsulation.

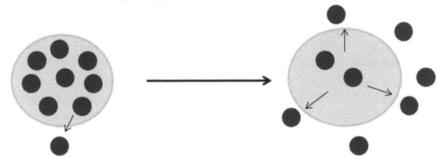

FIGURE 1.22   Nanoparticles of gels allow the drug diffusion from the polymer pores by swelling the structure.

1.5.2.2   NANO- AND MICROCAPSULES

The outer shell of polymer encapsulates active therapeutic agent and releases it through the degradation of polymeric matrix or a coat yielding nano- and microcapsules (Fig. 1.23). Usually, nano- or microcapsules are produced with hydrophilic polymers. Such capsules are generally used for transporting the drugs as protein, which is rapidly degraded in the body fluids. Liu et al.[162] reported that sulfopropyl dextran ion microparticles are used as drug carriers. It was loaded with DOX for evaluating its anti-cancer activity in vitro.

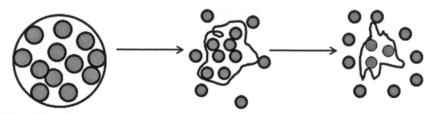

FIGURE 1.23   Nanocapsules allow the drug release through degradation of polymer matrix.

1.5.2.3   SMART POLYMERS

Recent research has captured the attention of smart polymers that can be tailored according to the requirement of drug delivery. For example, biocompatible hydrogels show satisfactory swelling properties in aqueous medium and therefore they can be used as controlled drug release.

1.5.2.4   CAPSOSOMES

Its structure has liposomal outer layer that is biodegradable and divides the interior part of capsules into compartments, which can hold same or different molecules. It shows that outer layer is permeable and allows the small size molecules to cross via passive diffusion.

1.5.2.5   MICELLES

The copolymers of individual linear polymers hold the hydrophobic and hydrophilic segments, which provide them capacity for the micellar structure formation in aqueous medium. These amphipathic polymers are arranged in such a way that the hydrophobic part is inside and the hydrophilic part outside. When amphiphilic block copolymers concentration rises above the critical micellar concentration (CMC),[163] micelles are form by self-assembling spontaneously in water. Micelles work as drug carriers because they have the capacity to encapsulate the hydrophobic drugs. They have high solubility and stability under physiological conditions. They facilitate circulation of drug through blood and cannot be removed by filtration through kidney because of their large size. Because of long half-life, the activity of the drug lasts for long period of time after single injection. As a result, therapeutic efficiency can be improved by incorporating low molecular weight drug inside micelles; thus, hydrophobic core of the polymeric micelles helps in incorporating drugs either by covalent or non-covalent interactions.

1.5.3 BIO-CPs

To prevent toxicity and impending exhaustion of some ligands even after coordinating to nontoxic metal ions, biologically and environmentally biocompatible biomolecules (as ligands) are used to produce bio-CPs particles. These bio-CPs particles generate inorganic oxides and sulfides as precursors.[164–167]

Metal histidine[168] or metal glutamate[169] based bio-CPs particles can be treated as model systems for investigating the metal-protein interaction to understand bio related processes. Some other bio-CP particles have good bio-compatibility and tunable porous structures and can adsorb and release drugs, thus can be used directly in organisms as a drug or drug carriers. Horcajada et al. recently reported $[Fe_3O(MeOH)_3(fumarate)_3(CO_2CH_3)]\cdot$ 4.5MeOH and $[Fe_3O(MeOH)(galactarate)_3Cl]\cdot6MeOH$, which produce endogenous substance on degradation. These bio-based MOFs can adsorb the significant amount of drugs such as azidothymidine triphosphate, busalfan, cidofovir, and others.[170] They can be loaded by soaking these MOFs in saturated solution of drugs such as azidothymidine triphosphate, busalfan, cidofovir, and others.

1.5.4 SPIN CROSSOVER

It is a transition from low-spin configuration to low lying metastable high-spin configuration due to external stimuli such as light irradiation or temperature. Among most widely reported spin crossover system, Fe (II) octahedral compound with 3d6 configuration has been extensively studied.

The low-spin nanoparticle, [CoIII (3,5-dbsq) (3,5-di-tert-butyl-1,2-catechol)], could be thermally transformed to material with high spin [CoIII (3,5-dbsq)$_2$]. Gaspar, Real, and coworkers explained the bimetallic synthesis of NMOFs [Fe (pyrazine) Pt (CN)$_4$]·xH$_2$O that exhibits magnetic, optical, and structural stability close to room temperature.[171] These spin crossover nanoparticles can be useful particularly in memory devices.

1.5.5   TEMPLATING WITH NMOFs

Lin et al. have explained that NMOFs can be used as a template for the synthesis of novel core shell nanostructure.[172] To synthesize it, NMOFs were firstly coated with polyvinylpyrollidone (PVP), which decrease the particle aggregation in solution. Then treat that PVP-coated intermediate with tetraethyl-orthosilicates (TEOS) in ethanol or ammonia solution, yielded to nanocomposites which have NMOFs core with silica shell.

Silica shell's thickness varies with the reaction time or the quantity of tetraethyl ortho-silicates used in the reaction mixture and thus thickness can be tuned. Silica can be additionally used as surface coating material thus enhanced biocompatibility, water dispersibility, and its further functionalization is easily possible with a derivative of silyl molecule. Thus, nanocomposites having NCPs or NMOFs cores and silica shells have been utilized for the multimodal imaging, biosensing, and anticancer drug delivery.

1.5.6   BIOSENSING AND MULTIMODAL IMAGING

Currently, for the recognition of cellular and sub-cellular actions, biosensing and multimodal imaging has played an elementary role. Its primary objective is to make available the information regarding molecular level, which helps in studying the complicated biological processes (as cancer) along with the stage of disease and also for finding the best curative approach to assess treatment with selectivity and specificity.

NCPs and NMOFs provide an important platform for making the multifunctional nanomaterials for biomedical and biosensing imaging. Most bioimaging technologies MRI and Optical Imaging (OI), using nanoparticles, are based on the usage of nanoparticles. For helping in the delivery of imaging agent to cancer cells, Linden et al. have investigated the functionalized Mesoporous Silica Nanoparticles (MSNPs).[173,174] Initially, they polymerized the MSNPs having amine functional group and hyper-branched poly-ethylene imine polymer on the surface and after labeling, targeted it with folic acid. Lin and coworkers[175] have reported the use of Polysilsesquioxane Nanoparticles (PSQNs) in cancer imaging by covalently linking the Gd (III) chelate with PSQNs with disulfide bond. By coating the Gd-PSQNs with PEG and anisamide ligand post synthesis, its biocompatibility and cell uptake in cancer cell can be enhanced. Their application includes engineering, chemistry, biology, and immunology helped in the development of techniques like MRI, optical imaging (OI), computed tomography imaging (CTI), and ultrasonographic imaging.[176]

1.5.6.1 MRI

It is a noninvasive imaging technique that can distinguish the diseased part (tissue) from the normal tissue on the basis of variations of ^{1}HNMR signal of water, present in high molar concentration in biological specimen.[177] These differences arise due to variation in density of water, tissue environment, and nuclear relaxation rate. It provides an excellent resolution, large penetration depth, and high soft tissue contrast. The efficacy of MRI contrast agent is mainly indicated by the relaxivity value. Larger relaxivity corresponds to more effective image contrast property.

By incorporating the highly paramagnetic metal ion (Gd^{3+} and Mn^{2+}) or metal ion complexes into the nanoparticles, image contrast enhanced because relaxation rate of water proton increases and rotational diffusion of contrast agent decreases,[108] for example, Gd_2 (1,4benzene-dicarboxylate)$_3$ $(H_2O)_4$. Zhou et al. reported that combining Gd (III) ions (magnetic) with carboxyl functionalized Ir (III) complexes (Phosphorescent), results in NCPs formation.[178] The presence of large number of Gd^{3+} centers in each particle extraordinarily increase the relaxivity per particle basis and can be used as site specific contrast agent after conjugating it to the appropriate targeting moieties.

1.5.6.2 OI

It is generally found everywhere for doing in vivo and in vitro biological studies; however, its in vivo application is restricted by the poor tissue penetration.[179] In such cases, the dye molecules within the tissue are excited by visible light, which fluoresce at longer wavelengths. A number of NMOFs have been produced that exhibit luminescence but these have not been applicable as biomedical imaging agent[129,180–183] because of their low quantum yield and non-optimum absorption properties. In a few cases, frameworks incorporate the optical dye either as a guest species or post synthetically.

Lin and coworkers synthesized NMOF containing Ruthenium (Ru) derivative as the bridging linker and Zn^{2+} and Zr^{4+} as metal connecting points.[184] To target the cancer cells proficiently, they coated these Zr based MOFs with amorphous silica layer and then functionalized it with poly ethylene glycol (PEG).

1.5.6.3   X-RAY COMPUTED TOMOGRAPHY (CT) IMAGING

This technique is based on specimen attenuation of X-ray and is able to provide 3D images having outstanding special resolution.[185,186] Barium, Iodine, and Bismuth are utilized as computed tomography contrast agent. To get adequate contrast, they must be used in large doses. Thus, superior contrast enhancement agent can be provided by the nanoparticle platform and metal centers contribute for the higher nanoparticle attenuations.

1.5.7   LUMINESCENCE

Luminescent CPs are typical organic chromophoric ligands, which absorb light and transmit the excitation energy to the metal ions. NMOFs have emission properties, which are considered to be the most versatile luminescent species, being coupled with guest. Photo luminescence can be induced by matrix excitation (generally oxides), which is followed by energy transfer to rare earth ions, then excite these ions directly. The excitation energy is then transferred to the emitting ions and leads to the emission.[187]

Aime et al. reported a method in favor of producing photofunctional nucleotide-lanthanide complex by introducing guest cofactor molecule.[188] By combining Tb (III) and 2-deoxyadenosine 5-monophosphate in water, the aggregated nanoparticles of average diameter 30 nm were synthesized. But Excitation of adenine chromospheres at 260 nm did not facilitate Tb (III) to show emission which confirmed that no energy transfer takes place from adenine to metal at that wavelength. Li et al. initiated and synthesized luminescent NMOFs specially for sensing and detection of the explosive compounds[189] such as DNT-2,4 dinitrotoluene (nitroaromatic explosive) and DMNB-2,3 dimethyl-2,3 dinitro butane (highly explosive taggant). For observing the nitroaromatic explosives in ethanol, luminescent NMOFs [Eu_2 (benzene-1,4 dicarboxylate)$_3$ $(H_2O)_2 \cdot (H_2O)_2$] have been reported. NMOFs dispersing in ethanol exhibit photoluminescence (PL) and fluorescence and the fluorescence peaks at 590, 617, and 698 nm may be ascribed to Eu^{3+} ions, agree to $^5D_0\text{-}^7F_1$, $^5D_0\text{-}^7F_2$, and $^5D_0\text{-}^7F_4$ transitions. After adding small amount of analytes (150 ppm) to the dispersed NMOFs in ethanol, luminescent intensity was affected but its intensity varies from one analyte to another, whereas some analytes such as benzene, toluene, chlorobenzene, phenol, o-cresol, and 4-bromophenol have no effect on the luminescence intensity. While luminescent intensity of NMOFs dispersed in ethanol was considerably quenched by nitroaromatic compounds such as DNT, TNT (2,4,6 trinitrotoluene). It indicates that NMOFs have sensing ability for nitroaromatic explosive.[190]

1.5.8 HETEROGENEOUS CATALYSIS

Heterogeneous catalyst's activity is based on the surface area as well as transport of the substrate; as a result, it shows size dependent chemical and physical properties.

Recently, the development of self-supported heterogeneous catalyst also becomes essential where NMOFs play an important part[191] as length, chirality, and pore dimensions (internal structure) of NMOFs help in making target reaction more substrate selective. The stereoselective nature of the catalysts arise from the less flexible geometries of the catalytic sites compared to the corresponding homogeneous system.

Sweigart et al. have reported the heterogeneous catalyst's example based on NMOFs. It was prepared by a combination of [($\eta^6$1, 4 hydroquinone) Rh (cyclooctadiene)] and Al $(OiPr)_3$ in tetrahydrofuran (THF); they examined its catalytic activity as compared to the polymerization of the phenylacetylene.[121] After combining the [($\eta^6$1,4 hydroquinone) Rh (cyclooctadiene)] with Al $(OiPr)_3$, its –OH groups are deprotonated and η^6 moiety of hydroquinone is converted into the η^4 moiety of quinine. The final structure of this heterogeneous NMOFs catalyst exhibited high stereoselectivity. A longer poly (phenylacetylene) may be obtained by decreasing the diameter of heterogeneous catalyst whereas by increasing the volume of the solvent, chain length of the poly (phenyacetylene) may be decreased dramatically. The mobilization of organometallic complexes occurs by incorporating it into self-supported network. To invent materials with high density catalytic active sites, NCP is particularly a promising strategy. The organometallic nano-catalysts of varying particle sizes were more stereoselective than molecular organo-Rhodium catalysts.

1.5.9   DRUG DELIVERY

Drug delivery is an advance process to transport curative agent in the body to achieve the target of interest. To develop a MOF for drug delivery, the carrier must be chosen such that it exhibits least toxicity in the human body. It is therefore essential that both the metal and bridging ligands must be biocompatible. For example, Fe is the component of hemoglobin and exists in appreciable amount in the body.

Recently, people are making advancements on the NCPs drug delivery system mainly in two directions:

- Stimuli responsive release of curative/therapeutic agent
- Combination of drugs with other nanomaterials

In drug delivery, procedure through which the drug is released has become the hot spot of the nanotechnology. The drug is released by hydrolytic degradation of the polymeric coating but degradation depends upon the polymer chain length and stability in the body fluid. Gombotz et al.[192] showed the ability of linkages against hydrolysis in aqueous medium as $1>2>3>4>5>6$ (Fig. 1.24).

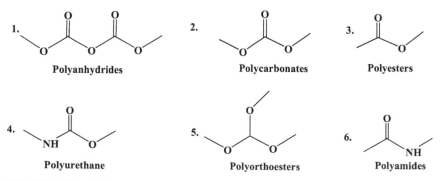

FIGURE 1.24   Linkage ability of polymers.

Ferey and coworkers[193] found first group of MOFs; Materials of Institute Lavoisier (MIL) that is used as a potential drug delivery system. It has carboxylic acid as a bridging ligand and trivalent metal centers. The great promise for the attractive characteristics of drug delivery held by MIL family is as: large pores (25–34A⁰), large surface area (3100–5900 m/g), and the capability of incorporating functional group into the MOFs. The drug loading and controlled drug release of Ibuprofen with chromium based MIL100 and MIL101[132] have been studied by Ferey and coworkers. They both showed high loading of Ibuprofen, as one gram of MOF load 0.347 g Ibuprofen for MIL 100 and 1.376 Ibuprofen for MIL 101. Drug loading property can be differentiated by the pore size; MIL 100 has small pore volumes of 8200 and 12700A⁰ whereas MIL101 has large pore volumes of 12700 and 20600A⁰. By suspending the Ibuprofen loaded materials in simulated fluid at 37°C, the delivery kinetics of Ibuprofen was investigated. For MIL 100, weakly bound drug molecules initially released within 2 h and entire cargo released within 3 days but for MIL101s within first 8 h and complete release after 6 days. The less toxic MIL 101 (Fe) should be more appropriate drug carrier and developed as a biocompatible alternative.[194] Xing et al. produced NCPs based on "host metal-ligand" and labile "metal-ligand" bond cleavage, which is initiated by acidic pH and thus fulfill the pH responsive drug release,[195] for example, incorporation of NCPs with gold nanorod. Many systems as dendrimers and polymer particles have been shown to hinder the broad applications of nanomedicines[196] as far as their capability of loading and releasing the drug is concerned. Various kinds of nanocarriers have been developed to deliver the drug to the target selectively and in a controlled manner.[197]

1.5.9.1 CONTROLLED RELEASE METHODS OF DRUGS

These systems tend to improve the effectiveness of drug therapy[198] by modifying various drug parameters such as release profile, ability for crossing the biological carriers, biodistribution, clearance, and the stability between others, as a result of pharmacodynamics and pharmacokinetics of the drugs. Control release decreases the side effects and increases the therapeutic activity, thus required number of dosages for the treatment decrease. It is highly useful for the drugs with poor bioavailability, as it is quickly metabolized and has narrow therapeutic window. Appropriate tools required for the site specific and time controlled drug delivery has been offered by the controlled release methods.

1.5.9.1.1   Time controlled-modified release formulation

Modified release formulations offer alternatives to the regular drug administration for improving management and optimizing its therapeutic activity. The drug is released through the system that protects and retains it. In this formulation tissues attain a therapeutic concentration of drug through controlled release. The normal dose of the drug in the modified formulation, releases active ingredients[199] easily. The delivery of the active ingredients occurs at the predetermined speed and at the site different from administration site. On the basis of drug release system, these formulations can be categorized into the followings:

1.5.9.1.2   Extended release formulation

In these formulations, active ingredient is released in sufficient amount for producing the therapeutic effects even though the release is not constant. Extended release formulation have been divided into two types, in first, polymeric matrix contains active ingredients and its delivery is controlled by diffusion through polymeric network of the system and presented in the form of hydrogels and nanoparticles. In second type, extended release formulation consists of polymer coated capsules forming a reserve deposit. The degradation and the permeability of polymer coatings control the drug release.

1.5.9.1.3   Sustained release formulation

In this case, therapeutic effect is maintained over a long period of time by releasing the active component regularly with zero order kinetic. In this type of system, osmotic pumps are used as the closest pharmaceutical formulations and control the drug solution's outflow through osmotic potential gradients across the semipermeable polymer barriers.

1.5.9.1.4   Pulsatile release formulation

This is the responsive delivery system in which body triggers drug release in pulsatile manner only when body feels its requirement in a definite lag time. Pulsatile drug delivery system releases the drug at right time, right place, and in right quantity. Generally, the two components, namely sensor and delivery device are used in these drug delivery systems. Environmental parameters are detected by sensors and stimulate the drug release. Pulsatile drug delivery systems are suitable for the patients suffering from chronic problems such as arthritis, asthma, diabetes, and hypertension.[200]

1.5.9.1.5 Delayed release formulation

In this process, active ingredients release does not overlap with the administration time and it does not extend its therapeutic action. In these, active ingredients are protected from the unfavorable media by coating it and further protect certain body parts from the antagonistic effects of active ingredients. But these coatings are sensitive to pH, due to which drug is released into small intestine, thereby checking its release to the stomach.

Modified release formulations have numerous drawbacks such as higher production cost, unpredictable in vitro or in vivo correlation, lack of reproducibility, improper handling, and others.

1.5.9.2 CONTROLLED DISTRIBUTION

A disease is treated by distributing the drug at targeted position, so use of drug carriers with controlled distribution system have become important and help in overcoming the hurdles produced by nonspecific drug delivery system. The functionalized nanoparticle surface contains receptor recognition elements which are present in the diseased tissue. The release of active ingredients can be controlled by associating them to polymer by particular linkers,[201] which can be degraded in the acidic medium or by using particular enzymes. These linkers have stability in plasma and degrade in tumor tissue or in lysosomal, endosomal[202] microenvironments. The most frequently used linkers are the peptides and oligosaccharides. Thus, polymer coated drug releases the drug when exposed to either of these two conditions; when pH of tumor tissues is lower than those of healthy ones and the pH changed as drug is sensitive to a change in pH.

1.5.10 THERANOSTIC

It is the treatment strategy that has the therapeutic modalities and diagnostic imaging capability (Fig. 1.25).[203–205] Generally, theranostic system depends on synergy among the metal complexes and nanoparticles.

Nanoparticles have progressively boosted their application in medicine and diagnostic therapy.

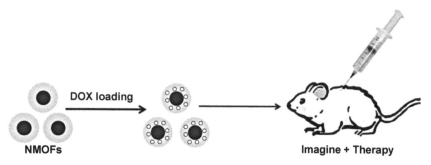

FIGURE 1.25   Theranostic treatment strategy.

They can be present as passive or active component.

1.5.10.1   NANOPARTICLES AS PASSIVE COMPONENTS

Nanoparticles, as passive components may have minimum three possibilities:

- Drug and metal complex can load it as the imaging component
- It can be used as metal complex carrier for the therapy and organic molecule for imaging
- Nanoparticles can incorporate one or two metal complexes for therapy and imaging

The most appropriate approach is the co-loading of Gd-chelates and organic drug on the different types of nanoparticles. Yeh et al. produced Gd-DOTA [DOTA = 1,4,7,10-tetraaza-1,4,7,10-tetra kis (carboxymethyl) cyclododecane] grafted silica nanotubes, which are loaded with DOX exhibiting promising contrast for MRI and anticancer activity (after incubation for 48 h, the viability of the cell reduced to 33 %).[206]

1.5.10.2 NANOPARTICLE AS ACTIVE COMPONENT

Guo and coworkers synthesized the gold nanorods having chitosan functionalities and loaded them with cisplatin, and can be applied in photothermal therapy. The consequences revealed that cancer cell death of these systems was stimulated upon irradiation with near infrared rays by attaching fluorescent organic dye to nanoparticles through covalent bond and make the system visible by fluorescence microscopically[207] and hence can be used in imaging. Silica-based hybrid materials have been used in photodynamic therapy (PDT). PDT is the light activated therapy for diseases like cancer. Prasad and coworkers stated that organically modified silica nanoparticles can be used in PDT.[208] It works by using the photosensitizers (that is light sensitive drugs) and these drugs can be localized in the malignant tissues. Its therapeutic effect is activated by exciting the localized photosensitizers with light which generate cytotoxic singlet oxygen ($^1O_2$) and destroy the diseased tissues without disturbing the normal healthy ones. But presently accepted PDT photosensitizers have a problem that they are absorbed in the visible spectral region (below 700 nm). But with the addition of dye two photons absorbing (TPA) to photosensitizer, this problem can be overcome where its indirect excitation takes place through fluorescence resonance energy transfer (FRET). Hai and coworkers used similar strategy for synthesizing silica particles (105 nm) by trapping the dye; methylene blue (MB) for making the use in near infrared imaging and photodynamic therapy.[209] MB can be used as effective photosensitizer because of high quantum yield of $^1O_2$ generation, near infrared therapeutic window and low dark toxicity. Very low toxicity was observed after treating cells either with nanoparticles or the laser alone but treating it with MB and laser irradiation, leads to the significant cell death.

Victor Lin and coworkers have reported numerous MSNPs based delivery systems having stimuli-responsive pore cap, for example, Au, CdS, and Fe_3O_4 nanoparticles for controlling the release of entrapped molecules.[210,211] For example, when gold nanoparticles conjugated with photolabile linker[212] are exposed to ultra violet light, Au nanoparticle pore cap is released. This system delivers paclitaxel to fibroblast cells and human liver. Considerable reduction in cell viability was examined after irradiating them with ultraviolet light. With the use of this strategy, some other drug molecules and neurotransmitters such as vanomycin, adenosine triphosphate (ATP) can be delivered.[210,211] Some other potential drug carriers like NMOFs were also reported as their pores can be loaded with different anticancer, antiviral drugs such as busalfan, azidothymidine triphosphate, DOX, and cidofovir by non-covalent interactions. Drug delivery system based on capped MSNPs was also reported.[213] It loaded the boronic acid functionalized MSNPs with cyclic adenosine monophosphate (cAMP), which is significant cellular signaling molecule. Then capped the material pores with insulin, which formed more stable conjugate with boronic acid on the nanoparticles and then saccharides were allowed to activate the drug release from material. Lin and coworkers synthesized an oxaliplatin prodrug taken with PSQNs and showed their enhanced accumulation in cancer cells[214] by using PEG and an active targeting ligand anisimide. These PSQNs possess better cytotoxicity (against four cancer cell lines in vitro) as compared to the drug free from oxaliplatin and after intravenous injection, it exhibits anticancer activity in human pancreatic xenograft murine models. In recent times, Lin and coworkers declared that PSQNs having prodrug cisplatin were utilized in chemoradiotherapy[215] using the human lung cancer as a disease modal. The PSQNs loaded with cisplatin exhibited improved anticancer efficiency, both in vitro and in vivo, compared to free cisplatin. Cheng and coworkers synthesized the PSQNs having controllable size, drug loading and release profiles. [216,217] The drugs having trialkoxysilane were manufactured by forming ester linkage between drug and trialkoxysilane group, condensed it with tetra-alkoxysilane so that the drug can be incorporated into the resulting nanoparticles. It has been observed that the particles with 20–50 nm diameters have improved anticancer activity and greater accumulation around tumor cells.[215]

1.6   CONCLUSION

The synthesis of nanoscale MOF by scaling down the MOF or porous CP to nanoscale region by using the variety of methods, including solvothermal, surfactant template solvothermal, nanoprecipitation, reverse microemulsions synthesis, has been witnessed in the past decades. New synthetic strategies are still required in order to overcome the limitations faced during formulating NMOFs and also for obtaining full advantages of NMOFs. NMOFs are increasingly finding their utility in a number of interesting applications from separation to targeted drug delivery, which allow the nanomaterials to explore other applications by taking advantage of the ability to tune the composition using perfect choice of building block.

1.7 ACKNOWLEDGMENTS

Laxmi and Shabnam Khan thank the UGC (New Delhi, India) for non-NET and Maulana Azad National Fellowship, ref # F1–17.1/2014–15/MANF-2014–15-MUS-UTT-36965/(SA-III/Website), respectively. Dr Fahmina Zafar is thankful to the UGC (New Delhi, India) for Dr D S Kothari fellowship, ref # F.4/2006 (BSR)/13–986/2013 (BSR) with Prof. Nahid Nishat (Mentor) and the Head, Dept. of Chemistry, Jamia Millia Islamia, for providing facilities to carry out their research work.

KEYWORDS

- **nano metal organic frameworks**
- **classification**
- **synthesis methods**
- **surfactant template solvothermal**
- **nanoprecipitation**

REFERENCES

1. Batten, S. R.; Neville, S. M.; Turner, D. R. *R. S. C.* **2009.**
2. Blake, A. J.; Champness, N. R.; Hubberstey, P.; Li, W. S.; Withersby, M. A.; Schroder, M. *Coord. Chem. Rev.* **1999,** *183,* 117.
3. Masoomi, M. Y.; Morsali, A. *Coord. Chem. Rev.* **2012,** *256,* 2921–2943.
4. Akhbari, K.; Morsali, A. *Coord. Chem. Rev.* **2010,** *254,* 1977.
5. Barnett, S. A.; Champness, N. R. *Coord. Chem. Rev.* **2003,** *246,* 145.
6. Roesky, H. W.; Andruh, M. *Coord. Chem. Rev.* **2003,** *236,* 91.
7. James, S. L. *Chem. Soc. Rev.* **2003,** *32,* 276.
8. Yaghi, O. M.; Li, H.; Davis, C.; Richardson, D.; Groy, T. L. *Acc. Chem. Res.* **1998,** *31,* 474.

9. Kitagawa, S.; Noro, S. In *Comprehensive Coordination Chemistry II*; McCleverty, J. A., Meyer, T. J., Eds.; Pergamon: Oxford, 2003; p 231.

10. Robin, A. Y.; Fromm, K. M. *Coord. Chem. Rev.* **2006**, *250*, 2127.

11. Hu, M. L.; Morsali, A.; Aboutorabi, L. *Coord. Chem. Rev.* **2011**, *255*, 2821.

12. Kamaci, M.; Kaya, I. *J. Inorg. Organomet. Polym.* **2013**, *23*, 1159–1171.

13. Zhang, Z.; Nguyen, H. T. H.; Miller, S. A.; Cohen, S. M. *Angew. Chem. Int. Edit.* **2015**, *54*, 1–6.

14. Ricco, R.; Malfatti, L.; Takahashi, M.; Hill, A. J.; Falcaro, P. *J. Mater. Chem. A.* **2013**, 113033.

15. Bell, A. T. *Science* **2003**, *299*, 1688.

16. Zhang, D. E.; Zhang, X. J.; Ni, X. M.; Zheng, H. G.; Yang, D. D. *J. Magn. Magn. Mater.* **2005**, *292*, 79.

17. Wang, J.; Gudiksen, M. S.; Duan, X.; Cui, Y.; Lieber, C. M. *Science* **2001**, *293*, 1455.

18. Fleischhaker, F.; Arsenault, A. C.; Kitaev, V.; Peiris, F. C.; von Freymann, G.; Manners, I.; Zentel, R.; Ozin, G. A. *J. Am. Chem. Soc.* **2005**, *127*, 9318.

19. Blanco, A.; Chomski, E.; Grabtchak, S.; Ibisate, M.; John, S.; Leonard, S. W.; Lopez, C.; Meseguer, F.; Miguez, H.; Mondia, J. P.; Ozin, G. A.; Toader, O.; van Driel, H. M. *Nature* **2000**, *405*, 437.

20. Salzemann, C.; Brioude, A.; Pileni, M. P. *J. Phys. Chem. B* **2006**, *110*, 7208.

21. Lee, J. H. *Sens. Actuators B* **2009**, *140*, 319.

22. Lu, W.; Qin, X.; Luo, Y.; Chang, G.; Sun, X. *Microchim. Acta.* **2001**, *1.*, 753–768.

23. Cao, Y. C.; Jin, R.; Mirkin, C. A. *Science* **2002**, *297*, 1536.

24. Bruchez, M.; Moronne, M.; Gin, P.; Weiss, S.; Alivisatos, A. P. *Science* **1998**, *281*, 2013.

25. Taton, T. A.; Mirkin, C. A.; Letsinger, R. L. *Science* **2000**, *289*, 1757.

26. Mirkin, C. A.; Letsinger, R. L.; Mucic, R. C.; Storhoff, J. J. *Nature* **1996**, *382*, 607.

27. Lee, J. H.; Huh, Y. M.; Jun, Y. W.; Seo, J. W.; Jang, J. T.; Song, H. T.; Kim, S.; Cho, E. J.; Yoon, H. G.; Suh, J. S. *J. Cheon. Nat. Med.* **2007**, *13*, 95.

28. Gao, X.; Cui, Y.; Levenson, R. M.; Chung, L. W. K.; Nie, S. *Nat. Biotechnol.* **2004**, *22*, 969.

29. Sakunthala, A.; Reddy, M. V.; Selvasekarapandian, S.; Chowdari, B. V. R.; Selvin, P. C. *Electrochim. Acta.* **2010**, *55*, 4441.

30. Saravanan, K.; Ramar, V.; Balaya, P.; Vittal, J. J. *J. Mater. Chem.* **2011**, *21*, 14925.

31. Sun, S.; Murray, C. B.; Weller, D.; Folks, L.; Moser, A. *Science* **2000**, *287*, 1989.

32. Batabyal, S. K.; Vittal, J. J. *Chem. Mater.* **2008**, *20*, 5845.

33. Schmid, G. *Nanoparticles from Theory to Application*; Wiley-VCH Verlag GmbH & Co. KGaA : Germany, 2005.

34. Chen, J.; Herricks, T.; Xia, Y. *Angew. Chem. Int. Ed.* **2005**, *44*, 2589.

35. Horn, D.; Rieger, J. *Angew. Chem. Int. Ed.* **2001**, *40*, 4330.

36. Peng, X.; Manna, L.; Yang, W.; Wickham, J.; Scher, E.; Kadavanich, A.; Alivisatos, A. P. *Nature* **2000**, *404*, 59.

37. Lin, H. Y.; Luan, J.; Wang, X. L.; Zhang, J. W.; Liu, G. C.; Tian, A. X. *RSC Adv.* **2014**, *448*(4), 62430–62445.

38. Fateeva, A.; Chater, P. A.; Ireland, C. P.; Tahir, A. A.; Khimyak, Y. Z.; Wiper, P. V.; Darwent, J. R.; Rosseinsky, M. J. *Angew. Chem. Int. Ed.* **2012**, *51*, 7440–7444.

39. Yaghi, O. M., Li, Q. *MRS Bull.* **2009**, *34*(9), 682–690.
40. Chen, Y. F.; Jiang, J. W. *Chem. Sus. Chem.* **2010**, *3*, 982–988.
41. Wu, C. D.; Li, L.; Shi, L. X. *Dalton Trans.* **2009**, *46*, 6790–6794.
42. Wang, M.; Xie, M. X.; Wu, C. D.; Wang, Y. G. *Chem. Commun.* **2009**, *60*, 2396–2398.
43. Rabone, J.; Yue, Y. F.; Chong, S. Y.; Stylianou, K. C.; Bacsa, J.; Bradshaw, D.; Darling, G. R.; Berry, N. G.; Khimyak, Y. Z.; Ganin, A. Y.; Wiper, P.; Claridge, J. B.; Rosseinsky, M. J. *Science* **2010**, *329*, 1053–1057.
44. Chen, X.; Ye, B.; Tong, M. *Coord. Chem. Rev. Elsevier.* **2005**, *249*, 545–565.
45. Kurimara, Y.; Tsuchida, E.; Kaneko, M. J. *J. Polym. Sci. Polym.* **1971**, *19*, 3511.
46. Jr. Pittman, C. V., Veges, R. L.; Jones, W. *J. Elder. Macromol.* **1971**, *4*, 302.
47. Kanda, S. *Nipp. Kag. Zass.* **1962**, *83*, 560.
48. Kaliyappan, T.; Kannan, P. *Prog. Polym. Sci.* **2000**, *25*, 343.
49. Sharpe, A. G. *The Chemistry of Cyano Complexes of the Transition Metals;* Academic Press: New York, 1976; p 275.
50. Krogmann, K.; Hansen, H. D.; Anorg, Z. *Allg. Chem.* **1968**, *67*, 358.
51. Miller, L. S.; Epstein, A. J.; Ann, N. Y. *Acad. Sci.* **1978**, 313.
52. Atoji, M.; Richardson, J. W., Rundle, R. E. *J. Am. Chem. Soc.* **1957**, *7a*, 3017.
53. Nguyen, P.; Paloma, G. E.; Manners, L. *Chem. Rev.* **1999**, *99*, 1515.
54. Takahashi, S.; Takai, Y.; Morimoto, H.; Murata, E.; Kataoka, S.; Sonogashira, K.; Nagihara, N. *J. Polym. Sci. Poly. Chem.* **1982**, *20*, 565.
55. Takahashi, S.; Takai, Y.; Morimoto, H.; Sonogashira, K. *J. Chem. Soc. Chem. Commun.* **1984**, 3.
56. Katano, N.; Sugihara, Y.; Ishii, A.; Nakayama, J. *Bull. Chem. Soc. Jpn.* **1998**, *71*, 2695.
57. Linsky, J. P.; Paul, T. R.; Nohr, R. S.; Kenny, M. E. *Inorg. Chem.* **1980**, *19*, 3131.
58. Hanack, M.; Mitulla, K.; Pawlowski, G.; Subramanian, L. R. *Organomet. Chem.* **1980**, *204*, 315.
59. Marks, T. J. *Angew. Chem. Int. Ed. Engl.* **1990**, *29*, 857.
60. Cassoux, P.; Valade, L.; Kobayashi, H.; Kobayashi, A.; Clark, R. A.; Underhill, A. E. *Coord. Chem. Rev.* **1991**, *110*, 115.
61. Jaykumar, R.; Nanjundan, S.; Prabaharan, M. *React. Funct. Polym.* **2006**, *66*, 299–314.
62. Jaykumar, R.; Lee, Y. S.; Nanjundan, S. *J. Appl. Polym. Sci.* **2004**, *92*, 710–721.
63. Prasath, R. A.; Nanjundan, S. *Eur. Polym. J.* **1999**, *35*, 1939–1948.
64. Reddys, T. A.; Srinivasan, M. *J. Polym. Sci., Part A* **1989**, 2805.
65. Hasnain, S.; Nishat, N. *Spectrochim Acta Part A.* **2012**, *95*, 452–457.
66. Hasnaina, S.; Zulfequarb, M.; Nishat, N. *Polym. Adv. Technol.* **2012**, *23*, 1002–1010.
67. Ahamad, T.; Kumar, V.; Nishat, N. *J. Biomed. Mater. Res. Part A.* **2008**, 288–294.
68. Hasnain, S.; Zulfequar, M.; Nishat, N. *J. Coord. Chem.* **2011**, *64*, 952–964.
69. Ahamad, T.; Nishat, N.; Parveen, S. *J. Coord. Chem.* **2008**, *61*, 1963–1972.
70. Laxmi, Khan, S.; Zafar, F.; Nishat, N. *RSC Adv.* **2016**, under review.
71. Tang, S. Y.; Bourne, R. A.; Smith, R. L.; Poliakoff, M. *Green Chem.* **2008**, *10*, 268–269.
72. Zafar, F.; Zafar, H.; Sharmin, E.; Nishat, N. *Development of Agro Byproduct Based Coordination Polymers for Biomedical Application.* International Symposium on

Advances in Biological & Material Sciences, organized by Humboldt Academy Lucknow & University of Lucknow, July 15, 2014.

73. Zafar, F.; Khan, S.; Zafar, H.; Sharmin, E.; Nishat, N. *Studies on Bio-Resource Derived Ligand And Transition Metal Ions-Based Coordination Complexes/Polymers for Biomedical Application.* APA 2014, International Conference organized by Asian Polymer Association (APA), New Delhi, India, February 19–21, 2014.

74. Zafar, F.; Zafar, H.; Sharmin, E.; Nishat, N. *Synthesis and Characterization of Biologically Active Coordination Complexes/Polymers from Agro-Byproduct.* POLYCHAR 22, World Forum on Advanced, Materials, organized by STIAS Research Centre, Stellenbosch, South Africa, April 7–11, 2014.

75. Zafar, F.; Zafar, H.; Sharmin, E.; Nishat, N. *CNSL Based Coordination Polymers as Drug-Carrier System.* 1st International conference on emerging trends of nanotechnology in drug discovery, organized by Sri Venkateswara College & Department of Biochemistry, University of Delhi, India in association with Centro de Quimica da Madeira, University of Madeira, Portugal, India, May 26–27, 2014.

76. Zafar, F.; Zafar, H.; Sharmin, E.; Nishat, N. *Synthesis and Characterization of Porous Coordination Complex/Polymer from Cashew Nut Shell Liquid (CNSL): A Sustainable Development.* 3rd International Conference on innovative approach in applied physical, mathematical/statistical, chemical sciences and emerging energy technology for sustainable development (APMSCSET-2014) organized by Social Welfare Foundation in association with Krishi Sanskriti, JNU, Delhi, India, September 27–28, 2014.

77. Zafar, F.; Zafar, H.; Sharmin, E.; Nishat, N. *Synthesis, Characterization and Antimicrobial Activity of Cardanol-Metal Ions Coordination Complexes/Polymers.* Jointly organized by Indian Institute of Technology (IIT) Delhi, ENEA, Rome, Italy and National research Council of Italy under the auspices of APA, India, October 27–30, 2014.

78. Zafar, F.; Zafar, H.; Sharmin, E.; Nishat, N. *Cashew Nut Shell Liquid Based Advanced Functional Materials.* International Conference on natural polymers, bio-polymers, bio-materials, their composites, nanaocomposites, blends, ipns, polyelectrolytes and gels: macro to nano scales (ICNP–2015) organized by International Unit on Macromolecular Science and Engineering (IUMSE) Kottayam, Kerala, India & Wroclaw Uniwersity of Technology, Faculty of Electrical Engineering 27 Wybrzeze Wyspianskiego St 50–370 Wroclaw, Poland & Laboratório de Biopolímeros e Sensores/LaBioS, Centro de Tecnologia [UTF-8] Cidade Universitária, AV Horácio Macedo 2030, Bloco J, Brazil, at Kottayam, Kerala, India, April10–12, 2015.

79. Zafar, F.; Kaur, B.; Khan, S.; Zafar, H.; Sharmin, E.; Nishat, N. Development of Mesoporous Nanocoordinated Polyurethanes from CNSL: Formaldehyde and Divalent Transition Metal Ions. Communicated (2015)

80. Zafar, F.; Khan, S.; Prashant, Zafar, H.; Sharmin, E.; Nishat, N. *Synthesis and Characterization of Nanocoordinated Polyurethanes from Agrobyproducts (CNSL & Furfuraldehyde) Derived Ligand and Divalent Transition Metal Ions.* To be communicated (2015)

81. Kahan, S.; Zafar, F.; Nishat, N. *Synthesis and Characterization of Coordination Polymers from Cardanol-Furfuraldehyde (Ligand) and Transition metal Ions.* To be communicated.

82. Zafar, F.; Khan, S.; Zafar, H.; Begum, M.; Zafar, H.; Sharmin, E.; Nishat, N. Synthesis and Characterization of Mg (II) Containing Nanocoordination Polymer Film Derived from Agrobyproduct (Cardanol and Furfuraldehyde). To be communicated (2015)

83. Zafar, F.; Khan, S.; Shabnam, Zafar, H.; Sharmin, E.; Nishat, N. *Development of Mg (II) Containing Nanocoordination Polymer Film Based on CNSL-Formaldehyde and HMTA.* To be communicated (2015).

84. Zafar, F.; Azam, M.; Sharmin, E.; Zafar, H.; Haq, Q. M. R.; Nishat, N. *RSC. Adv.* **2016,** *6,* 6607–6622.

85. Khan, S.; Laxmi, Zafar, F.; Nishat, N. *RSC. Adv.* **2016.** DOI: 10.1039/C6RA00849 F.

86. Raquez, J. M.; Deleglise, M.; Lacrampe, M. F.; Krawczak, P. *Prog. Polym. Sci.* **2010,** *35,* 487–509.

87. Rowsell, J. L.; Yaghi, O. M. *Angew. Chem. Int. Ed.* **2005,** *44,* 4670–4679.

88. Dinc, M.; Long, J. R. *Angew. Chem. Int. Ed.* **2008,** *47,* 6766–6779.

89. Jiang, H. L.; Tatsu, Y.; Lu, Z. H.; Xu, Q. *J. Am. Chem. Soc.* **2010,** *132,* 5586–5587.

90. Jiang, H. L.; Xu, Q. *Chem. Commun.* **2011,** *47,* 3351–3370.

91. Chen, B.; Xiang, S.; Qian, G. *Acc. Chem. Res.* **2010,** *43,* 1115–1124.

92. Rocca, J. D.; Liu, D.; Lin, W. *Acc. Chem. Res.* **2011,** *44,* 957–968.

93. Rieter, W. J.; Taylor, K. M L.; An, H.; Lin, W. *J. Am. Chem. Soc.* **2006,** *128,* 9024–9025.

94. Taylor, K. M. L.; Rieter, W. J.; Lin, W. *J. Am. Chem. Soc.* **2008,** *130,* 14358–14359.

95. Rieter, W. J.; Pott, K. M.; Taylor, K. M. L.; Lin, W. *J. Am. Chem. Soc.* **2008,** *130,* 11584–11585.

96. Stavila, Talin, A. A.; Allendorf, M. D. *Chem. Soc. Rev.* **2014,** *43,* 5994–6010.

97. Wanderley, M. M.; Wang, C.; Wu, C. D.; Lin, W. *J. Am. Chem. Soc.* **2012,** *134,* 9050–9053.

98. Kreno, E.; Leong, K.; Farha, O. K.; Allendorf, M.; Van Duyne, R. P.; Hupp, J. T. *Chem. Rev.* **2012,** *112,* 1105–1125.

99. So, M. C.; Wiederrecht, G. P.; Mondloch, J. E.; Hupp, J. T.; Farha, O. K. *Chem. Commun.* **2015,** *51,* 3501–3510.

100. Wang, J. L.; Wang, C.; Lin, W. *ACS Catal.* **2012,** *2,* 2630–2640.

101. Pettinari, C.; Tabacarub, A.; Galli, S. *Coord. Chem. Rev.* **2016,** *307,* 1–31.

102. Bohren, C. F.; Huffman, D. R. *Wiley-Interscience,* 1983.

103. Stewart, M. E., Anderton, C. R.; Thompson, L. B.; Maria, J.; Gray, S. K.; Rogers, J, A; Nuzzo, R. G. *Chem. Rev.* **2008,** *108,* 494.

104. Hirsch, L. R.; Stafford, R. J.; Bankson, J. A.; Sershen, S. R.; Rivera, B.; Price, R. E.; Hazle, J. D.; Halas, N. J.; West, J. L. *Proc. Natl. Acad. Sci. U. S. A.* **2003,** *100,* 13549.

105. Jain, P. K.; Huang, X.; El-Sayed, I. K.; El-Sayed, M. A. *Acc. Chem. Res.* **2008,** *41,* 1578.

106. Rieter, W. J.; Pott, K. M.; Taylor, K. M. L.; Lin, W. *J. Am. Chem Soc.* **2008,** *130,* 11584–11585.

107. Jung, S.; Oh, M. *Angew. Chem.* 2008, 120, 2079–2081.

108. Rieter, W. J.; Taylor, K. M. L.; An, H.; Lin, W. *J Am Chem Soc.* **2006,** *128,* 9024–9025.

109. Clark, D. E.; Sutton, W. H. *Annu. Rev. Mater. Sci.* **1996,** *26,* 299–331.
110. Zafar, F.; Sharmin, E.; Zafard, H.; Shah, M. Y.; Nishat, N.; Ahmad, S. *Ind. Crops. Prod.* **2015,** *67,* 484–491.
111. Klinowski, J.; Paz, F. A. A.; Silva, P.; Rocha, J. *Dalton Trans.* **2011,** *40,* 321.
112. Hu, Y. Y.; Liu, C.; Zhang, Y. H.; Ren, N.; Tang, Y. *Microporous Mesoporous Mater.* **2009,** *119,* 306–314.
113. Jhung, S. H.; Chang, J. S.; Hwang, J. S.; Park, S. E. *Microporous Mesoporous Mater.* **2003,** *64,* 33–39.
114. Hwang, Y. K.; Chang, J. S.; Park, S. E.; Kim, D. S.; Kwon, Y. U.; Jhung, S. H.; Hwang, J. S.; Park, M. S. *Angew. Chem. Int. Ed.* **2005,** *44,* 556–560.
115. Yang, G.; Kong, Y.; Hou, W. H.; Yan, Q. J. *J. Phys. Chem. B.* **2005,** *109,* 1371–1379.
116. Liao, J. H.; Chen, P. L.; Hsu, C. C. *J. Phys. Chem. Solids.* **2001,** *62,* 1629–1642.
117. Falcao, E. H. L.; Naraso, Feller, R. K.; Wu, G.; Wudl, F.; Cheetham, A. K. *Inorg. Chem.* **2008,** *47,* 8336–8342.
118. Liu, H. K.; Tsao, T. H.; Zhang, Y. T.; Lin, C. H. *Cryst. Eng. Comm.* **2009,** *11,* 1462–1468.
119. Sun, X. P.; Dong, S. J.; Wang, E. K. *J. Am. Chem. Soc.* **2005,** *127,* 13102–13103.
120. deKrafft, K. E.; Xie, Z. G.; Cao, G. H.; Tran, S.; Ma, L. Q.; Zhou, O. Z.; Lin, W. B. *Angew. Chem. Int. Ed.* **2009,** *48,* 9901–9904.
121. Horcajada, P.; Chalati, T.; Serre, C.; Gillet, B.; Sebrie, C.; Baati, T.; Eubank, J. F.; Heurtaux, D.; Clayette, P.; Kreuz, C.; Chang, J. S.; Hwang, Y. K.; Marsaud, V.; Bories, P. N.; Cynober, L.; Gil, S.; Ferey, G.; Couvreur, P.; Gref, R. *Nat. Mater.* **2010,** *9,* 172–178.
122. Park, K. H.; Jang, K.; Son, S. U.; Sweigart, D. A. *J. Am. Chem. Soc.* **2006,** *128,* 8740–8741.
123. Tanaka, D.; Kitagawa, S. *Chem. Mater.* **2008,** *20,* 922–931.
124. Miller, S. R.; Heurtaux, D.; Baati, T.; Horcajada, P.; Greneche, J. M.; Serre, C. *Chem. Commun.* **2010,** *46,* 4526–4528.
125. Imaz, I.; Hernando, J.; RuizMolina, D.; Maspoch, D. *Angew. Chem. Int. Ed.* **2009,** *48,* 2325–2329.
126. Imaz, I.; RubioMartinez, M.; GarciaFernandez, L.; Garcia, F.; RuizMolina, D.; Hernando, J.; Puntes, V.; Maspoch, D. *Chem. Commun.* **2010,** *46,* 4737–4739.
127. Nishiyabu, R.; Aime, C.; Gondo, R.; Kaneko, K.; Kimizuka, N. *Chem. Commun.* **2010,** *46,* 4333–4335.
128. Nishiyabu, R.; Aime, C.; Gondo, R.; Noguchi, T.; Kimizuka. *Angew. Chem. Int. Ed.* **2009,** *48,* 9465–9468.
129. Nishiyabu, R.; Hashimoto, N.; Cho, T.; Watanabe, K.; Yasunaga, T.; Endo, A.; Kaneko, K.; Niidome, T.; Murata, M.; Adachi, C.; Katayama, Y.; Hashizume, M.; Kimizuka, N. *J. Am. Chem. Soc.* **2009,** *131,* 2151–2158.
130. Roming, M.; Lunsdorf, H.; Dittmar, K. E. J.; Feldmann, C. *Angew. Chem. Int. Ed.* **2010,** *49,* 632–637.
131. Yan, X. H.; Zhu, P. L.; Fei, J. B.; Li. J. B. *Adv. Mater.* **2010,** *22,* 1283–1284.
132. Horcajada, P.; Serre, C.; Vallet-Regi, M.; Sebban, M.; Taulelle, F.; Ferey, G. *Angew. Chem. Int. Ed.* **2006,** *45,* 5974–5978.

133. Taylor Pashow, K.; Della Rocca, J.; Xie, Z.; Tran, S.; Lin, W. *J. Am. Chem. Soc.* **2009**, *131*, 14261–14263.
134. Nguyen, J. G.; Tanabe, K. K.; Cohen, S. M. *Cryst. Eng. Comm.* **2010**, *12*, 2335, 2338.
135. Zhang, D. E.; Zhang, X. J.; Ni, X. M.; Zheng, H. G.; Yang, D. D. *J. Magn. Magn. Mater.* **2005**, *292*, 79.
136. Wang, J.; Gudiksen, M. S.; Duan, X.; Cui, Y.; Lieber, C. M. *Science* **2001**, *293*, 1455.
137. Fleischhaker, F.; Arsenault, A. C.; Kitaev, V.; Peiris, F. C.; von Freymann, G.; Manners, I.; Zentel, R.; Ozin, G. A. *J. Am. Chem. Soc.* **2005**, *127*, 9318.
138. Blanco, Chomski, E.; Grabtchak, S.; Ibisate, M.; John, S.; Leonard, S. W.; Lopez, C.; Meseguer, F.; Miguez, H.; Mondia, J. P.; Ozin, G. A.; Toader, O.; van Driel, H. M. *Nature* **2000**, *405*, 437.
139. Salzemann, C.; Brioude, A.; Pileni, M. P. *J. Phys. Chem. B.* **2006**, *110*, 7208.
140. Lee, J. H. *Sens. Actuators B.* **2009**, *140*, 319.
141. Lu, W.; Qin, X.; Luo, Y.; Chang, G.; Sun, X. *Microchim. Acta* **2000**, *1*, 1791–1800.
142. Cao, Y. C.; Jin, R.; Mirkin, C. A. *Science* **2002**, *297*, 1536.
143. Bruchez, M.; Moronne, M.; Gin, P.; Weiss, S.; Alivisatos, A. P. *Science* **1998**, *281*, 2013.
144. Taton, T. A.; Mirkin, C. A.; Letsinger, R. L. *Science* **2000**, *289*, 1757.
145. Mirkin, C. A.; Letsinger, R. L.; Mucic, R. C.; Storhoff, J. J. *Nature* **1996**, *382*, 607.
146. Lee, J. H.; Huh, Y. M.; Jun, Y. W.; Seo, J. W.; Jang, J. T.; Song, H. T.; Kim, S.; Cho, E. J.; Yoon, H. G.; Suh, J. S.; Cheon, J. *Nat. Med.* **2007**, *13*, 95.
147. Gao, X.; Cui, Y.; Levenson, R. M.; Chung, L. W. K.; Nie, S. *Nat. Biotechnol.* **2004**, *22*, 969.
148. Sakunthala, A.; Reddy, M. V.; Selvasekarapandian, S.; Chowdari, B. V. R.; Selvin, P. C. *Electrochim. Acta* **2010**, *55*, 4441.
149. Saravanan, Ramar, V.; Balaya, P.; Vittal, J. J. *J. Mater. Chem.* **2011**, *21*, 14925.
150. Schmid, G.; Wiley-VCH Verlag GmbH & Co. KGaA. 2005.
151. Graf, N.; Lippard, S. J. *Adv. Drug Deliv. Rev.* **2012**, *64*, 993.
152. Horcajada, P.; Chalati, T.; Serre, C.; Gillet, B.; Sebrie, C.; Baati, T.; Eubank, J. F.; Heurtaux, D.; Clayette, P.; Kreuz, C.; Chang, J. S.; Hwang, Y. K.; Marsaud, V.; Bories, P. N.; Cynober, L.; Gil, S.; Ferey, G.; Couvreur, P.; Gref, R. *Nat. Mater.* **2010**, *9*(2), 172–178.
153. Imaz, I.; Hernando, J.; Ruiz-Molina, D.; Maspoch, D. *Angew. Chem. Int. Edit.* **2009**, *48*(13), 2325–2329
154. Imaz, I.; Rubio-Martínez, M.; García-Fernández, L.; García, F.; Ruiz-Molina, D.; Hernando, J.; Puntes, V.; Maspoch, D. *Chem. Commun.* **2010**, *46*, 4737.
155. Kelland, L. *Nat. Rev. Cancer* **2007**, *7*, 573.
156. Meerum Terwogt, J. M.; Groenewegen, G.; Pluim, D.; Maliepaard, M.; Tibben, M. M.; Huisman, A.; ten Bokkel Huinink, W. W.; Schot, M.; Welbank, H.; Voest, E. E.; Beijnen, J. H.; Schellens, J. M. *Cancer Chemother. Pharmacol.* **2002**, *49*, 201.
157. Sood, P.; Hurmond, K. B.; Jacob, J. E.; Waller, L. K.; Silva, G. O.; Stewart, D. R.; Nowotnik, D. P. *Bioconjugate Chem.* **2006**, *17*, 1270.
158. Feazell, R. P.; Nakayama-Ratchford, N.; Dai, H.; Lippard, S. J. *J. Am. Chem. Soc.* **2007**, *129*, 8438.
159. Green, J. R. *Oncologist* **2004**, *9*, 3.

160. Liu, D.; Kramer, S. A.; Huxford-Phillips, R. C.; Wang, S.; Della Rocca, J.; Lin, W. *Chem. Commun.* **2012,** *48,* 2668.
161. Morris, W.; Briley, W. E.; Auyeung, E.; Cabezas, M. D.; Mirkin, C. A. *J. Am. Chem. Soc.* **2014,** *136,* 7261–7264.
162. Liu, Z.; Cheung, R.; Wu, X. Y.; Ballinger, J. R.; Bendayan, R.; Rauth, A. M. *J. Control. Release* **2001,** *77,* 213–224.
163. Kwon, G. S.; Naito, M.; Kataoka, K.; Yokoyama, M.; Sajurai, Y.; Okano, T. *Colloids Surf. B.* **1994,** *2,* 429–434.
164. Ratanatawanate, C.; Chyao, A.; Balkus Jr, K. J. *J. Am. Chem.* Soc. **2011,** *133,* 3492.
165. Wu, L.; Quan, B. G.; Liu, Y. L.; Song, R.; Tang, Z. Y. *ACS Nano.* **2011,** *5,* 2224.
166. Nagarathinam, M.; Saravanan, K.; Leong, W. L.; Balaya, P.; Vittal, J. J. *Cryst. Growth Des.* **2009,** *9,* 4461.
167. Xiong, S.; Xi, B.; Wang, C.; Zou, G.; Fei, L. Wang, W.; Qian, Y. *Chem. Eur. J.* **2007,** *13,* 3076.
168. Anokhina, E. V.; Go, Y. B.; Lee, Y.; Vogt, T.; Jacobson, A. J. *J. Am. Chem. Soc.* **2006,** *128,* 9957.
169. Zhang, Y. G.; Saha, M. K.; Bernal, I. *Cryst. Eng. Commun.* **2003,** *5,* 34.
170. Horcajada, P.; Chalati, T.; Serre, C.; Gillet, B.; Sebrie, C.; Baati, T.; Eubank, J. F.; Heurtaux, D.; Clayette, P.; Kreuz, C.; Chang, J. S.; Hwang, Y. K.; Marsaud, V.; Bories, P. N.; Cynober, L.; Gil, S.; Fe´rey, G.; Couvreur, P.; Gref, R. *Nat. Mater.* **2010,** *9,* 172–178.
171. Boldog, I.; Gaspar, A. B.; Mart_nez, V.; Pardo-Ibanez, P.; Ksenofontov, V.; Bhattacharjee, A.; Gutlich, P.; Real, J. A. *Angew. Chem.* **2008,** *120,* 6533–6537. (*Angew. Chem. Int. Ed.* **2008,** *47,* 6433–6437).
172. Rieter, W. J.; Taylor, K. M. L., Lin, W. *J. Am. Chem. Soc.* **2007,** *129,* 9852–9853.
173. Rosenholm, J. M.; Meinander, A.; Peuhu, E.; Niemi, R.; Eriksson, J. E.; Sahlgren, C.; Linden, M. *ACS Nano.* **2009,** *3,* 197–206.
174. Rosenholm, J. M.; Peuhu, E.; Eriksson, J. E.; Sahlgren, C; Linden, M. *Nano Lett.* **2009,** *9,* 3308–3311.
175. Vivero-Escoto, J. L.; Rieter, W. J.; Lau, H.; Huxford-Phillips, R. C.; Lin, W. *Small.* **2013,** *9,* 3523–3531.
176. Kherlopian, A. R.; Song, T.; Duan, Q.; Neimark, M. A.; Po, M. J.; Gohagan, J. K.; Laine, A. F. *BMC Syst. Biol.* **2008,** *2,* 74.
177. Hashemi, R. H.; Bradley, W. G. Williams and Wilkins: Baltimore, 1997.
178. Zhou, Z.; Li, D.; Yang, H.; Zhu, Y.; Yang, S. *Dalton Trans.* **2011,** *40,* 11941.
179. Wessels, J. T.; Yamauchi, K.; Hoffman, R. M.; Wouters, F. S. *Cytometry Part A* **2010,** *77,* 667–676.
180. Taylor, K. M. L.; Jin, A.; Lin, W. *Angew Chem. Int Ed.* **2008,** *47,* 7722–7725**.**
181. Aime, C.; Nishiyahu, R.; Gondo, R.; Kimizuka, N. *Chem. Eur. J.* **2010,** *16,* 3604–3607.
182. Kerbellec, N.; Catala, L.; Daiguebonne, C.; Gloter, A.; Stephan, O.; Bunzli, J. C.; Guillou, O.; Mallah, T. *Cryst. Eng. Comm.* **2010,** *12,* 3959–3963.
183. Zhang, X. J.; Ballem, M. A.; Ahren, M.; Suska, A.; Bergman, P.; Uvdal, K. *J Am Chem Soc.* **2010,** *132,* 10391–10397.
184. Liu, D.; Huxford, R. C.; Lin, W. *Angew Chem. Int Ed.* **2011,** *50,* 3696–3700.
185. Brindle, K. *Nat Rev Cancer.* **2008,** *8,* 94–107.

186. Yu, S. B.; Watson, A. D. *Chem Rev.* **1999,** *99,* 2353–2378.
187. Bouzigues, C.; Gacoin, T.; Alexandrou, A. *ACS Nano.* **2011,** *5,* 8488.
188. Aimé, C.; Nishiyabu, R.; Gondo, R.; Kimizuka, N. *Chem. Eur. J.* **2010,** *16,* 3604.
189. Lan, A.; Li, K., Wu, H.; Olson, D. H.; Emge, T. J.; Ki, W.; Hong, M. C.; Li, J. *Angew. Chem. Int. Ed.* **2009,** *48,* 2334.
190. Yang, Y.; Turnbull, G. A.; Samuel, I. D. W. *Adv. Funct. Mater.* **2010,** *20,* 2093.
191. Dai, L. X. *Angew. Chem. Int. Ed.* **2004,** *43,* 5726.
192. Gombotz, W. R.; Pettit, D. K. *Bioconjug. Chem.* **1995,** *6,* 332–351.
193. Ferey, G.; Draznieks, C. M.; Serre, C.; Millange, F.; Dutour, J.; Surble, S.; Margiolaki, I. *Science* **2005,** *309,* 2040–2042.
194. Bauer, S.; Serre, C.; Devic, T.; Horcajada, P.; Morrot, J.; Ferey, G.; Stock, N. *Inorg Chem.* **2008,** *47,* 7568–7576.
195. Xing, L.; Zheng, H. Q.; Che, S. N. *Chem.–Eur. J.* **2011,** *17*(26), 7271–7275.
196. Howard, K. A.; Peer, D. *Nanomed.-UK.* **2013,** *8*(7), 1031–1033.
197. Peer, D.; Karp, J. M.; Hong, S.; FaroKHzad, O. C.; Margalit, R.; Langer, R. *Nat. Nanotechnol.* **2007,** *2*(12), 751–760.
198. Langer, R. *Nature* **1998,** *392*–395.
199. Wang, B.; Siahaan, T. J.; Soltero, R. A. In *Ed.* Wiley, Inc. 2005.
200. Reddy, J. R.; Veera, M.; Mohamed, T. S.; Madhu, C. S. *J. Pharm. Sci. Res.* **2009,** *1,* 109–115.
201. Brocchini, S.; Duncan, R. Polymer-Drug Conjugates: Drug Release from Pendent Linkers. In *Encyclopedia of Controlled Release*; Mathiowitz, E., Ed.; Wiley: NY, USA, 1999; pp 786–816.
202. Ferruti, P.; Marchisio, M. A.; Duncan, R. *Macromol. Rapid Commun.* **2002,** *23,* 332–355.
203. Doane, T. L.; Burda, C. *Chem. Soc. Rev.* **2012,** *41,* 2885.
204. Janib, S. M.; Moses, A. S.; MacKay, J. A. *Adv. Drug Delivery Rev.* **2010,** *62,* 1052.
205. Xie, J.; Lee, S.; Chen, X. *Adv. Drug Deliv Rev.* **2010,** *62,* 1064.
206. Hu, K. W.; Hsu, K. C.; Yeh, C. S. *Biomaterials* **2010,** *31,* 6843.
207. Guo, R.; Zhang, L.; Qian, H.; Li, R.; Jiang, X.; Liu, B. *Langmuir* **2010,** *26,* 5428.
208. Kim, S.; Ohulchanskyy, T. Y.; Pudavar, H. E.; Pandey, R. K.; Prasad, P. N. *J. Am. Chem. Soc.* **2007,** *129,* 2669–2675.
209. He, X. X.; Wu, X.; Wang, K. M.; Shi, B. H.; Hai, L. *Biomaterials* **2009,** *30,* 5601–5609.
210. Lai, C. Y.; Trewyn, B. G.; Jeftinija, D. M.; Jeftinija, K.; Xu, S.; Jeftinija, S.; Lin, V. S. Y. *J. Am. Chem. Soc.* **2003,** *125,* 4451–4459.
211. Giri, S.; Trewyn, B. G.; Stellmaker, M. P.; Lin, V. S. Y. *Angew. Chem., Int. Ed.* **2005,** *44,* 5038–5044.
212. Vivero-Escoto, J. L.; Slowing, I. I.; Wu, C. W.; Lin, V. S. Y. *J. Am. Chem. Soc.* **2009,** *131,* 3462–3463.
213. Zhao, Y.; Trewyn, B. G.; Slowing, I.; Lin, V. S. Y. *J. Am. Chem. Soc.* **2009,** *131,* 8398–8400.
214. Rocca, J. D.; Huxford, R. C.; Comstock-Duggan, E.; Lin, W. *Angew. Chem. Int. Ed.* **2011,** *50*(44), 10330–10334.

215. Rocca, J. D.; Werner, M. E.; Kramer, S. A.; Huxford-Phillips, R. C.; Sukumar, R.; Cummings, N. D.; Vivero-Escoto, J. L.; Wang, A. Z.; Lin, W. *Nanomed. Nanotechnol. Biol. Med.* **2014,** *11*(1), 31–38.

216. Tang, L.; Fan, T. M.; Borst, L. B.; Cheng, J. *ACS Nano.* **2012,** *6*, 3954–3966.

217. Tang, L.; Gabrielson, N. P.; Uckun, F. M.; Fan, T. M.; Cheng, J. J. *Mol Pharm.* **2013,** *10*, 883–892.

218. Rusanov, E. B.; Ponomarova, V. V.; Komarchuk, V. V.; Stoeckli-Evans, H.; Boldog, E. I.; Sieler, J.; Chernega, A. N.; Domasevitch, K. V. *Inorg. Chim. Acta.* **2002,** *69*, 338.

219. Ehlert, M. K.; Rettig, S. J.; Storr, A.; Thompson, R. C.; Trotter, J. *Acta Crystallogr. C* **1994,** *50*, 1023.

220. Ponomarova, V. V.; Komarchuk, V. V.; Boldog, I.; Chernega, A. N.; Sieler, J.; Domasevitch, K. V. *Chem. Commun.* **2002,** *436*.

221. Pettinari, C.; Tabacaru, A.; Boldog, I.; Domasevitch, K. V.; Galli, S.; Masciocchi, N. *Inorg. Chem.* **2012,** *51*, 5235.

222. Xie, Y. M.; Liu, J. H.; Wu, X. Y.; Zhao, Z. G.; Zhang, Q. S.; Wang, F.; Chen, S. C.; Lu, C. Z. *Cryst. Growth Des.* **2008,** *8*, 3914.

223. Rusanov, E. B.; Ponomarova, V. V.; Komarchuk, V. V.; Stoeckli-Evans, H.; Fernandez-Ibãnez, E.; Stoeckli, F.; Sieler, J.; Domasevitch, K. V. *Angew. Chem. Int. Ed.* **2003,** *42*, 2499.

CHAPTER 2

APPLICATION OF THERMODYNAMIC MODELS FOR PREDICTION OF EXPERIMENTAL SOLUBILITY OF ALKALI METAL HALIDES IN AQUEOUS ORGANIC SOLVENTS

SUSHMA P. IJARDAR[1,2,*], ARVIND KUMAR[2], DEBASHIS KUNDU[3], TAMAL BANERJEE[3] and NAVED I. MALEK[4]

[1]Department of Chemistry, Veer Narmad South Gujarat University, Surat 395007, India

[2]Salt and Marine Chemicals Division, CSIR—Central Salt and Marine Chemicals Research Institute (CSIR-CSMCRI), Council of Scientific & Industrial Research (CSIR), Bhavnagar 364002, India

[3]Department of Chemical Engineering, Indian Institute of Technology Guwahati, Guwahati 781039, Assam, India

[4]Applied Chemistry Department, S. V. National Institute of Technology, Surat 395007, India

*Corresponding author. E-mail: sushmaijardar@yahoo.co.in

CONTENTS

ABSTRACT

Aqueous electrolyte solutions have an important role in the chemical industry for various separation techniques. The introduction of inorganic salts has a dramatic effect on mutual solubility of organic solvent in water. The accurate knowledge of phase equilibria plays vital role in designing and selection of separation process. The solubility of alkali metal halides (AMHs), such as sodium fluoride (NaF), sodium chloride (NaCl), sodium bromide (NaBr), potassium chloride (KCl), potassium bromide (KBr), and potassium iodide (KI), in organic solvent and their aqueous binary mixtures have been studied. The experiments have been performed over full range of compositions and at temperature range from 308.15 to 328.15 K. An analytical gravimetric method has been used to measure solubility of studied AMHs. The effects of temperature, composition of binary mixture, and molecular interactions on the solubility have been discussed. Depending upon mixing ratio in binary mixture, the solubility of AMHs was expected to be controlled by molecular interactions existing within the mixture. The experimental solubility was correlated using non-random two-liquid (NRTL) and UNIversal QUAsi Chemical (UNIQUAC) models at all studied temperatures.

2.1   INTRODUCTION

An addition of an electrolyte in solvent mixtures or of an organic solvent to aqueous electrolyte solution has a remarkable effect on its phase equilibrium resulting in salting out or salting effect for solvent or electrolyte. Therefore, an accurate knowledge of phase equilibria is key toll for designing and optimization of various separation processes, such as isothermal crystallization, desalination process, liquid–liquid extraction (LLE), antisolvent crystallization, and azeotropic distillation, where accurate solubility data on temperatures is essential. The solubility of electrolytes in aqueous or nonaqueous systems also provides information regarding variation in boiling point of fluid, ion speciation, working temperature, and solvent composition, which is equally important for designing of chemical processes.[1–3] The solubility studies help us to understand nonideal behavior of solutions through solvent–solvent and ion–solvent interactions on molecular scale. At low salt concentration, solvent–solvent interactions were significant, which were dominated by ion association whereas as concentration of salt increases in mixture ion–solvent interactions dominate.[4,5] The thermodynamic modeling of solubility of salts in aqueous and nonaqueous solution is also important for industrial process. Debye and Hückel[6] first proposed a model to study the effect of salts on the phase behavior at very low concentration. This model has been extended for higher ionic strength by Bromley[7] and Pitzer.[8] Subsequently, several other Gibbs free energy models, such as UNIversal QUAsi Chemical (UNIQUAC),[9] non-random two-liquid (NRTL),[10] and UNIFAC[11] have been developed and verified using database of Dortmund Data Bank.[12]

Dimethyl sulfoxide (DMSO) is a dipolar aprotic solvent with two hydrophobic methyl moieties and strongly polar sulfoxide group. DMSO is most commonly used as a solvent in chemical processes. The boiling point of DMSO is high, and it contributes less in air pollution as compared to commonly used low-boiling-point alcohols, ketones, and ethers in industries. In biology, it is used as a cryoprotector in the denaturation of proteins, and as a drug carrier across cell membranes.[13,14] It possess good solvent scale values such as high dielectric constant ($\varepsilon = 47$) and hydrogen bond accepting value ($\beta = 0.76$) which makes it suitable for solubilization of several metal ions. The oxygen atom in DMSO can interact with positive charges and thus stabilize metal cation.[15] It has low hydrogen bond donating values ($\alpha = 0$). This indicates inability of solvent to solubilize anions. DMSO has infinite miscibility in water at ambient temperature and forms hydrogen bonds with water molecules. At 2:1 molar ratio, DMSO–water binary solution forms eutectic mixture, and low DMSO concentration acts as a cryoprotectant with low freezing point.[16] In spite of great industrial importance, there is no systematic data reported on solubility of alkali metal halides (AMHs) in DMSO–water system at varying temperatures which can furnish information about the recovery of DMSO and its ability as an antisolvent. The present solubility was initiated to get basic information regarding antisolvent crystallization of AMHs from water by DMSO, and the use of AMHs from recovery of DMSO from aqueous medium.

A detailed literature survey shows limited study on solubility of AMHs in aqueous organic system at different temperatures.[5,17–37] Pinho and Macedo reported solubility of KBr, NaCl, NaBr, and KCl in binary mixtures of water + methanol and water + ethanol.[5,17] Gomis and his coworkers studied solubility of NaCl and KCl in aqueous solutions of 1-propanol, 2-propanol, butanol,[18,19] and lithium chloride in water + pentanol.[20] The solubility of NaCl in binary mixtures of cyclohexanol, benzyl alcohol, and cyclohexanol + water has been reported by Wagner et al.[21] The liquid–liquid equilibria of the NaCl, NaBr, NaI, and KCl + 2-ethoxyethanol + H_2O at 298.15 K have been studied by Boruń et al.[22] The solubility of KCl, $MgCl_2$, and KBr in acetone + water at different temperatures have been reported by Wang et al.[23,24] The solubility of NaBr, NaCl, and KBr has also been reported in cationic and anionic surfactants.[25] Gmehling et al. have studied solubility of NaCl, KCl, LiCl, and LiBr in methanol, ethanol, acetone, and mixed solvents and effect of NaCl and KCl on solid liquid phase equilibria of DMSO + water.[26,27]

Taboda and her group investigated solubility and physicochemical behavior of lithium hydroxide in ethanol + water at different temperatures.[28] The solubility and density of KI in ethanol + water and NaI in water + methanol, water + ethanol, and water + 2-propanol at different temperatures have been reported by Pawar and his coworkers.[29,30] The phase equilibria of rubidium or cesium salts + monohydric alcohol or amides + water have been investigated at various temperatures by Hu et al.[31–36] Li et al., reported solid–liquid equilibrium of N, N-Dimethylacetamide + alkali metal chloride + water.[37]

This chapter presents the experimental solubility of AMHs, such as sodium fluoride (NaF), sodium chloride (NaCl), sodium bromide (NaBr), potassium chloride (KCl), potassium bromide (KBr), and potassium iodide (KI) in pure DMSO and DMSO–water binary solution at temperature ranges from 308.15 to 328.15 K over entire range of compositions. The change in solubility behavior is discussed as a function of strength of molecular interactions, nature of AMHs and temperature. Further, the experimental solubility was correlated employing local composition activity coefficient models UNIQUAC and NRTL at all studied temperatures.

2.2 EXPERIMENTAL SECTION

2.2.1 MATERIALS

NaF, NaCl, NaBr, KCl, KBr, and KI were purchased from Sisco Research Laboratories Pvt. Ltd. (SRL), India. The source and purity of AMHs and DMSO are given in Table 2.1. The studied AMHs (except KI) were dried in drying oven at 373.15 K for 3 days to avoid any hydrate formation. KI was dried at 323.15 K. After drying process, the water content in studied AMHs was below detectable limit. The purity of AMHs were checked by measuring concentration of Na^+ and K^+ by inductively coupled plasma (ICP)spectrometer Perkin Elmer, Optima 2000. DMSO was also purchased from SRL with purity better than 99.5 %. The purity of DMSO was checked by gas chromatography equipped with semi-capillary methyl silicone column (OD: 530 λ_m) and flame ionization detector. The water content in DMSO was 150 ppm as measured by Karl Fisher titration (Metrohm, 890 Titrando). Milli-Q distilled water was used for preparation of binary mixtures.

TABLE 2.1 CAS Number, Supplier, Purification Method, Purity Analysis Method and Final Purity of AMHs and DMSO.

Components	CAS Number	Supplier	Purification method	Purity analysis method	Final purity in mass (%)
DMSO	67-68-5	SRL	–	GC	99.5
NaF	7681-49-4	SRL	Drying at 373.15 K	ICP	99.0
NaBr	7647-15-6	SRL	Drying at 373.15 K	ICP	99.0
NaCl	7647-14-5	SRL	Drying at 373.15 K	ICP	99.9
KBr	7758-02-3	SRL	Drying at 373.15 K	ICP	99.5
KCl	7447-40-7	SRL	Drying at 373.15 K	ICP	99.5
KI	7681-11-0	SRL	Drying at 323.15 K	ICP	99.8

GC Gas chromatography, *ICP* Inductive coupled plasma spectrometer
All AMHs were dried in drying oven for 3 days in order to avoid for any hydrate formation.

2.2.2   MIXTURES PREPARATION

The binary mixtures of DMSO and water were prepared on salt free mass fraction using Mettler Toledo analytical balance B 204-S with an uncertainty of $\pm 1.10^{-7}$ kg.

2.2.3   SOLUBILITY MEASUREMENT

The solubility experiments were performed using similar setup and procedure adopted by Gmehling et al.[26] A four jacketed glass cell of 50 cc volume were placed in series attached to refrigeration and heating circulator (JULABO F 32-ME) to maintain the solutions temperatures. The temperatures were controlled by a built in Pt100 sensor with precision ± 0.1 K. The jacketed glass cells were placed over magnetic stirrer of 500 rpm. The set temperature was set slightly higher than working temperature of the solution. The desired quantity of salt was added into known concentration of DMSO–water binary mixture filled in glass cell. The glass cells were tightly capped with rubber septum. For sufficient contact time between mixture and metal halides, each mixture was stirred for 6 h at working temperature. The mixture was allowed to settle for 4 h and 3 ml of clear solution was withdrawn by thermostatic syringe into an empty glass vial. The weight of empty vial was denoted as W_1. The three samples were withdrawn for each concentration very cautiously so that no solid salt particles were drawn into clear solution. The weight of vials with clear solution was denoted as W_2. The glass vials were placed on the hot plate at around 363 K for evaporation of water and DMSO. The glass vials were kept in oven for 12 h at 450 K for removal of traces of the solvents. The final constant weight of vial with dry salt residue was denoted as W_3. The solubility of salts was calculated by following equation:

$$\text{Solubility [mol·kg}^{-1}] = (W_3 - W_1)/(W_2 - W_3) \times 1/M_{\text{salt}} \qquad (2.1)$$

where M_{salt} is the molar mass of the salt. The tabulated values in Tables 2.3 and 2.4 are the mean values of three solubility measurements at a constant temperature and salt free mole fraction. The standard deviation within different experimental results was defined in Equation 2.2.

$$\text{S. D.} = \left(\frac{1}{n-1} \sum (x_i - \bar{x})^2 \right)^{1/2} \tag{2.2}$$

x_i is the experimental solubility of AMHs i and $\bar{x}$ is mean of n solubility results. In each case standard deviations are less than 0.005. Two criteria were provided for data analysis: (i) if the experimental solubility is lower than 10 wt.%, the standard deviation should be lower than 0.005; and (ii) if the solubility was higher than 10 wt.%, the quotient $2s/\text{solubility} \times 100$, should be lower than 0.1.

2.2.4 COMPUTATIONAL DETAILS

Experimental solubility data was fitted to excess Gibbs free energy based NRTL[9] and UNIQUAC[10] activity coefficient models. These models rely on the experimental dataset and binary interaction parameters. The optimization problem requires an objective function which is nonlinear in nature and nonconvex in terms of optimization variables. Global optimization technique removes any local minima, maxima or saddle points and searches for global minimum or maximum within a specified boundary range. Here we have used genetic algorithm (GA)[38] to calculate the NRTL and UNIQUAC interaction parameters. GA has been successfully applied in the prediction of liquid–liquid equilibria systems[39,40] and also incorporates the successful application of NRTL and UNIQUAC models for ionic solutions. The objective function for GA is:

Maximize:

$$F_{\left(\substack{\text{with respect to } A_{ij} \\ \text{where } i,j=1,2,3 \\ \text{and } j \neq i}\right)} = -\sum_{k=1}^{m} \sum_{l=1}^{2} \sum_{i=1}^{c} w_{ik}^{l} \left(x_{pred,ik}^{l} - x_{expt,ik}^{l} \right)^2, \; w_{ik}^{l} = 1 \tag{2.3}$$

The NRTL and UNIQUAC interaction parameters are reported in Tables 2.5 and 2.6. Table 2.7 represents two structural parameters namely, volume and surface area that are required for UNIQUAC model. These structural parameters were predicted by polarizable continuum model (PCM) with the polyhedral algorithm (GEPOL) as described in the literature.[41] The solubility was predicted by modified Rachford-Rice algorithm.[42] Rachford-Rice algorithm is typically used for the prediction of phase behavior LLE process. Here we have considered the solute dissolved in aqueous DMSO solution as raffinate phase and pure salt as extract phase. Since, pure salt has no solvent or water, the mole fraction of salt in extract phase is 1 for all tie lines and mole fraction of solvents, that is, DMSO and water are 0. In raffinate phase, the mole fractions are taken from the experimental dataset.

2.2.4.1 PREDICTION OF SOLUBILITY BY MODIFIED RACHFORD-RICE ALGORITHM

Both pure solute-containing phase and liquid phase will be considered as liquid phases. Overall composition z_i and molar holdup L splits into two liquid phases (compositions are x_i^I and x_i^{II} molar holdups L^I and L^{II}, respectively). So, overall and component material balances are:

$$L = L^I + L^{II} \tag{2.4}$$

$$Lz_i = L^I x_i^I + L^{II} x_i^{II} \tag{2.5}$$

K_i is defined as distribution coefficient and LLE split of phase I as ψ, $\psi = L^I / L$. As the two phases are in phase equilibrium with each other, thus we have:

$$x_i^I \gamma_i^I = x_i^{II} \gamma_i^{II} \tag{2.6}$$

$$\frac{x_i^I}{x_i^{II}} = \frac{\gamma_i^{II}}{\gamma_i^I} = K_i \tag{2.7}$$

Here γ_i^{II} and γ_i^I (where i = number of compounds in a single phase) are calculated either NRTL or UNIQUAC model. So, the mole fraction in the liquid phase is given by:

$$x_i^I = \frac{K_i z_i}{\left[1 + \psi \left(K_i - 1\right)\right]}; \quad x_i^{II} = \frac{z_i}{\left[1 + \psi \left(K_i - 1\right)\right]} \tag{2.8}$$

ψ is calculated by modified Rachford-Rice equation (Eq. 2.9)

$$\sum_{i=1}^{n} \frac{z_i(1-K_i)}{\left[1+\psi(K_i-1)\right]} = 0 \tag{2.9}$$

Additionally, the following constraints are also to be satisfied

$$\sum_{i=1}^{n} x_i^I = 1, \quad \sum_{i=1}^{n} x_i^{II} = 1 \tag{2.10}$$

The goodness of fit is referred by the root mean square deviation (RMSD) and given by the following equation:

$$RMSD(\%) = \left[\sum_{k=1}^{m}\sum_{i=1}^{c}\sum_{l=1}^{2} \frac{\left(x_{pred,ik}^{I} - x_{expt,ik}^{I}\right)^2}{2mc}\right]^{1/2} \times 100 \tag{2.11}$$

where m is a number of tie-lines and c is number of compounds.

2.2.4.1.1   Non-random Two-Liquid (NRTL) Model

Nonideal liquid phase activity coefficient is given by the following equation:

$$\ln\gamma_i = \frac{\sum_{j=1}^{c}\tau_{ji}G_{ji}x_j}{G_{ki}x_k} + \sum_{j=1}^{c}\frac{G_{ij}x_j}{\sum_{k=1}^{c}G_{kj}x_k}\left(\tau_{ij} - \frac{\sum_{i=1}^{c}\tau_{ij}G_{ij}x_i}{\sum_{k=1}^{c}G_{kj}x_k}\right) \tag{2.12}$$

where, $G_{ji} = \exp\left(-\alpha_{ji}\tau_{ji}\right), \quad \tau_{ji} = \frac{g_{ji}-g_{ii}}{RT} = \frac{A_{ji}}{T}$

Value of τ_{ij} is reported in Table 2.5. The binary interaction parameter τ_{ij} is unitless, α_{ij} is taken as 0.2.

2.2.4.1.2   UNIversal QUAssi Chemical (UNIQUAC) Model

Nonideal liquid phase activity coefficient is given by the following equation:

$$\ln \gamma_i = \ln\left(\frac{\phi_i}{x_i}\right) + \frac{z}{2} q_i \ln\left(\frac{\theta_i}{\phi_i}\right) + l_i - \frac{\phi_i}{x_i}\sum_{j=1}^{c} x_j l_j$$

$$+ q_i \left(1 - \ln\sum_{j=1}^{c}\theta_j\tau_{ji} - \sum_{j=1}^{c}\frac{\theta_j\tau_{ij}}{\sum_{k=1}^{c}\theta_k\tau_{kj}} \right) \tag{2.13}$$

where,

$$\tau_{ij} = \exp\left(-\frac{A_{ij}}{T}\right), \quad \theta_i = \frac{q_i x_i}{\sum_{k=1}^{c} q_k x_k}, \quad \phi_i = \frac{r_i x_i}{\sum_{k=1}^{c} r_k x_k}, \quad l_i = \frac{z}{2}(r_k - q_k) + 1 - r_k$$

2.3   RESULTS AND DISCUSSIONS

2.3.1   SOLUBILITY OF ALKALI METAL HALIDES IN PURE DMSO

The experimental and literature value of solubility for NaF, NaCl, NaBr, KCl, KBr, and KI in pure DMSO at studied temperature are listed in Table 2.2.[43–45] In literature, most of the solubility data is reported at 298.15 K, a very limited literature data is available for NaCl, NaBr, and KCl at studied temperature range.[45] The solubility of NaCl and KCl matches with Unni et al.[43] The absolute deviation between solubility of NaCl and KCl was calculated around 0.003 and 0.0026, respectively. The deviation is higher around 0.03 and 0.017, respectively when compared with a solubility of NaCl and KCl reported by Long et al.[44] The solubility of KBr matches well with the values reported by Long et al.[44] with a maximum absolute deviation of 0.02. The higher deviation around 0.08 was observed with Gopal et al.[45] The average absolute deviation (AAD) at studied temperatures between experimental and literature values of solubility for NaCl, KCl, and KBr was 0.29, 0.35, and 0.36, respectively. The good agreements have been observed with literature in case of NaBr and KI, the

TABLE 2.2 Comparison Between Experimental and Literature Solubility of AMHs in DMSO at 100.7 kPa Pressure and T=308.15, 318.15, and 328.15 K.

Temp.	Experimental value	Literature value
NaF		
308.15	0.0054	–
318.15	0.0079	–
318.15	0.0104	–
NaCl		
308.15	0.07664	0.07923[a] 0.04802[b]
318.15	0.07729	0.08042[a] 0.05406[b]
328.15	0.07879	0.08162[a] 0.05868[b]
NaBr		
308.15	0.6825	0.6978[c]
318.15	0.8252	0.8300[c]
328.15	0.9784	
KCl		
308.15	0.0231	0.02296[a] 0.005615[b]
318.15	0.0259	0.02350[a] 0.01225[b]
328.15	0.0267	0.02404[a] 0.01588[b]
KBr		
308.15	0.4681	0.4448[b] 0.5437[c]
318.15	0.4792	0.4743[b] 0.5571[c]
328.15	0.4946	0.4974[b]
KI		
308.15	2.895	2.962[c]
318.15	3.075	3.096[c]
328.15	3.284	

[a]Ref 43

[b]Ref 44

[c]Ref 45

*Solubility was predicated at intermediate temperature considering linear fitting of solubility verses temperature in Ref 43.

#Solubility of salts was at ±1.0 K in Ref 44.

absolute deviations were found around 0.01 and 0.06, respectively.[44,45] The solubility of studied AMHs increases nonlinearly with temperature. In case of sodium metal halides (SMHs), the solubility decreases as NaBr > NaCl > NaF and similar solubility trend was observed for potassium metal halides (PMHs) that follows the order as KI > KBr > KCl. This trend is in accordance with the conclusion made by Miller and Parker.[46] The small anions are almost insoluble in dipolar aprotic solvents due to inability to form a hydrogen bond with it. Long[44] reported a similar trend for solubility of NaCl, NaBr, and KCl in DMSO. Recently, Nostro et al.[47,48] found a similar order for the salvation of anions (per fixed potassium cation) in ethylene carbonate and propylene carbonate. They have explained this trend considering Hofmeister series,[49] which was used to explain salting out of protein from aqueous solution by adding salts.

2.3.2   SOLUBILITY OF ALKALI METAL HALIDES IN BINARY MIXTURES OF DMSO–WATER

DMSO and water are completely miscible in all proportion. The solubility of NaF, NaCl, NaBr, KI, KCl, and KBr in the binary mixtures of DMSO-water at studied temperatures and compositions are listed in Tables 2.3 and 2.4. The comparisons between experimental and predicted solubility by NRTL and UNIQUAC at 308.15 K are presented in Figs. 2.1–2.6 at studied temperatures. The RMSDs and average RMSDs for the studied system by NRTL and UNIQAUC at all temperatures are given in Table 2.8. As depicted in Tables 2.3 and 2.4 and Figs. 2.1–2.6, the solubility of SMHs and PMHs decreases considerably with the addition of DMSO in binary mixtures. This trend is similar to results reported earlier with other organic solvents, like addition of alcohol[18,19,29,33] and DMA[37] to an aqueous solution of AMHs decreases the solubility of salts. At fixed concentration of DMSO, the solubility of SMHs and PMHs increases nonlinearly with increasing temperature. The solubility of SMHs decreases in order of NaBr > NaF > NaCl and PMHs decreases as KI > KBr > KCl at all temperatures (Tables 2.3 and 2.4). For fixed anion, the solubility of SMHs was higher as compared to PMHs.

TABLE 2.3 Solubility (mol·kg⁻¹) of SMHs in DMSO–Water at 100.7 kPa Pressure and T=308.15, 318.15, and 328.15 K.

DMSO (wt.%)	NaF			NaBr			NaCl		
	Temp.								
	308.15	318.15	328.15	308.15	318.15	328.15	308.15	318.15	328.15
10	0.6353	0.6661	0.6980	7.561	8.684	9.902	5.095	5.215	5.295
20	0.3980	0.4202	0.4428	6.565	7.456	8.466	4.433	4.459	4.489
30	0.2125	0.2299	0.2514	6.044	6.797	7.528	3.359	3.419	3.465
40	0.0959	0.1086	0.1293	5.604	6.223	6.887	2.436	2.490	2.5426
50	0.0438	0.0588	0.0740	5.125	5.692	6.203	1.855	1.912	1.965
60	0.0195	0.0289	0.0379	4.556	5.055	5.603	1.406	1.446	1.482
70	0.0102	0.0153	0.0209	4.092	4.560	5.124	0.8892	0.9255	0.9625
80	0.0071	0.0094	0.0139	3.458	3.853	4.268	0.6001	0.6286	0.6582
90	0.0060	0.0081	0.0115	2.379	2.778	3.183	0.3442	0.3559	0.3723

TABLE 2.4 Solubility (mol·kg⁻¹) of PMHs in DMSO–Water at 100.7 kPa Pressure and T =308.15, 318.15, and 328.15 K.

DMSO (wt.%)	NaF			NaBr			NaCl		
	Temp.								
	308.15	318.15	328.15	308.15	318.15	328.15	308.15	318.15	328.15
10	4.1227	4.646	5.133	5.162	5.678	6.230	8.330	8.868	9.614
20	3.1469	3.590	3.943	4.284	4.733	5.189	7.350	7.970	8.454
30	2.2881	2.715	3.134	3.529	3.872	4.213	6.416	6.921	7.327
40	1.5591	1.918	2.281	2.943	3.156	3.385	5.657	6.184	6.500
50	1.0072	1.284	1.529	2.426	2.565	2.693	4.954	5.301	5.621
60	0.6252	0.8556	1.017	1.888	1.999	2.122	4.433	4.773	5.106
70	0.3664	0.4804	0.5997	1.4368	1.5553	1.6438	4.014	4.393	4.618
80	0.21	0.2664	0.3218	1.0766	1.1626	1.2351	3.651	3.937	4.208
90	0.1069	0.141	0.1868	0.7265	0.8101	0.9087	3.299	3.533	3.753

The mixing of DMSO and water is an exothermic process. The partial negative charge on the oxygen atom of the DMSO favors the formation of the hydrogen bonds with water molecules.[50,51] The dissolution of AMHs in binary mixtures of DMSO+water may be governed by domination of DMSO–DMSO, DMSO–water, and water–water interactions by ion-DMSO/water interactions. As discussed in Section 2.1, DMSO is a good hydrogen bond acceptor. It can coordinate with metal ions through the oxygen atom of S–O dipole. However, the anion solvation was hindered by inductive effect due to the presence of two methyl ($-CH_3$) groups in DMSO and weak hydrogen bond donation capability.

In present study, the solubility of all AMHs in binary mixtures of DMSO-water is higher than pure DMSO which means water has an important role in solubility. The microhetrogenic nature (cluster formation) of DMSO–water mixture can shed more light on solubility of AMHs in a binary mixture. The microhetrogenity of a binary mixture of DMSO + water have been studied in detail by Washiska et al.[52,53] According to them, molecular clusters of DMSO and water were developed in DMSO–water binary mixture at particular mixing ratio. The DMSO clusters or DMSO cluster contain one or two water molecules which were formulated at $x_{H_2O} < 0.93$. The water clusters were developed at $x_{H_2O} > 0.93$. When NaCl was introduced into the binary mixture of DMSO–water, Na$^+$ preferentially interacted with DMSO cluster rather than with water cluster. DMSO has large donor number (29.8) than water (18). This conveys that DMSO can displace water from solvation shell of metal ion and is more capable in solvation of metal ion as compared to water.[54] This confirms that cations were solvated by DMSO cluster and anion solvation was facilitated by the addition of water. The overall solubility of AMHs was combined solvation of both cation and anion by DMSO or water.

Figure 2.1(a) represents solubility of NaF at 308.15 K. The solubility of NaF is less temperature dependent. The solubility of NaF is quite high up to 40 % DMSO concentration. After that very small increment in solubility was observed from 50–90 % DMSO concentration. Both UNIQUAC and NRTL show deviation with experimentally measured solubility of NaF in DMSO up to 50 wt.% (Fig. 2.1(a)). The deviation decreases significantly at higher concentration of DMSO and both models predict lower solubility of NaF with increasing concentration of DMSO. For NRTL prediction, the deviation increases significantly with temperature (Fig. 2.1(b, c)) resulting in RMSD of 0.0773 and 0.0352 %; but at 308.15 K, NRTL prediction gives an RMSD of 0.0472 %. UNIQUAC model predicts more accurate solubility of NaF with increase of temperature. It gives RMSD of 0.0416 % at

308.15 K whereas prediction accuracy increases to 0.0371% at 318.15 K and 0.0309% at 328.15 K. Thus, average RMSD of UNIQUAC-predicted solubility is 0.0365% whereas NRTL gives average RMSD of 0.0532%.

The solubility of NaCl is less temperature dependent as compared to KCl. The solubility of both NaCl and KCl decreases monotonously with addition of DMSO. The solubility of NaCl is slightly higher than KCl at all studied temperatures. The solubility of NaCl and KCl at 308.15 K is shown in Figure 2.2(a) and 2.3(a), respectively. As per the Table 2.8, RMSD of predicted solubility of NaCl by NRTL is higher (0.2396%) than UNIQUAC prediction (0.1884%). NRTL prediction gives higher RMSD values compared to UNIQUAC (Fig. 2.2(b, c)). In case of KCl also, NRTL prediction (0.2336%) is higher as compared to UNIQUAC prediction (0.1209%) (Fig. 2.3(b, c)).

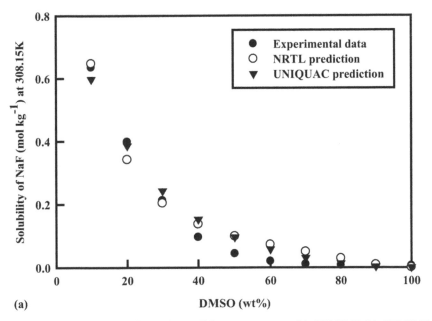

(a)

FIGURE 2.1 Solubility of NaF in DMSO–water system: (a) 308.15 K (b) 318.15 K (c) 328.15 K.

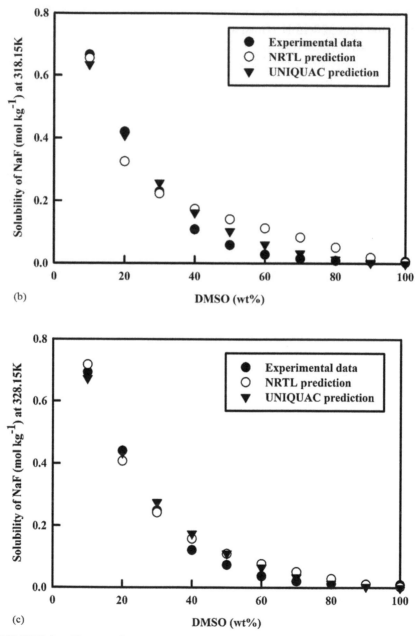

(b)

(c)

FIGURE 2.1 *(Continued)*

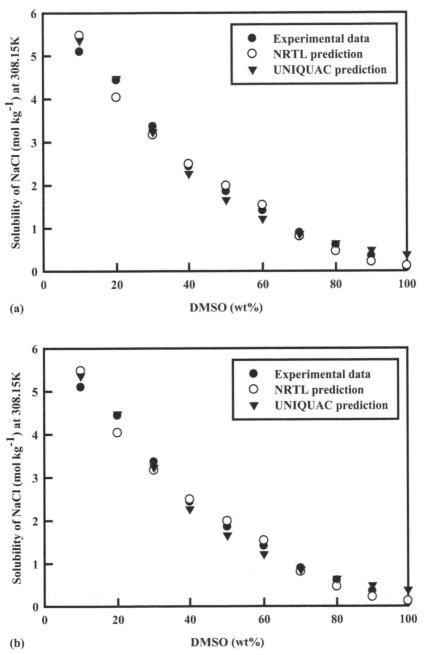

FIGURE 2.2   Solubility of NaCl in DMSO–water system: (a) 308.15 K (b) 318.15 K (c) 328.15 K.

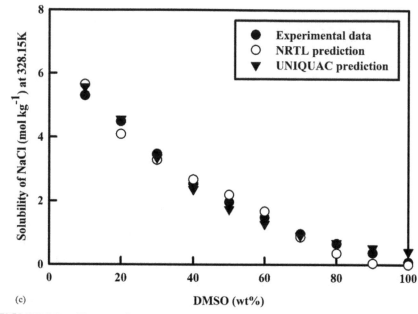

(c)

FIGURE 2.2   *(Continued)*

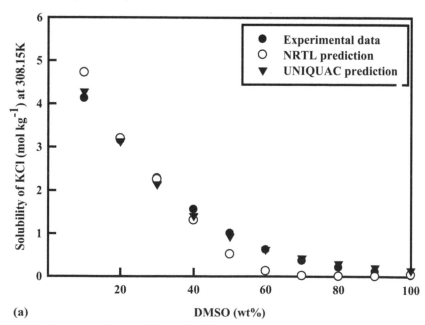

(a)

FIGURE 2.3   Solubility of KCl in DMSO–water system: (a)308.15 K (b) 318.15 K (c) 328.15 K.

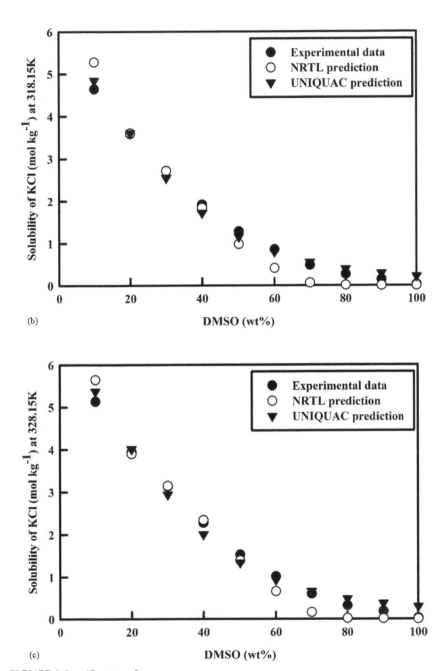

(b)

(c)

FIGURE 2.3 *(Continued)*

TABLE 2.5   NRTL Parameters for DMSO–Water–AMHs Systems. The Binary Interaction Parameters are Unitless.

AMHs	T/K	Salt–DMSO	Salt–water	DMSO–salt	DMSO–water	Water–salt	Water–DMSO
NaF	308.15	7.0418	9.634	11.592	87.163	3.0782	19.757
	318.15	5.4914	6.9487	7.3731	99.957	1.886	29.945
	328.15	6.9137	7.8709	7.7109	89.544	2.8067	18.365
NaCl	308.15	11.495	6.8673	35.729	82.857	24.872	87.819
	318.15	11.317	6.2273	25.182	98.457	27.079	98.839
	328.15	11.406	6.419	27.982	99.854	26.175	69.63
NaBr	308.15	10.347	5.7769	24.322	30.778	31.009	97.74
	318.15	10.872	5.9098	22.467	19.827	36.892	99.525
	328.15	11.358	6.3467	23.632	99.795	37.041	97.709
KCl	308.15	10.944	6.1347	43.008	0.20503	24.553	94.846
	318.15	11.19	6.1009	39.4	19.131	25.118	98.316
	328.15	11.486	6.1253	40.102	9.723	24.625	96.815
KBr	308.15	4.5979	6.6387	3.4528	−3.985	2.1594	13.632
	318.15	11.094	6.2385	30.546	6.8878	24.876	99.462
	328.15	9.6465	6.885	29.974	99.998	1.4451	13.896
KI	308.15	11.021	6.3442	23.388	-0.3034	24.566	99.699
	318.15	6.7328	5.558	2.2866	−4.0362	1.4807	10.245
	328.15	10.181	6.6839	22.905	88.912	0.3633	98.952

TABLE 2.6   UNIQUAC Parameters for DMSO–Water–AMHs Systems. The Binary Interaction Parameter τ_{ij} has a Unit of K^{-1}

AMHs	T/K	Salt–DMSO	Salt–water	DMSO–salt	DMSO–water	Water–salt	Water–DMSO
NaF	308.15	682.52	3719.3	5000	−342.04	464.42	5000
	318.15	717.34	3837.8	5000	−351.15	471.13	4999.9
	328.15	729.35	3851.5	5000	−341.65	462.47	5000
NaCl	308.15	501.06	3394.8	379.7	−525.21	266.44	498.59
	318.15	510.44	3333.5	388.13	−571	276.3	519.73
	328.15	534.12	3886	390.38	−549.21	288.73	591.21
NaBr	308.15	520.14	3304.5	222.27	−552.18	265.3	466.5

TABLE 2.6   *(Continued)*

AMHs	T/K	Salt–DMSO	Salt–water	DMSO–salt	DMSO–water	Water–salt	Water–DMSO
	318.15	532.04	3644.3	216.76	−572.88	270.96	484.52
	328.15	541.08	3647	212.3	−598.37	278.53	506.97
KCl	308.15	577.59	3364.1	322.88	−560.81	193.37	748.76
	318.15	576.61	3590	300.42	−585.97	198.14	759.15
	328.15	573.21	3537.8	280.35	−626.49	214.98	952.61
KBr	308.15	677.2	3738.5	182.88	−512.58	186.02	528.36
	318.15	688.76	3894.3	183.99	−496.58	188.9	547.89
	328.15	705.5	4120.9	184.42	−405.65	192.08	573.49
KI	308.15	730.93	3816.2	68.967	−422.51	196.77	964
	318.15	834.56	3916.1	58.644	−487.47	180.88	549.57
	328.15	850.67	3842.6	55.56	−484.35	185.97	581.06

TABLE 2.7   UNIQUAC Volume and Surface Area Structural Parameters for Components.

AMHs	Surface area parameter (q_{pred})	Volume parameter (r_{pred})
NaCl	2.4872	2.8366
NaBr	2.5962	2.9984
KCl	3.2167	4.35
KBr	3.3257	4.5117
KI	3.4764	4.7497
DMSO	2.4812	2.8439
Water	0.8679	0.7619

TABLE 2.8   Average RMSDs of DMSO–Water–AMHs Systems Predicted by NRTL and UNIQUAC Models.

AMHs	RMSD (%) for NRTL prediction			RMSD (%) for UNIQUAC prediction			Average RMSD (%)	
	308.15	318.15	323.15	308.15	318.15	323.15	NRTL	UNIQUAC
NaF	0.0472	0.0773	0.0352	0.0416	0.0371	0.0309	0.0532	0.0365
NaCl	0.2002	0.2761	0.2427	0.1822	0.1878	0.1952	0.2396	0.1884
NaBr	0.3513	0.3297	0.2935	0.337	0.3626	0.3919	0.3248	0.3639

TABLE 2.8   *(Continued)*

AMHs	RMSD (%) for NRTL prediction			RMSD (%) for UNIQUAC prediction			Average RMSD (%)	
KCl	0.2507	0.239	0.211	0.089	0.1189	0.1547	0.2336	0.1209
KBr	0.1248	0.1987	0.0861	0.0916	0.0975	0.103	0.1365	0.0974
KI	0.1606	0.1027	0.171	0.0738	0.0739	0.0781	0.1448	0.0753

The comparison of solubility data of NaCl and KCl at 308.15 K with literature data[27] at 298.15 and 312.15 K is presented in Figures 2.7(a) and 2.3(b). The concentration of DMSO was converted to mole fraction for the ease of comparison with the literature. It can be seen from Figure 2.7(a) that the solubility of NaCl from 298.15 to 318.15 K is close to each other but solubility increases with increase in temperature. The solubility of KCl is available at three different mole fractions and visible changes can be observed in solubility with rise in temperature (Fig. 2.7(b)).

Experimental solubility data of NaBr and KBr at 308.15 K are correlated with NRTL and UNIQUAC models and shown in Figures 2.4(a) and 2.5(a), respectively. NRTL model correlates with experimental data of NaBr more accurately than UNIQUAC model. For 20–40 wt.% of DMSO, both models predict solubility accurately. However, deviation increases significantly for UNIQUAC model from 50–80 wt.% of DMSO. Similar prediction trends are observed at 318.15 and 328.15 K (Fig. 2.4(b, c)). For KBr, UNIQUAC model predict solubility accurately, whereas deviation is observed from 60–80 wt.% of DMSO for NRTL prediction. Higher deviation obtained from NRTL was observed for all the three temperatures RMSD of 0.1248%, 0.1987%, and 0.0861%, respectively. The RMSDs predicted by UNIQUAC model are 0.0916%, 0.0975%, and 0.1030% at 308.15, 318.15, and 328.15 K, respectively (Fig. 2.5(b, c)).

Figure 2.6(a) represents the solubility of KI in DMSO at 308.15 K. NRTL model gives higher RMSD of 0.1606% compared to UNIQUAC model (0.0738%). KI has the highest solubility in almost all studied AMHs. At 318.15 and 328.15 K also (Fig. 2.6(b, c)), UNIQUAC model gives lesser RMSD (0.0739% and 0.0781%, respectively) and hence more accurate prediction.

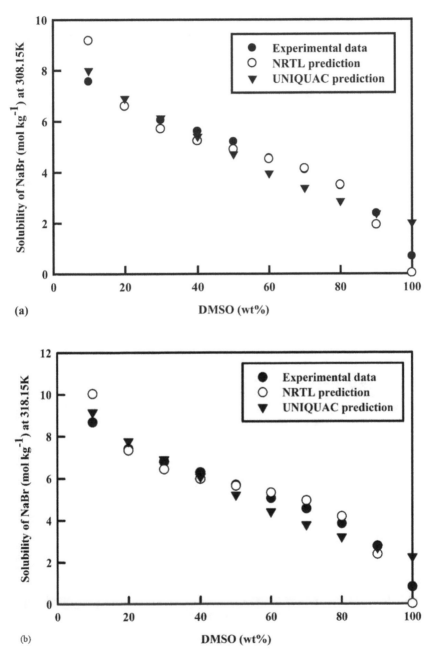

FIGURE 2.4 Solubility of NaBr in DMSO–water system: (a) 308.15 K (b) 318.15 K (c) 328.15 K.

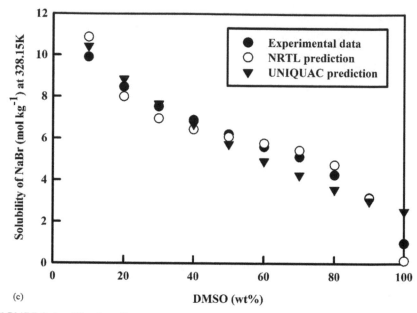

(c)

FIGURE 2.4   *(Continued)*

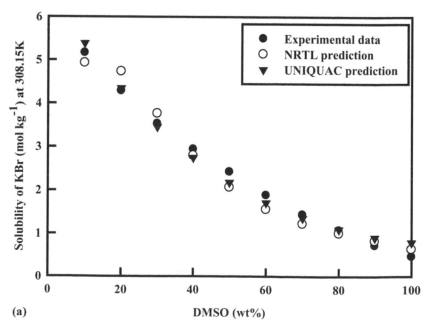

(a)

FIGURE 2.5   Solubility of KBr in DMSO–water system: (a) 308.15 K (b) 318.15 K (c) 328.15 K.

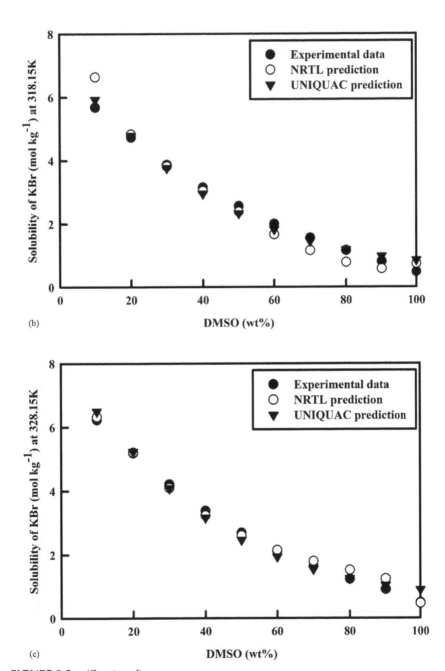

(b)

(c)

FIGURE 2.5 *(Continued)*

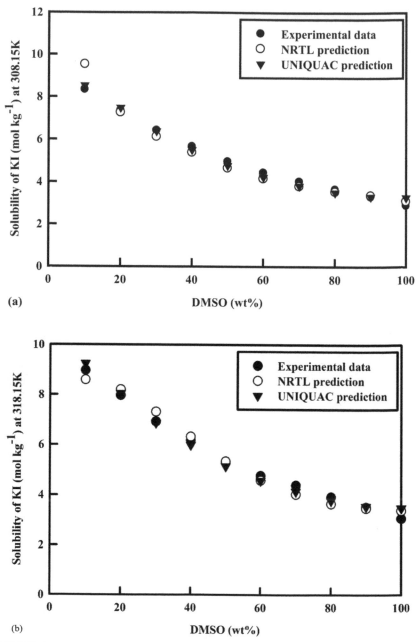

FIGURE 2.6   Solubility of KI in DMSO–water system: (a) 308.15 K (b) 318.15 K (c) 328.15 K.

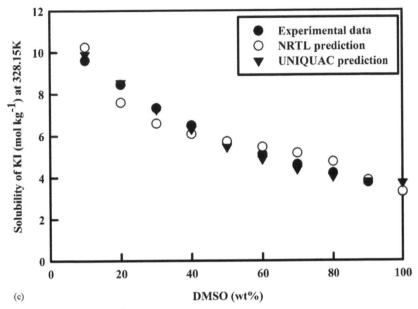

(c)

FIGURE 2.6　*(Continued)*

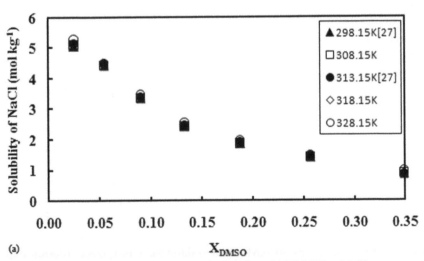

(a)

FIGURE 2.7　Comparison of experimental solubility of (a) DMSO + NaCl + water and (b) DMSO + KCl + water with literature.[27]

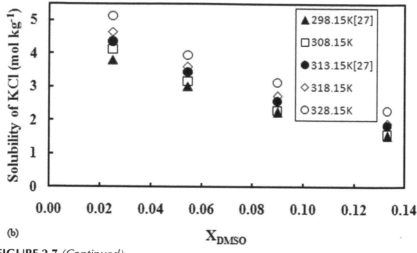

(b)

FIGURE 2.7 *(Continued)*

2.4 CONCLUSION

The experimental solubilities of seven AMHs in DMSO and DMSO + water were successfully determined using the analytical gravimetric method at three different temperatures, 308.15, 318.15, and 328.15 K, respectively. These results provide valuable information regarding designing of separation process for AMHs or DMSO from the aqueous medium. The solubility of AMHs decreases with increasing DMSO in the mixture while it increases with increasing temperature. For SMHs, the order of decreasing solubility is NaBr > NaCl > NaF whereas for PMHs, the order is KI >KBr > KCl. The overall solubility is a combined solvation of cation and anion in DMSO–DMSO and water–water cluster. The solubility data was successfully modeled using NRTL and UNIQUAC model. Both the models predict average deviations at all temperatures less than 1 %. NRTL model predicts lowest RMSD of 0.0532 % for solubility of NaF in DMSO. UNIQUAC model further improves the accuracy of prediction of solubility of NaF and gives an RMSD of 0.0365 %. UNIQUAC model also gives very low RMSD for KBr and KI systems (0.0974 % and 0.0753 %, respectively). As RMSD values of all the systems (Table 2.8) are very low, it can be concluded that both NRTL and UNIQUAC models can be applied to predict the solubility data of SMHs and PMHs in pure DMSO as

well as DMSO–water mixture. For SMHs and PMHs at studied temperature range, the minimum average RMSD predicted by NRTL is 0.0532%
and UNIQUAC predicts as low as 0.0365% for solubility of NaF. NRTL
predicts maximum RMSD of 0.3248% for solubility of NaBr in DMSO
and UNIQUAC predicts 0.3639% for the same system.

2.5 ACKNOWLEDGEMENT

Gratitude is expressed to CSIR-CSMCRI Supra Institutional Project
CSC-0203 to carry out this work.

KEYWORDS

- solubility
- alkali metal halides
- DMSO
- phase equilibria
- UNIQUAC
- NRTL

REFERENCES

1. Furter, W. F. *Chem. Eng. Comm.* **1992**, *116*, 35–40.
2. Korin, E.; Soifer, L. *J. Chem. Eng. Data.* **1997**, *42*, 1251–1253.
3. Seader, J. D.; Henley, E. J.; Roper, D. K. Separation Process Principles Chemical and Biochemical Operations; *Thermodynamics of Separation Operations*, John Wiley & Sons, Inc., 2011.
4. Wang, P.; Anderko, A.; Young, R. D. *Fluid Phase Equilib.* **2002**, *203*, 141–176.
5. Pinho, S. P.; Macedo, E. A. *J. Chem. Thermodyn.* **2002**, *34*, 337–360.
6. Debye, P.; Hückel, E. *Phys. Z.* **1923**, *24*, 185–206.
7. Bromley, L. A. *AIChE J.* **1973**, *19*, 313–320.
8. Pitzer, K. S. *Activity Coefficients in Electrolyte Solutions;* CRC Press: Boca Raton, FL, 1991.
9. Renon, H.; Prausnitz, J. M. *AIChE J.* **1968**, *14*, 135–144.
10. Abrams, D. S.; Prausnitz, J. M. *AIChE J.* **1975,** *21*, 116–128.

11. Thomsen, K.; Illiuta, M. C.; Rasmussen, P. *Chem. Eng. Sci.* **2004,** *59*, 3631–3647.
12. Dortmund Data Bank, DDB Software & Separation Technology, www.ddbst.de.
13. Reynolds, W. L. Dimethyl Sulfoxide in Inorganic Chemistry; *Progress in Inorganic Chemistry*, Vol 12; John Wiley & Sons: New York, 2007.
14. Wilhelm, E.; Letcher, T. Volume Properties: Liquids, Solutions and Vapours; *Excess Volumes of Liquid Nonelectrolyte Mixtures*, The Royal Society of Chemistry, 2015.
15. Zierkiewicz, W.; Privalov, T. *Organometallics* **2005,** *24*, 6019–6028.
16. Luzara, A.; Chandler, D. *J. Chem. Phys.* **1993,** *98*, 8160–8173.
17. Pinho, S. P.; Macedo, E. A. *J. Chem. Eng. Data.* **2005,** *50*, 29–32.
18. Gomis, V.; Ruiz, F.; DeVera, G.; Saquete, M. D. *Fluid Phase Equilib.* **1994,** *98*, 141–147.
19. Gomis, V.; Ruiz, F.; Asensi, J. C.; Saquete, M. D. *J. Chem. Eng. Data.* **1996,** *41*, 188–191.
20. Gomis, V.; Ruiz, F.; Boluda, N.; Saquete, M. D. *Fluid Phase Equilib.* **2004,** *215*, 79–83.
21. Wagner, K.; Friese, T.; Schulz, S.; Ulbig, P. *J. Chem. Eng. Data.* **1998,** *43*, 871–875.
22. Boruń, A.; Florczak, A.; Bald, A. *J. Chem. Eng. Data.* **2010,** *55*, 1252–1257.
23. Li, J.; Wang, J.; Wang, Y. *J. Chem. Eng. Data.* **2007,** *52*, 1069–1071.
24. Wang, Y.; Sha, Z.; Wang, Y.; Zheng, Q. *J. Chem. Eng. Data.* **2008,** *53*, 2547–2549.
25. Zhou, X.; Hao, J. *J. Chem. Eng. Data.* **2011,** *56*, 951–955.
26. Li, M.; Constantinescu, D.; Wang, L.; Mohs, A.; Gmehling, J. *Ind. Eng. Chem. Res.* **2010,** *49*, 4981–4988.
27. Mohs, A.; Decker, S.; Gmehling, J. *Fluid Phase Equilib.* **2011,** *304,* 12–20.
28. Taboada, M. E.; Veliz, D. M.; Galleguillos, H. R.; Graber, T. A. *J. Chem. Eng. Data.* **2005,** *50*, 187–190.
29. Pawar, R. R.; Nahire, S. B.; Hasan, M. *J. Chem. Eng. Data.* **2009,** *54*, 1935–1937.
30. Pawar, R. R.; Aher, C. S.; Pagar, J. D.; Nikam, S. L.; Hasan, M. *J. Chem. Eng. Data.* **2012,** *57*, 3563–3572.
31. Hu, M. C.; Zhai, Q. G., Liu, Z. H. *J Chem. Eng. Data.* **2004,** *49*, 717–719.
32. Hu, M. C.; Jin, L. H.; Jiang, Y. C.; Li, S. N.; Zhai, Q. G. *J. Chem. Eng. Data.* **2005,** *50*, 1361–1364.
33. Zhao, W. X.; Hu, M. C.; Jiang, Y. C.; Li, S. N. *Chin. J. Chem.* **2007,** *25*, 478–483.
34. Hu, M. C.; Jin, L. H.; Li, S. N.; Jiang, Y. C. *Fluid Phase Equilib.* **2006,** *242*, 136–140.
35. Guo, H. Y.; Hu, M. C.; Li, S. N.;Jiang, Y. C.; Wang, M. X. *J. Chem. Eng. Data.* **2008,** *53*, 131–135.
36. Hu, M. C.; Zhang, X. L.; Li, S. N.; Zhai, Q. G.; Jiang, Y. C.; Liu, Z. H. *Russ. J. Inorg. Chem.* **2005,** *9*, 1434–1440.
37. Zhao, D.; Li, S.; Zhai, Q.; Jiang, Y.; Hu, M. *J. Chem. Eng. Data.* **2014,** *59*, 1423–1434.
38. Goldberg, D. E. Genetic Algorithms in Search, Optimization and Machine Learning; *Computer implementation of a Genetic Alogritham*, Addison-Wesley Longman, 1989.
39. Rabari, D.; Banerjee, T. *Ind. Eng. Chem. Res.* **2014,** *53*, 18935–18942.
40. Bharti, A.; Banerjee, T. *Fluid Phase Equilib.* **2015,** *400*, 27–37.
41. Banerjee, T.; Singh, M. K.; Sahoo, R. K.; Khanna, A. *Fluid Phase Equilibria.* **2005,** *234*, 64–76.

42. Kundu, D.; Banerjee, T. *Ind. Eng. Chem. Res.* **2011,** *50*, 14090–14096.

43. Unni, A. K. R.; Sitaraman, N.; Menon, V. K. C. *Indian J. Chem. Soc.* **1977,** *12*, 1021–1023.

44. Long, B.; Zhao, D.; Liu, W. *Ind. Eng. Chem. Res.* **2012,** *51*, 9456–9467.

45. Gopal, R.; Jha, J. S. *Indian J. Chem.* **1974,** *12*, 618–619.

46. Miller, J.; Parker, A. J. *J. Am. Chem. Soc.* **1961,** *83*, 117–123.

47. Peruzzi, N.; Ninham, B.W.; Lo Nostro, P.; Baglioni, P. *J. Phys. Chem. B.* **2012,** *116*, 14398–14405.

48. Peruzzi, N.; Lo Nostro, P.; Ninham, B. W.; Baglioni, P. *J. Solution Chem.* **2015,** *44*, 1224–1239.

49. Hofmeister, F. *Arch. Exp. Pathol. Pharmakol.* **1888,** *24*, 247–260.

50. Luzara, A.; Chandler, D. *J. Chem. Phys.* **1993,** *98*, 8160–8173.

51. Wong, D. B.; Sokolowsky, K. P.; El-Barghouthi, M. I.; Fenn, E. E.; Giammanco, C. H.; Sturlaugson, A. L.; Fayer, M. D. *J. Phys. Chem. B.* **2012,** *116*, 5479–5490.

52. Nam Shin, D.; Wijnen, J. W.; Jan Engberts, B. F. N.; Wakisaka, A. *J. Phys. Chem. B.* **2001,** *105*, 6759–6762.

53. Nam Shin, D.; Wijnen, J. W.; Jan Engberts, B. F. N., Wakisaka, A. *J. Phys. Chem. B.* **2002,** *106*, 6014–6020.

54. Sekine, T.; Kusakabe, S. Solvent Extraction. 1990, Elsevier, 2012.

CHAPTER 3

ANNEALING INDUCED PHYSICOCHEMICAL AND OPTOELECTRONIC PROPERTY MODIFICATIONS IN ZNO THIN FILM

RAJESH A. JOSHI[*]

Department of Physics, Toshniwal Arts, Commerce and Science College, Sengaon, Dist. Hingoli, Maharashtra 431542, India

*Corresponding author. E-mails: urajoshi@gmail.com

CONTENTS

ABSTRACT

Zinc oxide (ZnO) thin films were deposited on a glass substrate using cost-effective chemical bath deposition (CBD) technique at room temperature. These deposited thin films were annealed in an air atmosphere at 100, 200, 300, and 400°C for 1 h; these pristine and annealed thin films were later characterized for structural, compositional, morphological, optical, and electronic properties. Peaks observed in X-ray diffraction (XRD) pattern at 31.71, 36.27, and 56.29° corresponds to orientation along (100), (101), and (110) plane of ZnO materials. Raman spectra obtained for the pristine ZnO thin films represents peak at 563 and 1091 cm^{-1} confirming longitudinal optical (LO) and transverse optical (TO) phonon modes in ZnO thin films. The energy dispersive X-ray (EDX) spectrum that is obtained from pristine thin films confirms expected elemental composition. Surface morphology observed through atomic force microscopy (AFM) shows grain growth improvement upon post-deposition annealing treatment. Optical absorbance coefficient and energy band gaps are observed to be blue shifted on annealing treatments which can be correlated to variation in defect density states of the thin film. I–V characteristics obtained from pristine and annealed thin film shows ohmic nature of the graph which infers the semiconducting behavior of synthesized thin films.

3.1   INTRODUCTION

Zinc oxide (ZnO) is an important II-VI group compound possessing potential physicochemical and optoelectronic properties which has attracted the attention of many researchers.[1] These significant characteristics of ZnO thin films such as direct band gap, large exciton binding energy, high conductivity, and high optical transparency in the visible and near infrared region has made it to be used for developing various optoelectronic devices like physical and chemical sensors, blue light emitting diodes,[2] solar build UV photo detectors,[3] buffer layers in solar cells, resonant tunneling devices,[4] and so forth.

These ZnO thin films can be synthesized by multiple ways using sophisticated costlier techniques like vacuum evaporation, thermal evaporation, spin coating, spray pyrolysis, and so forth, whereas chemical reaction-based synthesis methods like chemical bath deposition (CBD), successive ionic layer adsorption and reaction (SILAR), Sol gel, and so forth. are uniform, large area deposition, cost-effective, and user-friendly techniques.[5,6] These CBD techniques are more suitable for obtaining stoichiometry of material and that too at room temperature onto any substrate. Hence, considering the merits of chemical synthesis method we have deposited the ZnO thin film on a glass substrate using this potentially important CBD technique.

The device grade applications of these thin films are surface, interface, and stoichiometry dependent properties.[7] The material stoichiometry and substrate interface related aspects are synthesis controlled parameters, which can be optimized and configured using CBD techniques but surface and interface to some extent can be modified by providing post-deposition annealing treatment to thin films.[8] This post-deposition annealing treatment will naturally make an effect on physicochemical and optoelectronic properties of these ZnO thin films, hence, to understand the phenomenon and study the effect of annealing treatment on ZnO thin films post-deposition annealing at 100, 200, 300, and 400°C is provided under air atmosphere. The present article describes and highlights the comparative analysis of structural, optical, and electrical characteristics of these pristine and annealed ZnO thin films prepared by using well known CBD technique.

3.2   EXPERIMENTAL DETAILS

ZnO thin films were deposited onto glass substrates by CBD technique at room temperature using $ZnCl_4$ and H_2O_2 as precursors of Zn and O, respectively. The glass substrates were cleaned and washed with chromic acid and deionized water and later cleaned with acetone. The precursors used for CBD are 0.1 M concentration of the $ZnCl_4$ solution, triethanolamine (TEA) as a complexing agent and H_2O_2 as an anionic source. The synthesis of ZnO begins with mixing of these ingredients in the controlled proportion into a glass beaker dipping the glass substrates in it till the formation of white color thin films on the substrate surface which usually takes 1 h. These obtained thin films were then rinsed in deionized water for removing the excess loosely bonded chemical ingredients and later annealed at 100, 200, 300, and 400°C in an air atmosphere for about 1 h.

These pristine and annealed thin films were characterized for structural properties using XRD pattern obtained on Panalytical X'Pert Pro using Cu Kα radiation ($\lambda = 1.5405$ Å) in the range of 20–60°. Raman spectra of the pristine ZnO thin films observed on Renishaw Raman spectrometer RM 2000 in backscattering configuration at room temperature. The surface morphology of the thin films probed by atomic force microscope (AFM) images obtained on Bruker AXS multimode scanning probe microscope. The optical characterization performed using spectrophotometer Perkin Elmer LAMBDA 750 in absorbance mode. The electrical properties were studied using semiconducting device analyzer Agilent B1500A.

3.3   RESULTS AND DISCUSSION

3.3.1   STRUCTURAL ANALYSIS

The XRD pattern obtained from pristine and annealed ZnO thin films were represented in Figure 3.1. Peaks corresponding to (100), (101), and (110) planes were observed at 31.71, 36.27, and 56.29°, respectively, and it confirms ZnO (JCPDS data card 36-1451) along preferred C axis orientation possessing hexagonal Wurtzite structure.[9–11] The XRD pattern reveals the slight shift in (100) and (101) peaks which may correspond to annealing induced compositional variation in thin films, while a sharp rising of new peak is also observed in XRD pattern of thin film annealed at 400°C may be correlated to polygonization process that is material melting and resolidification. The inter-planner spacing (d) is found to be ≈2.8–3.83 Å for the preferred (100) orientation and the lattice parameters are found to be matching well with standard JCPDS data card.[12] The average crystallite size calculated using the Debye-Scherrer formula is found to be increasing from 22–50 nm with increase in annealing temperature may be a result of temperature-induced grain growth and resolidification.[13]

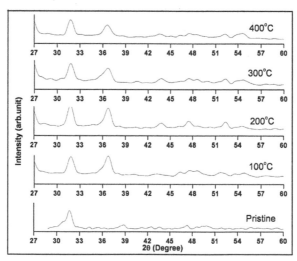

FIGURE 3.1   X-ray diffraction (XRD) pattern of pristine and annealed ZnO thin films prepared by chemical bath deposition method at room temperature.

3.3.2   *RAMAN SPECTRA*

Understanding the specifics of phonon spectrum both optical and acoustic of ZnO material can help in using ZnO for various optoelectronic applications. The Raman spectroscopy study carried on pristine ZnO thin films is as shown in Figure 3.2 which represents high peak at 563 and 1091 cm^{-1}. The Raman active zone-center optical phonons predicted by the group theory are $A_1 + 2E_2 + E_1$. The phonons of A_1 and E_1 symmetry are polar phonons and, hence, exhibit different frequencies for the transverse optical (TO) and longitudinal optical (LO) mode.[14] Nonpolar phonon modes with symmetry E_2 have two frequencies, E_2 high associated with oxygen atoms and E_2 low associated with Zn sublattice. The observed peak at 563 cm^{-1} corresponds to LO mode while the other high peak observed at 1091 cm^{-1} corresponds to TO mode of ZnO materials. Peak at 1372 cm^{-1} confirms the powder nature of the ZnO materials.[15]

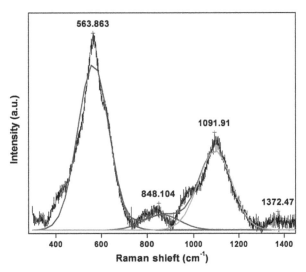

FIGURE 3.2   Raman spectrum obtained at room temperature from pristine ZnO thin films.

3.3.3   COMPOSITIONAL ANALYSIS

Figure 3.3 shows the energy dispersive X-ray spectrum (EDX) obtained from ZnO pristine thin films. From the figure, it can be seen that the peaks corresponding to Zinc (Zn) and Oxygen (O) are obtained which confirms the expected elemental tresses in thin films with nearly equal proportionate of elemental compositions.

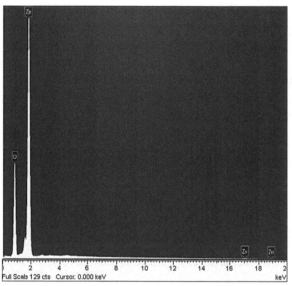

FIGURE 3.3   Dispersive X-ray spectrum (EDX) obtained from pristine ZnO thin films used for elemental analysis and compositional confirmation.

3.3.4   SURFACE MORPHOLOGY

Surface morphology is one of the major contenders for deciding the material applicability in an optoelectronic device, hence, the morphology is studied using AFM as shown in Figure 3.4a–e for pristine, 100, 200, 300, and 400°C, respectively. The homogenous granular distribution of grains can be seen on pristine thin films while on annealing treatments, the uneven homogenate granules are found to be grown which may be related to thermal polygonization.[16] The nature of grain growth seems to be following the nature as the annealing temperature is increasing.[17]

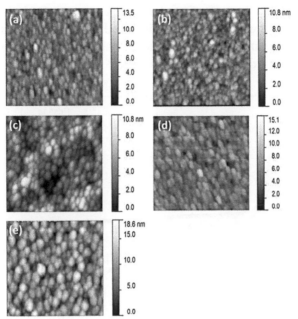

FIGURE 3.4a–e Atomic force microscopy (AFM) images obtained from pristine and annealed ZnO thin films deposited using chemical bath deposition method.

3.3.5 OPTICAL STUDY

Thin films of ZnO are multipurpose and multifunctional materials which can be used in many applications where the electronic transition needs to be studied well. Hence, the optical study of these pristine and annealed thin films carried out in absorbance mode is as represented in Figure 3.5. Spectroscopic absorbance measurement of pristine and annealed thin films reveals that there are significant differences in optical properties and electronic transitions amongst these ZnO thin films.[18] This difference can be explained on the basis of annealing-induced compositional modifications. The absorbance spectra show variation in absorbance peak with respect to annealed thin films this can be related to annealing driven exciton induction in ZnO thin films.[19] Figure 3.6 corresponds to transmittance spectra obtained from the pristine and annealed ZnO thin films. The transmittance is observed to be increasing as the annealing temperature is increased this may be related to annealing induced crystalline polygonization process, and alternation in stacking faults may result in proper orientation of crystallites and the formation of defect-free grain boundaries.[20] Post-deposition annealing treatment exhibits a red shift in optical absorbance and blue shift in transmittance spectrum may be due to the localization of charges in a crystal domain.

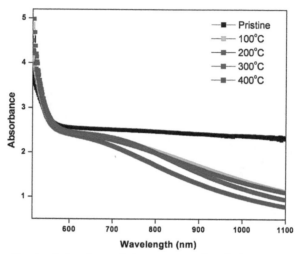

FIGURE 3.5 Graph of absorbance (αt) versus wavelength (nm) used for analysis of absorbance spectra of pristine and annealed ZnO thin films.

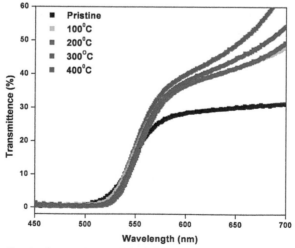

FIGURE 3.6 Graph of transmittance (%) against wavelength (nm) drawn as transmittance spectra of pristine and annealed ZnO thin films.

3.3.6 I–V STUDY

Figure 3.7 shows the current–voltage (I–V) response of the pristine and annealed ZnO thin films exhibiting the study of electrical properties. From the Ohmic nature of graph, it can be asserted that ZnO thin films show semiconducting nature while on annealing treatment it is observed that the I–V response is increasing which means an increase in the value of current (I) with respect to applied voltage (V) is observed. Since pristine thin films consist of fine particles with the large surface area and rigid grain boundaries, the I–V nature likely to be originated from donor–acceptor transitions, where the donor and/or acceptor defects are supposed to be located at surfaces or grain boundaries. As annealing treatment is provided and the temperature starts increasing, there is variation in physical topology as per Figure 3.4 and very least compositional orientation variation is observed as per Figure 3.1. It is considered that oxygen and zinc atoms at defect level start moving towards the lattice states, with an enhancement in crystallite size, this may be a favorable condition for exciton generation. Excitons in direct bandgap semiconductors are very luminescent and are widely used in optoelectronic devices.[21] The observed increment in I–V response confirms an increase in electrical conductivity of thin films from pristine to anneal.

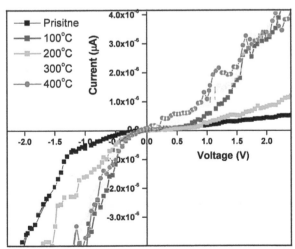

FIGURE 3.7   Current–voltage (I–V) response of pristine and annealed ZnO thin films.

3.4   CONCLUSION

The ZnO thin films have been successfully deposited on glass substrate by using large area depositing, cost-effective, and efficient CBD technique at room temperature. These pristine thin films are then annealed in an air atmosphere at 100, 200, 300, and 400°C, respectively. From the XRD pattern analysis, compositional modifications along with grain growth and improvement in crystallite size are observed. The elemental compositions of the pristine thin films are found to be in good correlation with expected ingredients. Surface morphology studied using AFM shows morphological enhancement and polygonization induced topological grain growth and improvements. The absorbance and transmittance spectra are observed to be red and blue shifted, respectively, which may be related to annealing induced defect state dismantling and grain boundary modifications. I–V characteristics represent semiconducting nature of thin films while on annealing treatment the conductivity is observed to be increasing which may be related to grain boundary charge generation and separation phenomenon.

KEYWORDS

- ZnO
- thin films
- chemical bath deposition (CBD)
- annealing treatment

REFERENCES

1. Krämer, A.; Engel, S.; Sangiorgi, N.; Sanson, A.; Bartolomé, J. F.; Gräf, S.; Müller, F. A. *Appl. Surf. Sci.* **2017,** *399,* 282.
2. Chowdhury, F.; Hasan, S. M. F.; Alam, M. S. *Turk. J. Phys.* **2012,** *36,* 1.
3. Wahab, H. A.; Salama, A. A.; Saeid, A. A.; Willander, O.; Battisha, I. K. *Res. Phys.* **2013,** *3,* 46.
4. Lupan, O.; Pauporte, T.; Chow, L.; Viana, B.; Pelle, F.; Ono, L. K.; Cuenya, B. R.; Heinrich, H. *Appl. Surf. Sci.* **2010,** *256,* 1895.

5. Azad, S.; Sadeghi, E.; Parvizi, R.; Mazaheri, A.; Yousefi, M. *Opt. Laser Technol.* **2017,** *90,* 96.

6. Rodrigues, A.; Castegnaro, M. V.; Arguello, J.; Alves, M. C. M.; Morais, J. *Appl. Surf. Sci.* **2017,** *402,* 136.

7. Yu, W.; Chen, X.; Mei, W.; Chen, C.; Tsang, Y. *Appl. Surf. Sci.* **2017,** *400,* 129.

8. Chithira, P. R.; John, T. T. *J. Lumin.* **2017,** *185,* 212.

9. Yusuf, G. T.; Efunwole, H. O.; Raimi, M. A.; Alaje, O. E.; Kazeem, A. K. *J. Nucl. Phys. Mater. Sci. Radiat. Appl.* **2014,** *2,* 73.

10. Zhang, X.; Ma, S.; Yang, F.; Zhao, Q.; Li, F.; Liu, J. *Ceram. Int.* **2013,** *39,* 7993.

11. Fan, H.; Xu, S.; Cao, X.; Liu, D.; Yin, Y.; Hao, H.; Wei, D.; Shen, Y. *Appl. Surf. Sci.* **2017,** *400,* 440.

12. Sandeep, K. M.; Bhat, S.; Dharmaprakash, S. M.; *J. Phys. Chem. Solids* **2017,** *104,* 36.

13. Mahajan, C. M., Takwale, M. G. *Curr. Appl. Phys.* **2013,** *13,* 2109.

14. Alim, K. A.; Fonoberov, V. A.; Shamsa, M.; Balandin, A. A. *J. Appl. Phys.* **2005,** *97,* 124313.

15. Rollo, A. G.; Vasilevskiy, M. I. *J. Raman Spectrosc.* **2007,** *38,* 618.

16. Shoushtari, M. Z.; Poormoghadam, A.; Farbod, M. *Mater. Res. Bull.* **2017,** *88,* 315.

17. Arunkumar, S.; Hou, T.; Kim, Y. B.; Choi, B.; Park, S. H.; Jung, S.; Lee, D. W. *Sens. Actuators. B.* **2017,** *243,* 990.

18. Carp, O.; Tirsoaga, A.; Ene, R.; Ianculescu, A.; Negrea, R. F.; Chesler, P.; Ionita, G.; Birjega, R. *Ultrason. Sonochem.* **2017,** *36,* 326.

19. Tian, X.; Pan, Z.; Zhang, H.; Xie, Y.; Zeng, X.; Xiao, C.; Hu, G.; Wei, Z. *Mater. Lett.* **2013,** *97,* 71.

20. Kondal, N.; Tiwari, S. K. *Mater. Res. Bull.* **2017,** *88,* 156.

21. Lu, P.; Zhou, W.; Li, Y.; Wang, J.; Wu, P. *Appl. Surf. Sci.* **2017,** *399,* 396.

CHAPTER 4

ELECTROCHEMICAL SENSING OF L-GLYCINE ON CARBON NANOTUBES

SOMA DAS[1,*] and MITALI SAHA[2]

[1]*Department of Chemistry, CMR Institute of Technology, Bangalore 560037, India*

[2]*Department of Chemistry, National Institute of Technology, Agartala 799055, India*

*Corresponding author. E-mails: somachem17@gmail.com, soma.d@cmrit.ac.in

CONTENTS

ABSTRACT

An electrochemical L-glycine biosensor was fabricated at the surface of carbon nanotube (CCNT) electrode, obtained from coconut oil. The investigation was done by linear sweep voltammetry at CCNT electrode in phosphate buffer solution at pH 6.5. The influence of the experimental parameters on the peak currents of L-glycine, such as pH, time interval, and scan rates, were optimized. Under optimum conditions, the peak current was found to be linear in the L-glycine concentration range from 1–100 μM with a sensitivity of ~ 2.953 μA·μM^{-1}·cm^{-2} (R=0.99698) and response time of about 5 s. Some characteristic studies of the nonenzymatic biosensor, such as reproducibility, substrate specificity, and storage stability, have also been studied. The results suggested that CCNT electrode is reliable and sensitive enough for the determination of L-glycine in standard solution as well as real sample too.

4.1 INTRODUCTION

Amino acids are biologically important organic compounds containing amine (–NH$_2$) and carboxyl (–COOH) functional groups, along with a side chain (R group) specific to each amino acid. The key elements of an amino acid are carbon, hydrogen, oxygen, and nitrogen, though other elements are found in the side chains of certain amino acids. About 500 amino acids are known (though only 20 appear in the genetic code) and can be classified in many ways.[1] They can be classified according to the core structural functional groups' locations as alpha- (α-), beta- (β-), gamma- (γ-), or delta- (δ-) amino acids; other categories relate to polarity, pH level, and side chain group type (aliphatic, acyclic, aromatic, containing hydroxyl, sulfur, etc.). In the form of proteins, amino acids comprise the second largest component (water is the largest) of human muscles, cells, and other tissues.[2] Outside proteins, amino acids perform critical roles in processes such as neurotransmitter transport and biosynthesis. Glycine is the smallest of the amino acids. This amino acid is essential for different muscle, cognitive, and metabolic functions. It helps break down and transport nutrients such as glycogen and fat to be used by cells for energy, and in the process, it supports strong immune, digestive, and nervous systems.[3] In the human body, glycine is found in high concentrations in the skin, connective tissues of the joints, and muscle tissue. One of the key amino acids used to form collagen and gelatin, glycine can be found in bone broth and other protein sources. In fact, glycine (along with many other nutrients such as proline and arginine) is part of what gives "superfood" bone broth its amazing healing ability.[4,5]

Amino acids are usually analyzed by liquid chromatographic methods,[6] Fourier transform infrared spectroscopy (FTIR) studies,[7] differential capacitance, radioactive indicators, solid-phase extraction, flow injection[8,9] electrochemiluminescence, and so forth.[10] These methods are quite accurate, dependent on multistep sample cleanup procedures, so are relatively expensive and time-consuming. For this reason, there is an interest in developing faster, simpler, and low-cost procedures for the analysis of amino acids. In recent years, electrochemical detection of amino acids has gained importance, as a sensitive and selective detection technique for the electroactive compounds.[11–17] Mahmoud et al.[15] fabricated a glassy carbon electrode modified with nickel oxide nanoparticles to investigate the electrochemical oxidation of glycine, L-serine, and L-alanine in an alkaloid solution. Under optimized conditions, the calibration curves are linear in the concentration range of 1–400 μM for L-serine. Voltammetric determination of tyrosine based on an L-serine polymer film electrode has been reported by Li.[16] The results showed linearity in the concentration range of $2.0 \times 10^{-6} - 5.0 \times 10^{-4}$ mol·L^{-1}. Soma et al. have studied cyclic voltammetry (CV), differential pulse voltammetry (DPV), square wave voltammetry (SWV), and linear sweep voltammetry (LSV) for the detection of L-serine and L-phenylalanine in phosphate buffer solution (PBS) at pH 6.8 and 7, respectively. A linearity between the oxidation peak current and the concentration of both amino acids were obtained in the range of 1–100 μM ($R^2 = 0.99783$) for L-serine, 0.99618 for L-phenylalanine with lower detection limit of 0.54 μM for L-serine and 1 μM for L-phenylalanine.[18]

In this chapter, we have used carbon nanotubes (CCNT), obtained from pyrolysis of coconut oil for the fabrication of electrode. The electrochemical experiments have been carried out using LSV for the detection of L-glycine in PBS at pH 6.5. A linearity between the oxidation peak current and the concentration of both amino acids were obtained in the range of 1–100 μM (R = 0.99698) with lower detection limit of 1 μM. The studies revealed that this particular electrode possessed excellent sensitivity, selectivity, high stability, and low potential along with a fast response toward the detection of L-glycine.

4.2 EXPERIMENT

4.2.1 REAGENTS AND APPARATUS

L-glycine, sodium dihydrogen phosphate (NaH$_2$PO$_4$), disodium hydrogen phosphate (Na$_2$HPO$_4$), and phosphoric acid (H$_3$PO$_4$) were purchased from

Sigma Aldrich. Pharmaceutical samples (Medett Products, India of L-glycine was used for real sample analysis. Electrochemical studies were performed using a mini potentiostat (Dropsens μStat 100). Pocket-sized pH meter (HANNA instrument) was used to maintain the pH of the sample solution. A solution of 250 ml 0.1 M PBS (pH 6.5) was prepared by mixing 0.21 g of Na_2HPO_4 and 0.27 g of NaH_2PO_4 in 250 ml deionized water and adjusted the pH by the addition of H_3PO_4. The stock solution of 100 ml 10^{-5} M L-glycine was prepared by dissolving 0.015 g L-glycine in 100 ml of PBS (pH 6.5). Standard solutions were prepared by diluting the stock solution in PBS by maintaining the pH. Deionized water was used throughout this study.

## 4.2.2	FABRICATION OF CCNT ELECTRODE

Carbon nanotubes (CCNT) was prepared by burning coconut oil under insufficient air, in an oil lamp at around 650°C and then the soot was collected and purified in soxhlet extractor using petroleum ether, acetone, alcohol, and finally by water to remove any unburnt oil and other soluble impurities. The residue was dried and then functionalized.[19] CCNT electrode was fabricated using the same method as mentioned in our published paper.[19,20] For the fabrication of the electrode, polystyrene solution was first prepared in chloroform (9:1 ratio). Then CCNT was mixed with polystyrene solution using mechanical stirrer followed by sonication. A drop of the slurry was then deposited as a very fine thin film on the two silver wires, serving as working and counter electrodes. The third silver wire was used as a reference electrode.

## 4.2.3	DETECTION OF L-GLYCINE

For the detection of L-glycine, LSV studies were performed with the sample solutions in PBS at CCNT electrode. The pH level of 6.5 was maintained for L-glycine. To optimize the conditions of electrochemical detection of both the amino acids at CCNT electrode, effect of pH, scan rate, and time interval were studied in detail. Then, the linearity, detection limit, sensitivity, reproducibility, and stability of the sensor were also investigated. To determine the selectivity of the sensor, the effect of the presence of some small biomolecules on the current responses of L-glycine at

CCNT electrode was evaluated under optimized experimental conditions. The utility of the CCNT electrode was tested by determining the amino acids in some pharmaceutical samples.

4.3 RESULTS AND DISCUSSIONS

4.3.1 EFFECT OF pH

The effect of pH on the oxidation of 10^{-5} M (10 μM) solutions of L-glycine at CCNT electrode was studied by LSV in the pH range from 6.5 at 100 m·Vs^{-1}. Figure 4.1 showed that there was a gradual decrease in the oxidation peak current with the increasing pH in case of both amino acids. I/μA versus pH graph showed that the maximum peak current was observed at pH 6.5 for L-glycine. Therefore, the pH 6.5 was chosen for the subsequent analytical experiments.

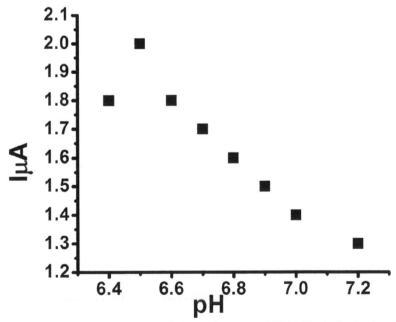

FIGURE 4.1   Effect of pH on the oxidation peak current of 10^{-5} M L-glycine in phosphate buffer solution (PBS) (pH 6.5) at 100 m·Vs^{-1} on carbon nanotube (CCNT) electrode.

4.3.2   EFFECT OF SCAN RATE

The effect of scan rate on the electrochemical detection of L-glycine at the CCNT electrode was investigated by LSV. Initially, LSV was performed with PBS solution on CCNT electrode at the scan rate of 100 m·Vs⁻¹ (Blank) (Fig. 4.2(a)). No peak current was observed at the potential range of −0.04–0.08 V, which indicated that CCNT electrode did not undergo any reaction with PBS. Then LSV was performed with 10^{-5} M L-glycine (pH 6.5) solutions in PBS on bare silver electrode at the scan rate of 100 m·Vs⁻¹ (Blank) (Fig. 4.2(b)). No peak current was observed at the potential range of −0.04–0.08 V, which indicated that bare silver electrode did not undergo any reaction.

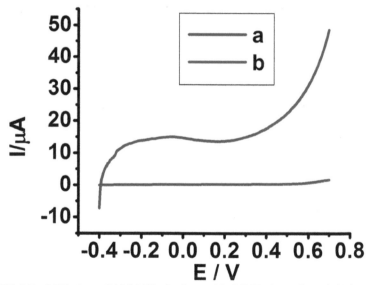

FIGURE 4.2   LSV plots of 10^{-5} M L-glycine at (a) CCNT electrode and (b) bare silver electrode in PBS at 100 m·Vs⁻¹.

The influence of scan rate was investigated in the range of 50–110 m·Vs⁻¹ for L-glycine. Figure 4.3 displayed LSV of 10^{-5} M solution of L-glycine (pH 6.5) at various scan rates. The current (I/μA) versus scan rate (m·Vs^{-1}) plot shown in the insets exhibited a linear relationship in both cases. The regression equations for L-glycine was calculated as, I/ μA = 1.76193 + 0.00835 m·Vs^{-1} with R value of 0.99444 and standard deviation of 0.0284 when N = 4.

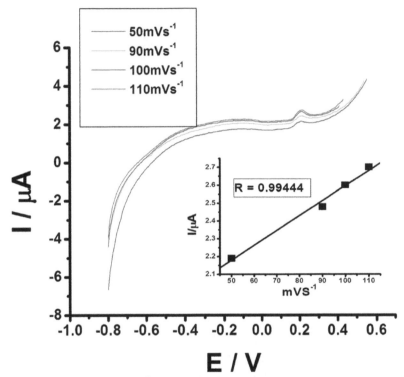

FIGURE 4.3   LSV plots of 10^{-5} M L-glycine in PBS (pH 6.5) at various scan rates (50, 90, 100, and 110 m·Vs^{-1}) at CCNT electrode. Inset: The plot of peak current (I/μ A) versus scan rate (v/m·Vs^{-1}).

The potential required for the detection of L-glycine at CCNT electrode was found to be 0.2 V. The linearity observed over the entire scan rates studied indicated that the electrochemical reaction was adsorption-controlled.[21]

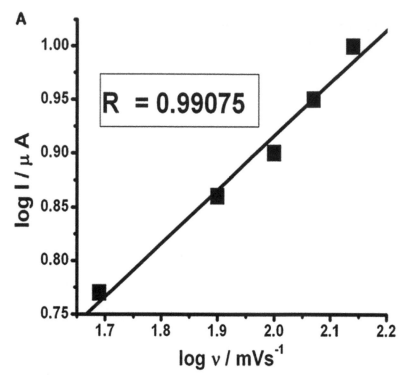

FIGURE 4.4   Linear relation between logarithm of peak current (log I/μA) and logarithm of scan rate (log v/m·Vs^{-1}) of 10^{-5} M L-glycine at CCNT electrode.

Figure 4.4 showed linear relationship between logarithm of peak current (log I/μA) versus logarithm of scan rate (log v/m·Vs^{-1}). Slope value for L-glycine was 0.99075, which is very close to the theoretical value of 1 for a purely adsorption-controlled process.[22]

4.3.3   EFFECT OF TIME INTERVAL

LSV study was also performed to study the nature of peak current and peak potentials as well as maximum accumulation time required for L-glycine, and it was observed that sharp intense peaks were obtained at the same peak potential. Figure 4.5 showed the linear relation between current and time interval during the analysis at $100 \ \text{m} \cdot \text{Vs}^{-1}$.

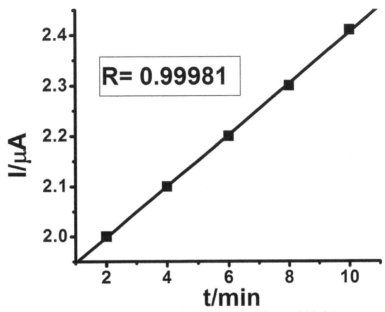

FIGURE 4.5 The plot of peak current (I/μA) versus time interval (t/min).

The regression equation in case of L-glycine was found to be

$$I / \mu A = 1.896 + 0.051 \ \text{min,} \qquad (4.1)$$

where $R = 0.99981$, $SD = 0.0038$, and $N = 5$.

The analysis was conducted up to a certain period of time (0–10 min) because it was observed that the peak current increased linearly with the time up to 10 min, but when this study was conducted for more than 10 min, then a breakdown in the linearity relationship was observed which may be due to the stabilization of current with time. Therefore, the maximum accumulation time was found to be 10 min for 10^{-5} M L-glycine.

4.3.4   LINEARITY, DETECTION LIMIT, AND SENSITIVITY OF THE SENSOR

Figure 4.6 showed the LSV of different concentrations of L-glycine in PBS at pH 6.5. The figure showed that the current increased linearly with the increase of concentrations of the amino acid. The calibration plots (inset) showed a linear dependence of the anodic peak current in the concentrations range of 1–100 μM (10^{-6}–10^{-4} M). The linear regression equations were found to be,

$$I / \mu A = 2.2725 + 0.022 \, \mu M, \qquad (4.2)$$

which gave R value of 0.99698 with SD=0.05643 (N=10).

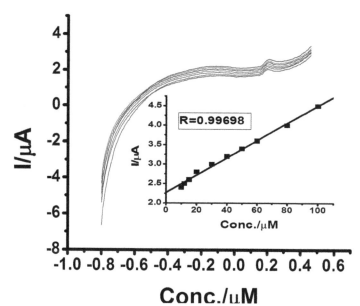

FIGURE 4.6   Plots of LSV of different concentrations of L-glycine (1–100 μM) in PBS (pH 6.5) on CCNT electrode at 100 m·Vs⁻¹. Inset: Calibration curve of response current (I/μA) versus concentration (Conc. /μM).

The active surface area of CCNT electrode was calculated using Randles--Sevcik equation:

$$I_P = (2.69 \times 10^5) + n^{3/2} AD^{1/2} Cv^{1/2}$$

where n is the number of electrons participating in the redox reaction, A is the electroactive surface area (cm^2), D is the diffusion coefficient (cm^{2}s^{-1}), C is the concentration of the redox probe molecule (molcm^{-3}), and v is the scan rate (mVs^{-1}), and the calculated electroactive surface area of CCNT electrode was found to be 0.0765 cm^2, where $C = 5 \times 10^{-4}$ M, $D = 7.1 \times 10^{-6}$cm^2/s, and n = 1 for [Fe (CN)$_6$]$^{3-/4-}$system.[23] The sensitivity was calculated from the slope of the current versus concentration in the calibration plot (Fig. 4.6 inset) divided by the active surface area of CCNT, according to the following formula:[24]

Sensitivity = slope of the plot/active surface area of the electrode,

and the sensitivity of the CCNT-based L-glycine sensor was calculated to be ~2.953 μA·μM^{-1}·cm^{-2}.

Limit of detection (LOD) and limit of quantification (LOQ) were calculated using the formulas, LOD = 3 s/m; LOQ = 10 s/m, where s is the standard deviation of the peak currents of the blank (five runs) and m is the slope of the calibration curve.[23] The values were found to be 1 and 8.17 μM, respectively. CCNT-based glucose sensor showed a short response time of 5 s.

4.3.5   REPRODUCIBILITY AND STABILITY OF THE SENSOR

A series of five successive LSV measurements were carried out with 10^{-5} M L-glycine (pH = 6.5) in PBS on five fabricated CCNT electrodes, which gave relative standard deviations of 3.1% (Fig. 4.7). The results indicated that the CCNT electrode provided good reproducibility toward oxidation of both L-glycines.

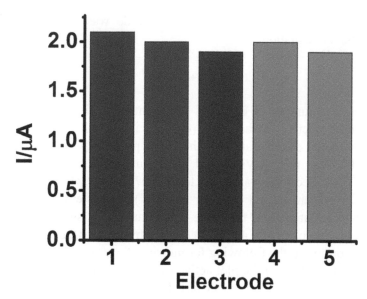

FIGURE 4.7 Current responses of 10^{-5} M L-glycine obtained at five different CN electrodes. For L-glycine, N=5, RSD=3.1%.

The stability of this sensor was studied by storing the electrode in air for 20 days, where the current response of 10^{-5} M L-glycine was found to be stable, maintaining ~80% of its initial intensity (Fig. 4.8).

4.3.6 INTERFERENCE

Under optimized experimental conditions described above, the effects of some small biomolecules on the current responses of 10^{-5} M L-glycine have been evaluated. Vitamin C, dopamine, L-alanine, L-serine, L-phenyl-alanine, tryptophan, and tyrosine had no influence on the current response of L-glycine at CCNT electrode at the working pH of 6.5. The experimental results (Table 4.1) showed that ten times of each substance had almost no interference with the determination of L-glycine. Thus, the proposed method was able to assay L-glycine in presence of interfering substances. The average signal change was found to be 0.7051%

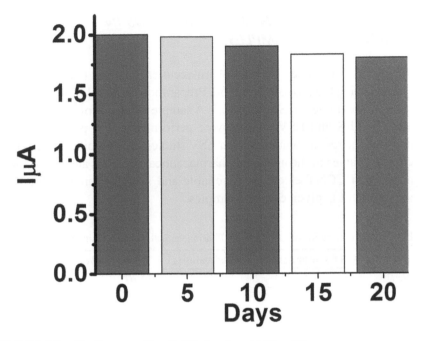

FIGURE 4.8 (I/μA) versus t/day (0–20) showing stability of the sensor.

TABLE 4.1 Influence of Interfering Species on the Voltammetric Response of 10^{-5} M L-Glycine.

L-glycine $(10^{-5}$ M$)^+$	Observed	Signal	Average
Interfering species $(10^{-4}$ M$)$	Potential (V)	Change (%)	Signal change (%)
L-glycine	0.2	0	
L-glycine + vitamin C	0.21	5	
L-glycine + dopamine	0.19	5	2.85
L-glycine + L-alanine	0.2	0	
L-glycine + L-serine	0.2	0	
L-glycine + L-phenylalanine	0.21	5	
L-glycine + tryptophan	0.2	0	
L-serine + tyrosine	0.19	5	

4.3.7 DETERMINATION OF AMINO ACIDS IN PHARMACEUTICAL SAMPLES

L-glycine was determined in some pharmaceutical samples (Medett Products, India) using the proposed method. Preparation of sample solution was the same as mentioned in Section 4.2.1. A sample solutions of 10^{-5} M were prepared in PBS and LSV studies were performed at 6.5 pH. Table 4.2 summarizes the results obtained from LSV studies of L-glycine along with the certified values of the analyzed pharmaceutical products and the results suggested that CCNT electrode is reliable and sensitive enough for the determination of L-glycine in real samples.

TABLE 4.2   Determination of L-Glycine in Pharmaceutical Samples Using CN Electrode.

Sample	CCNT sensor (g)	Certified value (g)	Recovery (%)	Bias (%)
L-glycine	2.2 ± 0.03^a	2.4	91.67	8.33

[a]Average of five determinations.

4.4 CONCLUSION

In this chapter, we have described the fabrication of CCNT electrode for the electrochemical detection of L-glycine. LSV showed that the oxidation peak current of 10^{-5} M L-glycine was linearly proportional to its concentration over the range from 1–100 μM, with correlation coefficient of 0.99698. This sensor showed good sensitivity, selectivity, and strong stability. The results also demonstrated the suitability of CCNT electrode for fast analysis of L-glycine in standard solutions as well as in commercial pharmaceutical products.

4.5 ACKNOWLEDGMENT

The authors are thankful to principal, CMRIT, and director, NIT Agartala for allowing to publish the result.

KEYWORDS

- **L-glycine**
- **biosensor**
- **carbon nanotube**
- **linear sweep voltammetry**

REFERENCES

1. Wagner, I.; Musso, H. New Naturally Occurring Amino Acids. *Angew. Chem. Int. Ed. Engl.* **1983,** *22*(11), 816–28. DOI: 10.1002/anie.198308161.
2. Latham, M. C. *Body Composition, the Functions of Food, Metabolism and Energy.* Human Nutrition in the Developing World. Food and Nutrition Series–No. 29. Rome: Food and Agriculture Organization of the United Nations.
3. Amino. Dictionary.com. 2015 (accessed July 3, 2015).
4. Amino acid. Cambridge Dictionaries Online. Cambridge University Press, 2015 (accessed July 3, 2015).
5. Amino. FreeDictionary.com. Farlex, 2015 (accessed July 3, 2015).
6. Heftmann, E. *Chromatography, Fundamentals and Applications of Chromatography and Related Differential Migration Methods, Part B: Applications,* 5th ed.; Elsevier: Amsterdam, 1992.
7. Li, H. Q.; Chen. A.; Roscoe, S. G.; Lipkowski, J. Electrochemical and FTIR Studies of L-Phenylalanine Adsorption at the Au (111) Electrode. *J. Electroanal. Chem.* **2001,** *500*, 299–310.
8. Grudpan, K.; Kamfoo, K. Flow Injection Dialysis for The Determination of Anions Using Ion Chromatography. *Talanta* **1999,** *49*, 1023–1026.
9. Alwarthan, A. A. Determination of Ascorbic-Acid by Flow-Injection with Chemiluminescence Detection. *Analyst* **1993,** *118*, 639–642.
10. Agater, I. B.; Jewsbury, R. A. Direct Chemiluminescence Determination of Ascorbic Acid Using Flow Injection Analysis. *Anal. Chim. Acta.* **1997,** *356,* 289–294.
11. Keyvanfard, M.; Shakeri, R.; Maleh, H. K.; Alizad, K. Highly Selective and Sensitive Voltammetric Sensor-Based on Modified Multiwall Carbon Nanotube Paste Electrode for Simultaneous Determination of Ascorbic Acid, Acetaminophen and Tryptophan. *Mater. Sci. Eng. Carbon.* **2013,** *33*, 811–816.
12. Daud, N.; Yusof, N. A.; Tee, T. W.; Abdullah, A. H. Electrochemical Sensor for As (III) Utilizing CNTs/Leucine/Nafion Modified Electrode. *J. Electrochem. Sci.* **2012,** *7*, 175–185.

13. Akhtar, P.; Too, C. O., Wallace, G. G. Detection of Amino Acids at Conducting Electroactive Polymer Modified Electrodes Using Flow Injection Analysis. Part II. Use of microelectrodes. *Anal. Chim. Acta.* **1997,** *339,* 211–223.

14. Li, H.; Li, T.; Wang, E. Electrocatalytic Oxidation and Flow Detection of Cysteine at an Aquocobalamin Adsorbed Glassy Carbon Electrode. *Talanta* **1995,** *42,* 885–888.

15. Mahmoud, R.; Mojtaba, S.; Seied, M. P. Amprometric Detection of Glycine, L-Serine, and L-Alanine Using Glassy Carbon Electrode Modified by NiO Nanoparticles. *J. Appl. Electrochem.* **2012,** *42,* 1005–1011.

16. Chunya, L. Voltammetric Determination of Tyrosine-Based on an L-Serine Polymer Film Electrode. *Colloids Surf. B* **2006,** *50,* 147–151.

17. Hu, Y. F.; Zhang, Z. H.; Zhang, H. B.; Luo, L. J.; Yao, S. Z. Electrochemical Determination of L-Phenylalanine at Polyaniline Modified Carbon Electrode-Based on β-Cyclodextrin Incorporated Carbon Nanotube Composite Material and Imprinted Sol–Gel Film. *Talanta* **2011,** *84,* 305–313.

18. Soma, D.; Mitali, S. Electrochemical Detection of L-Serine And L-Phenylalanine at Bamboo Charcoal-Carbon Nanosphere Electrode. *J. Nanostruct. Chem.* **2014,** *4,* 102–110.

19. Soma, D.; Mitali, S. Electrochemical Studies of Carbon Nanotube Obtained from Coconut Oil as Non Enzymatic Glucose Biosensor. *Adv. Sci., Eng. Med.* **2013,** *5,* 645–648.

20. Soma, D.; Mitali, S. Potato Starch-Derived Carbon Nano Almond for Non Enzymatic Detection of Sucrose. *New Res. Carbon Mater.* **2014,** *30*(3), 244–251.

21. Tian, H.; Jia, M.; Zhang, M.; Hu, J. Nonenzymatic Glucose Sensor-Based on Nickel Ion Implanted-Modified Indium Tin Oxide Electrode. *Electrochim. Acta.* **2013,** *96,* 285–290.

22. Gosser, D. K. J. *Cyclic Voltammetry: Simulation and Analysis of Reaction Mechanisms.* Wiley-VCH: NewYork, 1993.

23. Dar, G. N.; Umar, A.; Zaidi, S. A.; Ibrahim, A. A.; Abaker, M.; Baskoutas, S.; Al-Assir, M. S. Ce Doped ZnO Nanorods for the Detection of Hazardous Chemical. *Sensors and Actuators B.* **2012,** *173,* 72–75.

24. Soma, D.; Mitali, S. Potato Starch-Derived Carbon Nano Almond for Non Enzymatic Detection of Sucrose. *New. Carbon Mater.* **2014,** *30*(3) 244–251.

CHAPTER 5

AN OVERVIEW OF PROSPECTS OF SPINEL FERRITES AND THEIR VARIED APPLICATIONS

ANN ROSE ABRAHAM[1], SABU THOMAS[2] and NANDAKUMAR KALARIKKAL[1,2,*]

[1]School of Pure and Applied Physics, International & Inter University Centre for Nanoscience and Nanotechnology, Mahatma Gandhi University, Kottayam, Kerala 686560, India

[2]International & Inter University Centre for Nanoscience and Nanotechnology, Mahatma Gandhi University, Kottayam, Kerala 686560, India

*Corresponding author. E-mail: nkkalarikkal@mgu.ac.in

CONTENTS

ABSTRACT

Magnetic particles in the nanosize regime are the topic of extreme scientific and technical attention due to the array of mesmerizing properties exhibited by them. Nanosized spinel ferrite particles have always been a subject of wide curiosity. The wonderful properties of nanoferrites endow them with unique status in power electronics, nonvolatile memory devices, and biomedical applications. The primary endeavor of this chapter is to highlight the potential of spinel ferrites as radar-absorbing material (RAM), electromagnetic interference (EMI) shielding materials and also in spintronics, power and in biomedical fields. The state of the art techniques for the development of spinel ferrites by solgel and other innovative methods are also discussed. The numerous process parameters that influence the structure, properties, and functionalities of ferrites are detailed. After a brief and concise preface to nanomagnetism, spinel ferrites and their main characteristics, the chapter focuses on recent studies, investigations, and advancements in the field of ferrites. Novel fabrication techniques to develop ferrites and ferrite-based composites are briefly explained. A detailed description of the use of such materials for diversified applications with particular emphasis to EMI suppression and biomedical applications is given in the chapter.

5.1   INTRODUCTION

The magnetic attributes of a material appear extensively diverse from that of the bulk counterpart when reduced to the nanoscale. The unique properties of the magnetic materials at the nanoscale are dominated by two features: (1) finite size effects[1] such as, high surface to volume ratio and (2) surface effects, influenced by the presence of interparticle interactions (exchange and/or dipolar),[2] magnetization is affected by anisotropy. Magnetic behavior of nanoparticles (NPs) is commonly explained by the anisotropy energy per particle, given by

$$E = K_{eff} V \sin^2 \theta$$

Where, V is the average nanoparticle volume, K_{eff} is the effective anisotropy constant and its value depends on contribution of the (i) bulk (magnetocrystalline) anisotropy that arises from spin-orbit coupling, (ii) shape anisotropy, (iii) stress anisotropy, (iv) externally-induced anisotropy, and (v) exchange anisotropy.[2] θ denotes the angle between the magnetization and the easy magnetization axis of the particle. V decreases with a decrease in particle size, and hence the anisotropy energy decreases to a small value. Below a critical volume, additional energy is required to generate a domain wall. The domain walls formation becomes energetically unfavorable, as the particle size reduces to a critical particle diameter D_c, and, hence the particles form a single domain. Variation in magnetization does not occur through domain wall motion anymore and, hence requires the coherent rotation of spins and as a consequence larger coercivities. As the particle size decreases below the single domain value, the spins become progressively more affected by thermal fluctuations and the system turns out to be superparamagnetic (SPM). If temperature increases, the thermal energy causes the particle magnetization to rotate freely, leading to the diminishing of magnetism. This spin flipping occurs at the *blocking temperature*, T_B. The magnetization decreases above the blocking temperature, and the system acts like a paramagnetic material. The single-domain particle turns superparamagnetic at $T > T_B$.

The superparamagnetic behavior[3] is explained by the Neel–Brown relation as

$$\tau = \tau_0 \exp\left(E_A \middle/ K_B T \right)$$

τ is the relaxation time, τ_0 is the relaxation time constant ($\sim 10^{-9}$ s) and T is the temperature.

Stoner–Wohlfarth (SW) theory[4] describes the effect of different types of anisotropy on magnetic properties, like coercivity and remanence. SW theory states that blocking temperature follows the relation,

$$T_B = \frac{KV}{25\,K_B}$$

Where, K is the effective magnetic anisotropy constant, V is the mean volume of the NPs, and K_B is the Boltzmann constant. In case of a particle with uniaxial anisotropy, $\Delta E = KV$ (at $H=0$) and the condition for superparamagnetism becomes $KV = 25 K_B T$.

Thus, blocking temperature (T_B) increases with increase in particle size. The magnetic nanoparticle system appears to be superparamagnetic,[5] above blocking temperature.[6] Below blocking temperature T_B, magnetic moments of SPM particles cannot rotate freely as they remain "frozen" in random orientation, and the free movement of the magnetic moment is blocked by the anisotropy as the thermal fluctuations do not dominate.[7]

The critical diameter[8] for a magnetic particle to reach the single domain limit is defined by

$$D_c = \frac{36\sqrt{AK}}{\mu_0 M_S^2}$$

Where, A is the exchange constant, K is the effective anisotropy constant and M_s is the saturation magnetization. The variation of coercivity with particle size is shown in Figure 5.1 below.

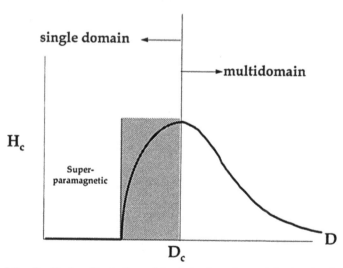

FIGURE 5.1   Qualitative illustration of the behavior of coercivity in ultrafine particle systems as the particle size changes.

Source: Reprinted (adapted) with permission from Leslie-Pelecky, D.L.; Rieke, R.D. Magnetic Properties of Nanostructured Materials. *Chem. Mater.* **1996,** *8*(96), 1770–1783.Copyright (1996) American Chemical Society.

The field-cooled zero-field-cooled (FC-ZFC) curves that indicate the temperature dependence of the magnetization, $M(T)$ in a system consisting of Co nanoparticles randomly oriented in a polystyrene matrix is shown in Figure 5.2 below.

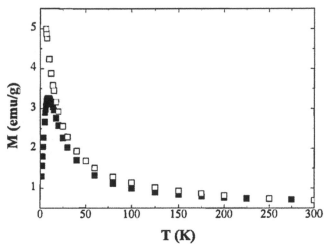

FIGURE 5.2   Magnetization as a function of temperature measured in the zero-field-cooled (solid symbols) and field-cooled (open symbols) cases for a nanocomposite consisting of cobalt particles in a polystyrene/triphenylphosphine matrix.

Source: Reprinted (adapted) with permission from Leslie-Pelecky, D.L.; Rieke, R.D. Magnetic Properties of Nanostructured Materials. *Chem. Mater.* **1996**, *8*(96), 1770–1783.Copyright (1996) American Chemical Society.

The coercive field (H_c) values can be calculated using the equation,

$$H_c = 0.48 \frac{2K}{M_S} 1 - 2\sqrt{\frac{T}{T_B}}$$

Where, T_B is the blocking temperature.

5.2   SPINEL FERRITES

Ferrites are a large class of oxides, investigated intensively due to their remarkable magnetic properties.[9] Ferrites are classified mainly into three groups with different crystal types. They are spinel, garnets, and magneto-plumbite. Spinel ferrites have a cubic structure with general formula $MO.Fe_2O_3$, where M is a divalent metal ion like Mn, Ni, Fe, Co, Mg, and so forth. Garnets have a complex cubic structure whereas magneto-plumbite has a hexagonal structure.

Spinel ferrites are represented by the formula unit AB_2O_4.[10] Spinel ferrites are attractive due to their scientific and technological significance in magnetic memories, electronic circuits as inductors, electromagnetic interference suppression, radio frequency applications, magnetic energy storage, magnetocaloric refrigeration systems,[11] and microwave frequency applications. The feasibility to prepare ferrites by various methods by means of different precursors offers the opportunity to tailor their properties for desired applications. There are many instances where ferrites cannot be replaced by ferromagnetic metals. The financial viability of ferrites due to their cost-effectiveness helps them in competing with other metals.

5.2.1   STRUCTURE OF SPINEL FERRITES

Materials which crystallize in the spinel structure have the general formula AB_2O_4 or $(AO)(B_2O_3)$ in which A and B are the cations at the tetrahedral and octahedral sites respectively and O indicates the oxygen anions. A represents a divalent metal cation such as Mg, Fe, Co, Ni, Cu, Zn, Cd, Mn, and B is the iron cation.

The spinel structure is derived from that of the mineral spinel $MgAl_2O_4$. The unit cell consists of eight formula units $(8 \times AB_2O_4)$ where A and B are the divalent and trivalent metal ions. The comparatively larger 32 oxygen ions[12] form face-centered cubic (FCC)[11] lattice. In a cubic unit cell, two kinds of interstitial sites are present, namely: a) 64 tetrahedral sites and b) 32 octahedral sites, out of which only 8 and 16 sites are occupied by metal ions. The tetrahedral sites are surrounded by four oxygen atoms (A sites) and octahedral sites are surrounded by six oxygen ions (B sites).

5.2.1.1   NORMAL AND INVERSE SPINEL STRUCTURE

In the normal or regular spinel, the divalent (A^{2+}) metal ions occupy the tetrahedral sites and the trivalent (B^{3+}) metal ions occupy the octahedral sites. The stoichiometry is $A_8B_{16}O_{32}$. Examples are $ZnFe_2O_4$, $CdFe_2O_4$ and so forth.

The inverse spinel is one in which half of the number of octahedral sites are occupied by the divalent (A^{2+}) metal ions, and the trivalent (B^{3+}) metal ions are equally divided between the tetrahedral and the remaining octahedral sites. The stoichiometry is $B_8(A_8B_8)O_{32}$ or $B(AB)O_4$. Here, the A sites are occupied solely by trivalent metal ions and the B sites by equal numbers of trivalent and divalent metal ions. Examples are magnetite (Fe_3O_4) and ferrites like $NiFe_2O_4$, $CoFe_2O_4$, and $CuFe_2O_4$.

5.3   APPLICATIONS OF SPINEL FERRITES

The wonderful properties enjoyed by the ferrites endow them with incomparable application potential. Greater than before interest is being put into tailoring of attributes of magnetic nanoparticles by manipulation of their size, composition, and morphology, for the desired application.[13] The opportunity of tailoring ferrites to nanoparticle size regime has helped to realize revolutionary applications in the electronics, spintronics, magnonics and also in the biomedical field. Nanosized spinel ferrite particles have engrossed significant research interest for multi-functional applications. Here in this chapter, the broad applications of spinel ferrites are classified into various groups.

5.3.1   ELECTROMAGNETIC INTERFERENCE (EMI) SUPPRESSION

With the recent widespread utilization of electrical and electronic devices, electromagnetic interference (EMI) is a significant threat to electronic applications[14] and human health.[15] Hence, the inevitability of microwave absorbing material is escalating day by day,[16] in order to shield or suppress the electromagnetic interference. Microwave-reflective and absorbent properties of spinel ferrites were reported by Shen et al.[17] The nanocomposites of conductive polymer and magnetic particles have a variety of advantages such as low density, high hardness, structural diversity, and improved electromagnetic properties.[18] Electromagnetic properties of zinc ferrite/expanded graphite composites were reported.[19]

The EMI shielding effectiveness (SE) of a material is defined as the ratio of transmitted power to incident power,

$$SE(dB) = -10 \log\left(\frac{P_t}{P_0}\right)$$

Shielding effectiveness (SE) of a system relies on three processes, reflection, absorption,[14] and multiple internal reflections and also on various parameters such as permittivity, permeability, conductivity, and thickness.

For a shielding material, if SE_R is due to reflection, SE_A owes to absorption and SE_M is the contribution from multiple reflections, the total shielding is given by,

$$SE = SE_R + SE_A + SE_M$$

The nanocomposites of $CuFe_{10}Al_2O_{19}$/multiwall carbon nanotubes were developed for microwave-absorbing applications and reported by.[20] Composite of CNT with M type hexaferrite ($CuFe_{10}Al_2O_{19}$) is fabricated with an objective to successfully enhance their reflection loss value over a broad frequency range in the X-band (8.2–12.4 GHz) region. Composite materials containing both dielectric and magnetic components are of interest as microwave absorbers since a microwave absorber absorbs electromagnetic energy and it is dissipated as heat energy by both dielectric and magnetic losses. A magnetic M-type hexaferrite ($CuFe_{10}Al_2O_{19}$) was synthesized and coated on the acid-modified multiwall carbon nanotube (MWCNT) by an in situ technique. For the fabrication of microwave test plates, thermoplastic polyurethane (TPU)/$CuFe_{10}Al_2O_{19}$/MWCNT nanocomposites were prepared via the solution mixing process. The nanocomposites were found to exhibit astonishing and superior microwave absorption properties than pristine MWCNT and $CuFe_{10}Al_2O_{19}$. The enhanced microwave absorption in the nanocomposites is achieved by the dielectric loss of MWCNT and the magnetic loss of $CuFe_{10}Al_2O_{19}$. The relative complex permittivity and permeability also contribute to the improved microwave absorption property of the composites. The nanocomposite displayed a better specific capacitance of 269 F/g, and superior electrochemical impedance properties than those of the pristine MWCNT and $CuFe_{10}Al_2O_{19}$. The results indicate the effective practical utility of the developed ferrite/CNT nanocomposites for microwave absorbing and supercapacitor applications.

Microwave absorbent and reflective properties of spinel ferrites were reported by Shen et al.[17] Composite of ferrite powder and silicon rubber is produced. By reflection/transmission technique, dielectric constant and magnetic permeability are determined. Absorption and reflection loss which contribute to the total shielding effectiveness are calculated from the material constants. Manganese zinc ferrite is reported to exhibit the highest absorption and reflection loss, attributed to the high dielectric constant and dielectric loss properties enjoyed by the Mn-Zn ferrite filler.

The electromagnetic properties of Fe_3O_4 dispersed in oleic acid solution were reported by Kuanr et al.[20] Fe_3O_4 nanoparticles were synthesized by a seed-mediated technique, using Fe $(acac)_3$, 1,2-hexadecanediol, phenylether, oleic acid, and oleylamine. The mixture was magnetically stirred under argon flow, heated to 200°C for 2 h and again heated to reflux at 265°C for 30 min under nitrogen atmosphere and cooled to room temperature. Ethanol was added to the mixture, centrifuged and the black precipitate obtained was washed with ethanol to obtain Fe_3O_4 nanoparticles of 4 nm. The obtained particles were redispersed in hexane along with oleic acid and oleylamine finally. Similarly, Fe_3O_4 nanoparticles of 6 and 8 nm were prepared and characterized. The X-ray diffraction pattern clearly showed the presence of magnetite. Transmission electron microscopy (TEM) images reveal that some of the nanoparticles were congregated, due to the large specific surface area and high surface energy of Fe_3O_4 nanoparticles. A Cu coplanar waveguide structure on GaAs substrate was fabricated and the Iron oxide nanoparticles (Fe_3O_4) with different particle sizes were spin-coated on the top of the transmission line, to analyze the microwave properties of Fe_3O_4. Using network analyzer, the transmission parameters were measured. The magnetic field dependence of the resonance frequency (*fr*) and frequency linewidth (Δf) was achieved from Lorentzian fits to the experimental data. Using a vector network analyzer, it is observed that with an increase in the applied field, the resonance frequency increases for all particle sizes and Δf decreases with the increase in the particle size.

The nanoparticle layer is assumed to be an effective medium of spherical magnetic particles embedded in a thin-film of the dielectric matrix. In case of spherical nanoparticles, the magnetic permeability tensor is described by the magnetic permeability tensor of a bulk material with demagnetization factors, N_x, N_y, and N_z. If N^e is the demagnetization factor of the effective medium, the effective demagnetization field is estimated as,

$$N^e = \left(1 - f_P\right)N^P + f_P N$$

Where, N^p is the demagnetization factor of the single spherical particle, $N_x = N_y = N_z = \frac{1}{3}$, is the demagnetization factor for a thin film ($N_x=0$, $N_y=0$, and $N_z=1$), and f_p is the filling fraction. It is observed that the magnetization values are different for the different samples with varied particle sizes. M_s values are found to be 0.14, 0.19, 0.25, and 0.29 kg for the samples with a particle size of 4, 6, 8, and 10 nm, respectively, if we assume a filling fraction of 0.3. The values are consistent with previous reports that indicate a change in Ms with particle size. From the calculations, f_p is found to be about 0.3 for the 4 nm particles and 0.5 for the 10 nm particles. The results prove that as the particle size increases, M_s values increase. The data points out a novel finding, that with an increase in the size of the particles, there is an increase in the filling fraction.

A theoretical study was carried out using the power absorbed by the different regions of the coplanar waveguide. The transmitted power in the coplanar waveguide per unit area was calculated from the Poynting vector. The power transmitted in the dielectric and air was calculated from the relation,

$$\langle P \rangle = \frac{c}{8\pi\sqrt{\varepsilon_{d,a}}} \oint h^2 dx dy$$

Where, ε_d and ε_a represent the relative permittivities of the dielectric medium and air, respectively. The transmission characteristics of the magnetic nanoparticle layer on the coplanar waveguide were obtained using the law of conservation of power. The results were found to be in accordance with the experiment. The resonance absorption for ferrite particles is analyzed from the ferromagnetic resonance (FMR) experiments carried out in frequency domain on ferrite nanoparticles-based coplanar transmission lines. The resonant frequency and the line width as a function of applied field are observed to analyze the effect of the interactions between particles of FMR spectra. At a fixed magnetic field, with increase in particle size the resonance frequency was observed to increase and attain a peak value at around particle size of 14 nm and then decreases with particle size. The increase in the magnetization as the particles become larger must be the reason for this increase in the resonance frequency.

One dimensional nanofibers of $Mn_{0.5}Zn_{0.5}Fe_2O_4$ ferrite-grafted poly-aniline (PANI) nanocomposites were reported to be good electromagnetic shielding materials.[18] Electrical and optical properties of nickel ferrite/polyaniline nanocomposite were reported.[22] Ferrite-flake composites were reported to be effective for the suppression of broadband and high-frequency noise.[23] Microwave electromagnetic and absorbing properties of Dy^{3+}-doped Mn-Zn ferrites were reported by Song et al.[24] Spinel ferrite films[25] and high resistive Mn-Zn ferrite films[26] were reported to be effective for electromagnetic compatible (EMC) devices. The electromagnetic interference shielding effectiveness of ~ 12.7 dB (94.6% shielding) was reported for Cobalt ferrite sphere-coated buckhorn-like barium titanate.[27] Spinel ferrite materials are extensively used in nonvolatile memory device applications based on their resistive switching performances.[28]

5.3.2 BIOMEDICAL APPLICATIONS

Augmented interest in magnetic nanoparticles has led to noteworthy advancements in the field of ferrites for biomedical applications. The entry of magnetic nanoparticles into the biomedical sciences has created a revolution in speedy and effective diagnosis and treatment of cancer. Nanoparticles are striking for cancer therapy and also for treatment of other ailments due to their unique attributes together with negligible side effects. Among all, surface-engineered superparamagnetic iron oxide nanoparticles (SPIONs) have attracted significant attention for cancer therapy applications.[29]

Size reduction to the nanometric scale leads to interesting magnetic properties, such as superparamagnetism, enhanced anisotropy, and surface effects which are of great interest in biomedicine for magnetic resonance imaging or thermotherapy.[30] Particle size plays a major role in the tuning of properties of magnetic nanoparticles. Magnetic properties of the ferrites rely on the particle size and the uniformity of response to the external magnetic field. Spinel ferrites with superparamagnetic behavior and size preferably less than 30 nm are desirable as magnetic drug delivery systems for biomedical applications. These parameters play an important role in the biomedical application as transport systems and drug delivery.[31]

The high magnetic moment ($\sim 10^4$ Bohr magnetons, μ_B) enjoyed by nano ferrites, their chemical stability and reactive surface that permits surface engineering make them good candidates for biomedical purposes.[8]

A nanoparticle system based on monodisperse nickel ferrites was developed with the intention of enhanced response to magnetic hyperthermia treatments and other biomedical applications.[32] Monodisperse stable nickel ferrite nanoparticles with different proportions of Ni^{2+} ions (nickel percentages varying from 3 to 20%) and sizes have been produced by optimization of the thermal decomposition method and the seed-growth technique sample has been transferred to water by surface coating with poly (maleic anhydride-alt-1-octadecene) (PMAO) polymer. Good control of the size, high homogeneity, and controlled nickel doping were achieved by this method by varying the temperature and reactant concentrations. Ni^{2+} ions were varied to modulate the magnetic properties for future hyperthermia applications. The monocrystalline nature of these nanoparticles was assured form the x-ray diffraction (XRD) and TEM images. Mean sizes calculated from XRD and TEM micrographs are in good agreement. Ni^{2+} content seems to play an important role in the magnetic behavior of the samples, affecting the saturation magnetization, anisotropy constant, and g_{eff} values. It has been found that the heating capacity measured by magnetic hyperthermia in vitro experiment decreases at higher Ni proportion of the samples. For all these reasons, the seed growth sample with the lowest fraction of Ni^{2+} has proved to be the best candidate for biomedical applications. 3-(4,5-dimethylthiazol-2-yl)-2,5-diphenyltertrazolium bromide (MTT) cytotoxicity assay was used to analyze their biocompatibility. Their potential use as magnetic resonance imaging (MRI) contrast agent was studied by relaxivity in vitro proof (Fig. 5.3).

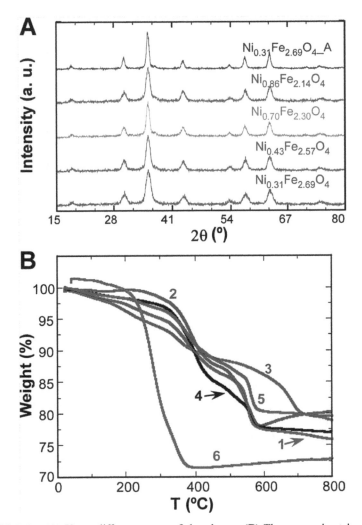

FIGURE 5.3 **(A)** X-ray diffractograms of the phases. **(B)** Thermogravimetric analysis of the samples (1: $Ni_{0.31}Fe_{2.69}O_4$, 2: $Ni_{0.43}Fe_{2.57}O_4$, 3: $Ni_{0.64}Fe_{2.36}O_4$, 4: $Ni_{0.86}Fe_{2.14}O_4$, 5: $Ni_{0.31}Fe_{2.69}O_4$ A, and 6: $Ni_{0.31}Fe_{2.69}O_4\_A\_PMAO$) in Ar atmosphere.

Source: Reprinted (adapted) with permission from Lasheras, X. et al. Chemical Synthesis and Magnetic Properties of Monodisperse Nickel Ferrite Nanoparticles for Biomedical Applications. *J. Phys. Chem. C.* 2016. Copyright (2016) American Chemical Society.

The specific absorption rate (SAR) was studied to estimate their potential applications for hyperthermia treatments. Measurements of SAR versus frequency indicate that the SAR values increase with magnetic frequencies and particle size under a constant field (Fig. 5.4).

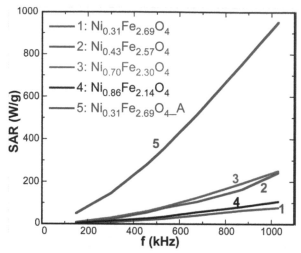

FIGURE 5.4   Specific absorption rate (SAR) values as a function of frequency at constant ac excitation amplitude of 20 kA·m⁻¹.

Source: Reprinted (adapted) with permission from Lasheras, X. et al. Chemical Synthesis and Magnetic Properties of Monodisperse Nickel Ferrite Nanoparticles for Biomedical Applications. *J. Phys. Chem.C,* **2016**. Copyright (2016) American Chemical Society.

The magnetic behavior of the samples was analyzed by means of field and temperature dependent magnetization measurements and electronic magnetic resonance. Magnetization as a function of temperature after cooling at ZFC-FC (10 Oe) was measured in a commercial superconducting quantum interference device (SQUID) magnetometer. Hysteresis loops at room temperature and at 5 K were done in a vibrating sample magnetometer (VSM).

All samples exhibit superparamagnetic nature, whose most distinctive features are the convergence of FC and ZFC curves above the blocking temperature (T_B) and the increase of the T_B with the particle size (Fig. 5.5A). These results follow the Stoner–Wohlfarth theory. For small ferrite samples, narrow ZFC signals were obtained due to the homogeneity of particle sizes, but a broadening of the maximum of the ZFC branch is observed in $Ni_{0.31}Fe_{2.69}O_4$A ferrite due to the strong dependence of T_B with particle diameter (T_B is proportional to D^3). The coercive field (H_c) values at 5 K are calculated to be around 200 Oe for all samples and no major changes are observed in the H_c values for different samples, as the parameters associated with rotation of nanoparticles about the easy magnetization axis did not considerably modify the H_c value.

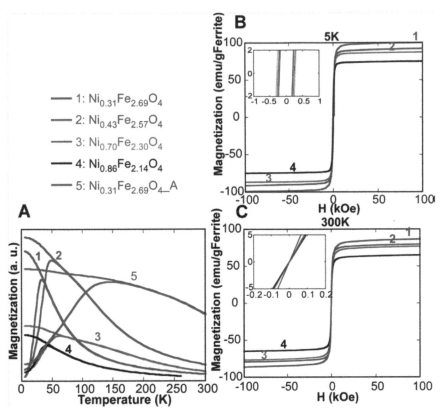

FIGURE 5.5 **(A)** ZFC/FC curves of nickel ferrite nanoparticles at an applied field of 10 Oe, **(B)** M(H) measurements at 5 K, and **(C)** M(H) measurements at room temperature.

Source: Reprinted (adapted) with permission from Lasheras, X. et al. Chemical Synthesis and Magnetic Properties of Monodisperse Nickel Ferrite Nanoparticles for Biomedical Applications. *J. Phys. Chem.C*, **2016.** Copyright (2016) American Chemical Society.

The in vitro cytotoxicity assay (analyzed in African green monkey kidney epithelial Vero cells) shows that these $Ni_{0.31}Fe_{2.69}O_4$_A_PMAO nickel ferrite nanoparticles are not cytotoxic even at 0.5 mg/ml concentration, as not many changes are observed in the cell metabolic activity compared with control cells (incubated without nanoparticles). Thus, the nickel ferrite nanoparticles system exhibit preliminary biocompatibility and nontoxicity and enhanced magnetic properties, proving themselves to be admirable candidates for biomedical applications such as hyperthermia or MRI contrast agents (Fig. 5.6).

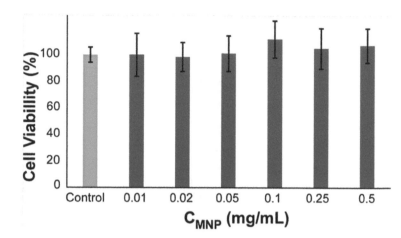

FIGURE 5.6 Cytotoxicity experiment of $Ni_{0.31}Fe_{2.69}O_4$-PMAO sample at different nanoparticle concentrations made in Vero cells.

Source: Reprinted (adapted) with permission from Lasheras, X. et al. Chemical Synthesis and Magnetic Properties of Monodisperse Nickel Ferrite Nanoparticles for Biomedical Applications. *J. Phys. Chem.C*, **2016**. Copyright (2016) American Chemical Society.

Cytotoxicity assays performed in Vero cells show that nickel ferrite nanoparticles are not cytotoxic at concentrations up to 0.5 mg/ml, and relaxivity measurements showed an interesting response of the sample at T_2, and are, hence, suitable MRI contrast agents. The enhanced hyperthermia response is attributed to higher crystallinity, bigger particle size that contributes to the highest specific absorption rate, and lower nickel proportion in ferrite structure. The ferrite systems have proved to be promising for magnetic hyperthermia applications and are an appealing alternative for developing diagnosis or therapeutic active agents. Magnetic nanoparticles like SPIONs and ferrites are remarkably auspicious for diagnosis and treatment of cancer,[29] medical imaging applications,[33] biomedical diagnoses and treatment,[34] and other biomedical applications[35] owing to their multifunctionality and lower toxicity. Hence, ferrites are widely used in cancer theranostics.[36] Ferrites are loaded with drugs for cancer therapy.[37] Therapies with targeted and image-guided approaches were also reported.[38]

5.3.3 NONLINEAR OPTICAL APPLICATIONS OF FERRITES

Spinel ferrites are known for their exciting optical limiting performances. Optical limiters[39] exhibit an induced reduction in transmittance at higher light fluences. These are very useful for protecting sensitive devices and eyes from laser-induced damage. Nonlinear optical properties[40] of (1-x) $CaFe_2O_4$–$xBaTiO_3$ composites[41] have been reported. In the case of spinel cadmium ferrites,[42] synthesized by a combustion method, observed nonlinearity was found to arise from the two-photon absorption behavior. Heat-treated magnesium ferrite ($MgFe_2O_4$) was reported to exhibit third-order nonlinear optical response.[43] The optical limiting properties of spinel ferrites, $NiFe_2O_4$, $Ni_{0.5}Zn_{0.5}Fe_2O_4$, $ZnFe_2O_4$, $Ni_{0.5}Co_{0.5}Fe_2O_4$, and $CoFe_2O_4$ were investigated by the open aperture Z-scan technique and compared.[44] The optical limiting curves of ZFO samples for different input laser energies are shown in Figure 5.7. The nonlinearity was found to fit a two photon-like absorption process.[44] From the z-scan measurement performed at four different pulse energies, excited state absorption[45] was found to contribute to the nonlinear optical response. $ZnFe_2O_4$ is established to be the better choice than others for the optical limiting applications. With the increase in particle size, the nonlinearity was also observed to increase.[44] Thus, as the particle size of the ferrites increases, the optical limiting threshold reduces and hence optical limiting performance enhances.

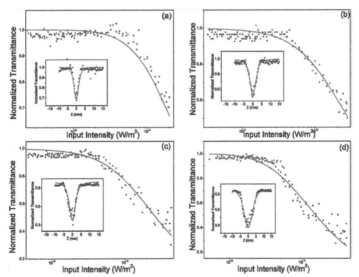

FIGURE 5.7   Nonlinear absorption in ZFO samples for input laser energies of (a) 40 mJ, (b) 60 mJ, (c) 80 mJ, and (d) 100 mJ. Insets show the corresponding open aperture z-scan curves.

Source: Reprinted from Thomas, J. J., Krishnan, S., Sridharan, K., Philip, R.;Kalarikkal, N. A comparative study on the optical limiting properties of different nano spinel ferrites with Z-scan technique. *Mater. Res. Bull.* **2012**, *47*, 1855–1860. Copyright (2012), with permission from Elsevier.

The two-photon absorption coefficient β values against laser pulse energies were plotted (Fig. 5.8). β value is found to increase substantially as the input laser pulse energy increases beyond 80 mJ and becomes a nonlinear function of pulse energy indicative of the higher order nonlinear processes such as free-carrier absorption that occurs at higher energies.

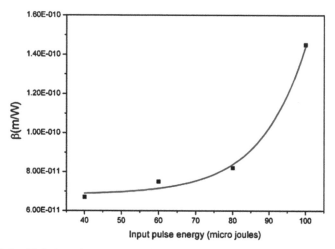

FIGURE 5.8   Variation of two-photon absorption coefficient of $ZnFe_2O_4$ with input pulse energy.

Source: Reprinted from Thomas, J. J., Krishnan, S., Sridharan, K., Philip, R.;Kalarikkal, N. A comparative study on the optical limiting properties of different nano spinel ferrites with Z-scan technique. *Mater. Res. Bull.* **2012,** *47,* 1855–1860. Copyright (2012), with permission from Elsevier.

5.3.4   RADIO FREQUENCY APPLICATIONS

Ferrites are supreme materials for radio frequency applications. Ferrites possess wonderful properties like relatively good permeability and permittivity, small electrical conductivity,[46] reasonable magnetization, low magnetic and dielectric losses,[46,47] and narrow ferromagnetic resonance line width that enable them for varied device applications. Ferrites are of great significance in electromagnetic applications because they can absorb electromagnetic radiation in microwave bands. Ferrites that exhibit promising magnetic property are attractive to examine the radar absorption. The high saturation magnetization of zinc ferrite makes it a paramount radar absorbing material. The radar absorbing performance of the Zn ferrite nanoparticles has been investigated by both experimental measurement and computational studies to exemplify this aspect.

Spinel ferrite nanocrystals (NCs) guarantee a diverse range of electro-magnetic and AC magnetic applications.[48] Ferrite systems exhibit losses at microwave frequencies that facilitate device applications such as filters, phase shifters, isolators, and so forth. Ferrites have proved to be exten-sively useful for design and development of devices for high-frequency radio frequency (RF) applications like telecommunications and radar systems that facilitate transfer and exploitation of electromagnetic signals. Microwave technologies necessitate higher frequencies and bandwidth up to 100 GHz and control components below 40 GHz. Ferrites being nonconducting oxides, allow total penetration of electromagnetic fields, unlike metals. At high frequencies, dispersion of domain walls occur (at about 10 GHz) and domain walls are unable to follow the fields and hence, absorption of microwave power occurs by spin dynamics.

Ferrites are indispensable for signal processing devices due to their nonreciprocity effects[49] that originate from the non-diagonal nature of the ferrite's permeability tensor and gyromagnetic resonance effects.[50] Ferrites are employed in microwave integrated systems that include nonre-ciprocal structures like isolators, phase shifters, circulators, and antennas operating over a broad frequency band. Recently, slot ferrite-coupled line sections were developed to realize integrated nonreciprocal devices. Highly crystalline spinel MnZn-ferrite films were reported to be devel-oped by a novel solution process for high-frequency applications.[25]

5.3.5   POWER APPLICATIONS

Ferrites usually exhibit minimum power losses at around 80°C and are the future magnetic materials for power electronics.[51] The losses are proved to be inversely proportional to resistivity. The high electrical resistivity of the ferrites, low dielectric constant, low Eddy current and dielectric losses contribute to the extensive application of ferrites in high-frequency magnetic components. The conductivity of ferrites is proportional to dielectric constant. Ferrites are the best choice as core material for frequencies from 10 kHz to a few hundred MHz owing to their low cost, high Q (inductor quality), high stability, and low volume. Soft magnetic materials (like Zn–Ni ferrites) are exploited tremendously by the modern electronics industry due to their unique attribute of high electrical resistivity. The low Eddy current losses over wide frequency ranges, stability over a wide temperature range and high permeability facilitate the design of ferrite cores for power supplies of a large variety of devices like computers, microwave devices, TV, and video systems. Power delivery and efficiency can be enhanced by increasing the working frequency of the ferrite transformer. Three-dimensional (3-D) ferrite cores are developed from ferrite wafers of 1 mm thickness by a micropowder blasting process, at working frequencies up to 1 MHz for low-power applications.[9] Manganese-substituted nickel–zinc ferrites have been developed as power core materials for applications in switched-mode power supplies (SMPS).[52] A very low power loss value of 500 mW/cc was obtained at a frequency of 500 kHz, temperature of 100°C, and a driving flux density of 50 mT. Broadband, low-cost, and low-loss microwave devices (like circulators, phase shifters, isolators, absorbers) are required for signal processing. Ferrites are ideal for microwave applications[53] because of their very high specific resistance and high performance. The nanocomposite of $ZnFe_2O_4$ and carbon[54] has been reported to be a proficient anode material for lithium-ion batteries,[54] that is a promising capable electrochemical power source. The highly superior electrochemical performance, cycling stability, and capacity retention exhibited by the ferrite nanocomposite reveal its potential for electrochemical energy storage application.

5.3.6   FERRITES FOR ENHANCED MAGNETOELECTRIC COUPLING AND MAGNETOCAPACITANCE EFFECTS

Spinel ferrites in combination with perovskites are exciting due to the induced magnetoelectric coupling,[55] owing to their multiferroic nature and applications in memory devices, optical-memory switching, multistate memory system, photo-induced devices, and so forth.[56] Multiferroics are those materials in which ferromagnetism and ferroelectricity coexist.[57] Multiferroic heterostructures or artificial multiferroics composed of ferrite-ferroelectrics are of enormous significance in this era, due to the increased requirement for room temperature multiferroics, due to greater than ever longing for multifunctional smart devices.[58] Ferrite–ferroelectric-based multiferroics exhibit enhanced magnetoelectric coupling at room temperatures that enable practical device applications.59 Integration of ferrites with ferroelectrics leads to a novel class of multi-functional materials known as multiferroics with excellent magnetic and dielectric performances.[60] It gives rise to remarkable properties like the magneto-dielectric (MD) effect and multiferroicity. Hence, meticulous attention is given to the development of ferrimagnetic-ferroelectric composites with multifunctional properties. They have extensive applications in magnetic field sensors, spintronic devices,[56] and multiple-state data storage. Sreenivasulu et al. have reported the enhanced magneto-capacitance response displayed by the $BaTiO_3$-ferrite multiferroic nanocomposite systems.[61] Enhanced magnetoelectric effect was observed in core-shell particulate composites with magnetic cobalt ferrite core and a shell of barium titanate,[58] $BaTiO_3$–$CoFe_{1.8}Zn_{0.2}O_4$ multiferroic composites,[62] $xBaTiO_3$–$(1-x)ZnFe_2O_4$ nanostructures.[63] Enhanced magnetocapacitance has been reported by ferrites in combination with ferroelectrics.[64,65,66]

Pachari et al. have reported enhanced magneto-capacitance effect in $BaTiO_3$–ferrite composite systems.[64] Composites of (1-X) $BaTiO_3$: X $(CoFe_2O_4/ZnFe_2O_4/Co_{0.5}Zn_{0.5}Fe_2O_4)$ (Where, X=20, 30, and 40 wt %) were prepared by conventional solid-state mixing route. The existence of two different morphologies says, plate-like (~5 μm with a thickness ~1 μm) and spherical shape of tetragonal $BaTiO_3$ along with polyhedral morphology of cubic ferrites in the prepared composite systems. The percentage of ferrite phase is observed to determine the random orientation of $BaTiO_3$ with plate-like morphology in these systems. The magnetoresistance effect was analyzed from the Cole-Cole plot. The magnetoresistance effect is greatly influenced by the type and percentage of ferrites. The magneto-capacitance response depends strongly on magnetostriction, the concentration of ferrite phase and magnetoresistance of grain or grain boundary. Depending on the percentage of the ferrite phase, the magnetocapacitance values were observed to vary in the range between −3 to−9, and for $BaTiO_3$: $CoFe_2O_4$, −0.5−−7 for $BaTiO_3$: $ZnFe_2O_4$ and from +1.5 to −1.5 for $BaTiO_3$:$Co_{0.5}Zn_{0.5}Fe_2O_4$ composite. The combined effects of phase morphology and magnetoresistance in these composites have contributed to the enhancement of magnetocapacitance effect.

5.3.7   OTHER BROAD APPLICATIONS

High-performance ferrite nanoparticles were obtained through nonaqueous redox phase tuning.[67] Rapid wireless control of intracellular calcium was enabled by the enhanced crystallinity of the nanoparticles. Redox tuning during solvent thermolysis could produce effective theranostic agents through selective phase control in ferrites.[67]

Ferrites such as $NiFe_2O_4$, $CoFe_2O_4$, and $MnFe_2O_4$ with a much higher T_C have promising applications in the field of spin filtering and magnetic energy storage applications. A $CoFe_2O_4$-based spin-filter has reported the highest spin-polarization (-8%) value at room temperature. The spin filtering nature of an ultrathin $Sm_{0.75}Sr_{0.25}MnO_3$ manganite film in a tunnel junction has been reported.[68]

Ferrites are favored because of their amazing electrical properties and exploited for an inspiring range of applications extending from milli-meter wave integrated circuitry,[9] radio frequency circuits, ferrofluids, electronics,[69] read/write heads in high-speed digital tapes, high-density storage,[69] magnetic recording, magneto-optical recording,[69] magnetic separation, ferrofluids, high-quality filters, and also in the field of tele-communication industry.[69]

Ferromagnetic nanostructures have wide applications in nanode-vices [70]and have attracted huge interest. $BaFe_{12}O_{19}$/NPR composite (nano-sized barium hexaferrite ($BaFe_{12}O_{19}$) in novolac phenolic resin (NPR)) is developed as microwave absorber for X-band application in the frequency range of 8.2–12.4 GHz.[71]

5.4   CONCLUSION

Ferrites are of vital importance in contemporary engineering and scientific applications. After a brief introduction to nanomagnetism, recent advances in the synthesis and potential applications of ferrite nanoparticles are briefly described. The amazing properties demonstrated by the ferrite-based composite system, say, dielectric resonance, microwave attenuation properties, nonlinear optical properties, and antimicrobial properties are discussed. Attention is given to briefly describe the varied applications of ferrites in all spheres of life, with a special focus on EMI shielding and biomedical applications of spinel ferrites. Ferrites in combination with carbon nanotubes (CNTs) are efficient microwave absorbers. Ferrite-ferro-electric-based multiferroics that facilitate practical device applications are of wide interest due to the demand for power efficient multifunctional smart devices. Thin films of ferrites are highly appealing for spintronics applications, as they have a high Curie temperature and yield large tunnel magnetoresistance (TMR) effects. The emergence of ferrite nanoparticles as a potential theranostic tool in biomedical applications is discussed. A brief attempt is made in this chapter to exemplify the significant aspects of spinel ferrites that make them marvelous among other potential candidates.

KEYWORDS

- ferrites
- superparamagnetism
- microwave frequencies
- radar absorption
- EMI shielding
- biomedical
- multiferroics

REFERENCES

1. Issa, B.; Obaidat, I. M.; Albiss, B. A.; Haik, Y. Magnetic Nanoparticles: Surface Effects and Properties Related to Biomedicine Applications. *Int. J. Mol. Sci.* **2013,** *14*, 21266–21305.
2. Jovic, N.; Antic, B.; Goya, G. F.; Spasojevic, V. Magnetic Properties of Lithium Ferrite Nanoparticles with a Core/Shell Structure. *Curr. Nanosci.* **2012,** *8*, 651–658.
3. Sharma, S. K.; Kumar, R.; Siva Kumar, V. V.; Dolia, S. N. Size Dependent Magnetic Behavior of Nanocrystalline Spinel Ferrite Mg0.05Mn0.05Fe2O4. *Indian J. Pure Appl. Phys.* **2007,** *45*, 16–20.
4. Leslie-Pelecky, D. L.; Rieke, R. D. Magnetic Properties of Nanostructured Materials. *Chem. Mater.* **1996,** *8*, 1770–1783.
5. Thomas, J. J.; Kalarikkal, N.; Garg, A. B.; Mittal, R.; Mukhopadhyay, R. Mossbauer Study of Ni, Ni-Co, and Co Ferrite Nanoparticles. *AIP Conf. Proc.* **1176,** 1175–1176 (2011).

6. Raghasudha, M.; Ravinder, D.; Veerasomaiah, P. Investigation of Superparamagnetism in MgCr0.9Fe 1.1O4 Nano-ferrites Synthesized by the Citrate-gel Method. *J. Magn. Magn. Mater.* **2014**, *355*, 210–214.

7. Vejpravová, J. P.; Sechovský, V. Superparamagnetism of Co-Ferrite Nanoparticles. *Proc. 14th Annu. Conf. Dr. Students—WDS Prague 2005* 518–523, 2005.

8. Cheng, K.; et al. Magnetic Nanoparticles: Synthesis, Functionalization, and Applications in Bioimaging and Magnetic Energy Storage. *Chem. Soc. Rev.* **2009**, *38*, 2532–2542.

9. Valenzuela, R. Novel Applications of Ferrites. *Phys. Res. Int.* **2012**, 2012.

10. Muthuselvam, I. P.; Bhowmik, R. N. Structural phase stability and magnetism in Co 2 FeO 4 spinel oxide. *Solid State Sci.* **2009**, *11*, 719–725.

11. Thomas, J. J.; Shinde, a. B.; Krishna, P. S. R.; Kalarikkal, N. Temperature Dependent Neutron Diffraction and Mössbauer Studies in Zinc Ferrite Nanoparticles. *Mater. Res. Bull.* **2013**, *48*, 1506–1511.

12. Thankachan, R. M.; et al. Cr^{3+}Substitution Induced Structural Reconfigurations in the Nanocrystalline Spinel Compound $ZnFe_2O_4$ as Revealed from X-ray Diffraction, Positron Annihilation and Mössbauer Spectroscopic Studies. *RSC Adv.* **2015**, *5*, 64966–64975.

13. El-Toni, A. M.; et al. Design, Synthesis and Applications of Core–Shell, Hollow Core, and Nanorattle Multifunctional Nanostructures. *Nanoscale* **2016**. DOI:10.1039/C5NR07004J.

14. Luo, J.; Shen, P.; Yao, W.; Jiang, C.; Xu, J. Synthesis, Characterization, and Microwave Absorption Properties of Reduced Graphene Oxide/Strontium Ferrite/Polyaniline Nanocomposites. *Nanoscale Res. Lett.* **2016**, *11*, 141.

15. Polley, D.; Barman, A.; Mitra, R. K. EMI Shielding and Conductivity of Carbon Nanotube-Polymer Composites at Terahertz Frequency. *Opt. Lett.* **2014**, *39*, 1541–1544.

16. Qin, F.; Brosseau, C. A Review and Analysis of Microwave Absorption in Polymer Composites Filled with Carbonaceous Particles. *J. Appl. Phys.* **2012**, *111*.

17. Kim, Y.; Kim, S. Microwave Reflective and Absorbent Properties of Spinel Ferrite Composites. *J. Magn. Soc. Jpn.* **1998**, *22*(1), 375–377.

18. Wang, W.; Gumfekar, S. P.; Jiao, Q.; Zhao, B. Ferrite-grafted Polyaniline Nanofibers as Electromagnetic Shielding Materials. *J. Mater. Chem. C.* **2013**, *1*, 2851.

19. Shen, G.; Yu, S.; Cao, Y. Preparation and Electromagnetic Properties of Zinc Ferrite/Expanded Graphite Composites. *Mater. Sci.* **2014**, *32*, 470–474.

20. Bhattacharya, P.; Das, C. K. In Situ Synthesis and Characterization of CuFe10Al2O19/MWCNT Nanocomposites for Supercapacitor and Microwave-Absorbing Applications BT—Industrial & Engineering Chemistry Research. *Ind. Eng. Chem. Res.* **2013**, *52*, 9594–9606.

21. Kuanr, B. K.; et al. Size Dependent Microwave Properties of Ferrite Nanoparticles: Application to Microwave Devices. *J. Appl. Phys.* **2009**, *105*, 5–8.

22. Khairy, M.; Gouda, M. E. Electrical and Optical Properties of Nickel Ferrite/Polyaniline Nanocomposite. *J. Adv. Res.* **2014**, *6*, 555–562.

23. Yun, Y. W.; et al. Electromagnetic Shielding Properties of Soft Magnetic Metal and Ferrite Composites for Application to Suppress Noise in a Radio Frequency Range. *J. Electroceramics.* **2006**, *17*, 467–469.

24. Song, J.; Wang, L.; Xu, N.; Zhang, Q. Microwave Electromagnetic and Absorbing Properties of Dy^{3+} Doped MnZn Ferrites. *J. Rare Earths.* **2010,** *28,* 451–455.

25. Subramani, A. K.; et al. Spinel Ferrite Films by a Novel Solution Process for High Frequency Applications. *Mater. Chem. Phys.* **2010,** *123,* 16–19.

26. Subramani, A. K.; et al. High Resistive Ferrite Films by a Solution Process for Electromagnetic Compatible (EMC) Devices. *J. Magn. Magn. Mater.* **2009,** *321,* 3979–3983.

27. Ji, R.; Cao, C. Cobalt Ferrite Sphere-Coated Buckhorn-like Barium Titanate: Fabrication, Characterization, its Dielectric Resonance, and Microwave Attenuation Properties. *J. Appl. Phys.* **2014,***116.*

28. Hu, W.; et al. Opportunity of Spinel Ferrite Materials in Nonvolatile Memory Device Applications Based on Their Resistive Switching Performances. *J. Am. Chem. Soc.* **2012,** *134,* 14658–14661.

29. Laurent, S.; Mahmoudi, M. Superparamagnetic Iron Oxide Nanoparticles: Promises for Diagnosis and Treatment of Cancer. *Int. J. Mol. Epidemiol. Genet.* **2011,** *2,* 367–390.

30. Gomes, D. A.; et al. Synthesis of Core-Shell Ferrites Nanoparticles for Ferrofluids : Chemical and Magnetic Analysis. *J. Phys. Chem. C.* **2008,** *112,* 6220–6227.

31. Dumitrescu, A. M.; et al. Advanced Composite Materials Based on Hydrogels and Ferrites for Potential Biomedical Applications. *Colloids Surfaces A Physicochem. Eng. Asp.* **2014,** *455,* 185–194.

32. Lasheras, X.; et al. Chemical Synthesis and Magnetic Properties of Monodisperse Nickel Ferrite Nanoparticles for Biomedical Applications. *J. Phys. Chem. C.* **2016.** Doi:10.1021/acs.jpcc.5b10216.

33. Fang, C.; Zhang, M. Multifunctional Magnetic Nanoparticles for Medical Imaging Applications. *J. Mater. Chem.* **2009,** *19,* 6258.

34. Yan, K.; et al. Recent Advances in Multifunctional Magnetic Nanoparticles and Applications to Biomedical Diagnosis and Treatment. *RSC Adv.* **2013,** *3,* 10598.

35. Li, X.; et al. Current Investigations into Magnetic Nanoparticles for Biomedical Applications. *J. Biomed. Mater. Res. Part A.* **2016,** *104,* 1285–1296.

36. Gobbo, O. L.; Sjaastad, K.; Radomski, M. W.; Volkov, Y.; Prina-Mello, A. Magnetic Nanoparticles in Cancer Theranostics. *Theranostics* **2015,** *5,* 1249–1263.

37. Jurgons, R.; et al. Drug Loaded Magnetic Nanoparticles for Cancer Therapy. *J. Phys. Condens. Matter.* **2006,** *18,* S2893–S2902.

38. Huang, J.; et al. Magnetic Nanoparticle Facilitated Drug Delivery for Cancer Therapy with Targeted and Image-Guided Approaches. *Adv. Funct. Mater.* **2016.** Doi:10.1002/adfm.201504185.

39. Ramakanth, S.; Hamad, S.; Venugopal Rao, S.; James Raju, K. C. Magnetic and Nonlinear Optical Properties of $BaTiO_3$Nanoparticles. *AIP Adv.* **2015,** *5,* 057139.

40. Raneesh, B.; et al. Composition-Structure–Physical Property Relationship and Nonlinear Optical Properties of Multiferroic Hexagonal $ErMn_{1-x}Cr_xO_3$Nanoparticles. *RSC Adv.* **2015,** *5,* 12480–12487.

41. Woldu, T.; et al. Nonlinear Optical Properties of $(1-x)$ $CaFe_2O_4$–$xBaTiO_3$Composites. *Ceram. Int.* **2016,** *42,* 11093–11098.

42. Saravanan, M.; Girisun, T. C. S. Nonlinear Optical Absorption and Optical Limiting Properties of Cadmium Ferrite. *Mater. Chem. Phys.* **2015,** *160,* 413–419.

43. Saravanan, M.; Sabari Girisun, T. C.; Vinitha, G. Third-order Nonlinear Optical Properties and Power Limiting Behavior of Magnesium Ferrite Under CW Laser (532 nm, 50 mW) Excitation. *J. Mater. Sci.* **2016,** *51,* 3289–3296.

44. Thomas, J. J.; Krishnan, S.; Sridharan, K.; Philip, R.; Kalarikkal, N. A Comparative Study on the Optical Limiting Properties of Different Nano Spinel Ferrites with Z-scan Technique. *Mater. Res. Bull.* **2012,** *47,* 1855–1860.

45. Krishnan, S.; Suchand Sandeep, C. S.; Philip, R.; Kalarikkal, N. Two-Photon Assisted Excited State Absorption in Multiferroic YCrO$_3$ Nanoparticles. *Chem. Phys. Lett.* **2012,** *529,* 59–63.

46. Trivedi, U. N.; Chhantbar, M. C.; Modi, K. B.; Joshi, H. H. Frequency Dependent Dielectric Behaviour of Cadmium and Chromium Co-substituted Nickel Ferrite. *Indian J. Pure Appl. Phys.* **2005,** *43,* 688–690.

47. Krishna, K. R. Dielectric Properties of Ni-Zn Ferrites Synthesized by Citrate Gel Method. *World J. Condens. Matter Phys.* **2012,** *02,* 57–60.

48. Li, D.; et al. Synthesis and Size-Selective Precipitation of Monodisperse Nonstoichiometric M$_x$Fe$_{3-x}$O$_4$ (M = Mn, Co) Nanocrystals and Their DC and AC Magnetic Properties. *Chem. Mater.* **2016,** *28,* 480–489.

49. Schloemann, E. Advances in Ferrite Microwave Materials and Devices. *J. Magn. Magn. Mater.* **2000,** *209,* 15–20.

50. Yadav, G. S.; Dey, P. K.; Ganapati; Kumari, A.; Dey, T. K. Application of Ferrite Medium in Microwave Devices. 60th CONGRESS ISTAM,2016.

51. Nikolov, G. T.; Valchev, V. C. Nanocrystalline Magnetic Materials Versus Ferrites in Power Electronics. *Procedia Earth Planet Sci.* **2009,** *1,* 1357–1361.

52. Verma, A.; Alam, M. I.; Chatterjee, R.; Goel, T. C.; Mendiratta, R. G. Development of a New Soft Ferrite Core for Power Applications. *J. Magn. Magn. Mater.* **2006,** *300,* 500–505.

53. Pardavi-horvath, M. Microwave Applications of Soft Ferrites. *J. Magn. Magn. Mater.* **2000,** *216,* 171–183.

54. Thankachan, R. M.; et al. Enhanced Lithium Storage in ZnFe2O4-C Nanocomposite Produced by a Low-energy Ball Milling. *J. Power Sources.* **2015,** *282,* 462–470.

55. Woldu, T.; Raneesh, B.; Reddy, M. V. R.; Kalarikkal, N. Grain Size Dependent Magnetoelectric Coupling of BaTiO$_3$ Nanoparticles. *RSC Adv.* **2016,** *6,* 7886–7892.

56. Mukherjee, S.; Mitra, M. K. Effect of Nickel Ferrite on Bismuth Ferrite to generate Nanocomposite in Relation to Structure, Characterization, Magnetic properties and Band Gap Evaluation2015. DOI:10.5185/amlett.2015.5833.

57. Hur, N.; et al. Electric Polarization Reversal and Memory in a Multiferroic Material Induced by Magnetic Fields. *Nature* **2004,** *429,* 392–395.

58. Corral-Flores, V.; Bueno-Baques, D.; Carrillo-Flores, D.; Matutes-Aquino, J. A. Enhanced Magnetoelectric Effect in Core-Shell Particulate Composites. *J. Appl. Phys.* **2006,** *99,* 1–4.

59. Abraham, A. R.; Raneesh, B.; Das, D.; Kalarikkal, N. Magnetic Response of Superparamagnetic Multiferroic Core-Shell Nanostructures. **2016,** *050151,* 050151.

60. Stingaciu, M.; Reuvekamp, P. G.; Tai, C.-W.; Kremer, R. K.; Johnsson, M. The Magnetodielectric Effect in $BaTiO_3$–$SrFe_{12}O_{19}$Nanocomposites. *J. Mater. Chem. C.* **2014,** *2,* 325.

61. Sreenivasulu, G.; Petrov, V. M.; Chavez, F. A.; Srinivasan, G. Superstructures of Self-Assembled Multiferroic Core-Shell Nanoparticles and Studies on Magneto-Electric Interactions. *Appl. Phys. Lett.* **2014,** *105,* 10–15.

62. Sharma, R.; Pahuja, P.; Tandon, R. P. Structural, Dielectric, Ferromagnetic, Ferro-electric and ac Conductivity Studies of the $BaTiO_3$–$CoFe_1$.8 ZnO.2 O_4Multiferroic Particulate Composites. *Ceram. Int.* **2014,** *40,* 9027–9036.

63. Chand Verma, K.; Tripathi, S. K.; Kotnala, R. K. Magneto-electric/Dielectric and Fluorescence Effects in Multiferroic $xBaTiO_3$–(1 − x)$ZnFe_2O_4$Nanostructures. *RSC Adv.* **2014,** *4,* 60234–60242.

64. Pachari, S.; Pratihar, S. K.; Nayak, B. B. Enhanced Magneto-capacitance Response in $BaTiO_3$–Ferrite Composite Systems. *RSC Adv.* **2015,** *5,* 105609–105617.

65. Trivedi, H.; et al. Local Manifestations of a Static Magnetoelectric Effect in Nano-structured BaTiO3-BaFe12O9 Composite Multiferroics. *Nanoscale* **2015,** *7,* 4489–4496.

66. Das, A.; Chatterjee, S.; Bandyopadhyay, S.; Das, D. Enhanced Magnetoelectric Properties of BiFeO3 on Formation of BiFeO3/SrFe12O19 Nanocomposites. *J. Appl. Phys.* **2016,** *119,* 234102.

67. Chen, R.; et al. High-Performance Ferrite Nanoparticles Through Nonaqueous Redox Phase Tuning. *Nano Lett.* **2016,** *16,* 1345–1351.

68. Prasad, B.; et al. Nanopillar Spin Filter Tunnel Junctions with Manganite Barriers. *Nano Lett.* **2014,** *14,* 2789–2793.

69. Pathan, A. T. Dielectric Properties of Co-Substituted Li-Ni-Zn Nanostructured Ferrites Prepared Through Chemical Route. *Int. J. Comput. Appl.* **2012,** *45,* 24–28.

70. Yao, Z. N.; et al.Detection of Domain Wall Distribution and Nucleation in Ferromag-netic Nanocontact Structures by Magnetic Force Microscopy. *J. Magn. Magn. Mater.* **2013,** *342,* 1–3.

71. Ozah, S.; Bhattacharyya, N. S. Nanosized Barium Hexaferrite in Novolac Phenolic Resin as Microwave Absorber for X-band Application. *J. Magn. Magn. Mater.* **2013,** *342,* 92–99.

CHAPTER 6

EVALUATION OF AN IMMOBILIZED TITANIUM DIOXIDE NANOCATALYST FOR PHOTOCATALYTIC PERFORMANCE

SRIMANTA RAY[1,*] and JERALD A. LALMAN[2]

[1]*Department of Chemical Engineering, National Institute of Technology Agartala, Jirania, West Tripura, Tripura 799046, India*

[2]*Department of Civil and Environmental Engineering, University of Windsor, Windsor, Ontario N9B 3P4, Canada*

Corresponding author. E-mail: rays.nita@gmail.com, srimanta,chemical@nita.ac.in

CONTENTS

ABSTRACT

An immobilized titanium dioxide (TiO_2) photocatalyst composed of stacked nanofibers on surface etched aluminum foil was evaluated in the present study for photocatalytic (PC) performance. TiO_2 nanofibers were produced by electrospinning and subsequent controlled calcination. Decrease in specific surface area of the TiO_2 photocatalyst was observed with increase in calcination temperature from 400°C to 500°C due to sintering of pores and surface aggregation. Increase in rutile crystalline phase and decrease in bandgap energy (E_g) was noted in TiO_2 nanofibers calcined at temperature higher than 400°C. A maximum specific surface area (259 ± 23 $m^2 \cdot g^{-1}$) and highest E_g (3.24 eV) was recorded for TiO_2 nanofibers calcined at 400°C (NF). The PC degradation rate of the nanofiber catalyst was twice that observed for TiO_2 nanoparticles (of comparable specific surface area) in slurry. The PC degradation rate of the immobilized TiO_2 nanofiber photocatalyst was not noted to change significantly after repeated use.

6.1 INTRODUCTION

In recent years, oxidative degradation in aqueous phase using a photo-illuminated catalyst surface has provided a potential alternative for the treatment of effluents rich in organic pollutants.[30,31] Photo-initiated catalysis on catalyst surface otherwise known as heterogeneous photocatalysis offers a green treatment approach by degrading the toxic organic pollutants into carbon dioxide (CO_2) and water using photonic energy.[25] Among the reported photocatalysts which have been used, titanium dioxide (TiO_2) has received the most attention of the research due to its high oxidative potential.[4] The oxidative potential of TiO_2 originates from its semiconductor bandgap. The oxidizing power of TiO_2 is revealed when radiation with wavelengths less than 380 nm is used to illuminate the surface.[25] Photo-illuminated TiO_2 surface generates an electron–hole pair, which migrates to the surface of the photocatalyst and reacts with surface hydroxyl group to form hydroxyl radical ('OH).[18] The 'OH radicals subsequently mediate the degradation of organic molecules.[25]

The specific surface area and crystal structure are two important parameters controlling the photocatalytic (PC) performance of TiO_2.[16,20]

For TiO_2 particles, specific surface area is function of particle size. Globally, TiO_2 within the micrometer range is utilized in paint manufacturing.[1] The recombination of charge carriers en route to the catalyst surface and inefficient light scattering are the main reasons for poor PC activity of the pigmentary grade TiO_2 particles.[1,7] The crystal structure dictates the bandgap energy (E_g) and the oxidative potential of TiO_2. Rutile, anatase, brookite, and monoclinic are four common TiO_2 structures.[18] Among the different crystal forms of TiO_2, anatase has the highest E_g and more PC activity than rutile and other crystal form of TiO_2.[4] Rutile is the more stable form; however, for particle sizes less than 14 nm in diameter, anatase is thermodynamically more stable.[46] Thus, anatase TiO_2 with stabilized form of nanostructures are desirable for PC applications.

Increasing innovations in manufacturing have permitted processes to produce particle sizes in nanometer range. Several nanometer size TiO_2 formulations have been synthesized and evaluated for their PC potential.[5,4] Various physical techniques, such as splluttering and vapor deposition, as well as chemical methods, for instance, hydrothermal and glycothermal crystallization, have been tested for synthesizing TiO_2 nanoparticles.[5,7] However, the most successful method for preparing TiO_2 nanoparticles is the sol–gel method.[38] In the sol–gel method, a titanium alkoxide (sol precursor) is hydrolyzed to produce nano-sized high surface area TiO_2 particles. Homogeneity of the nanoparticles, well-defined fine structure of TiO_2, high surface area, and ease of coupling with catalyst immobilization techniques, are some of the advantages of the sol–gel techniques over other methods.[7,38]

Sol–gel-derived TiO_2 nanoparticles are used as an aqueous dispersion or slurry for PC studies. However, the use of TiO_2 nanoparticles in form of slurry is associated with several limitations related to the practical application of the catalyst. Nanoparticles tend to aggregate when wet, resulting in loss of surface area; therefore, nanoparticles slurries require vigorous mechanical agitation in order to minimize particle aggregation during the PC reaction.[20] The PC efficiency of nanoparticle slurry is dependent on the penetration depth of incident radiation, which is a function of solution turbidity. Increasing TiO_2 nanoparticle concentration causes higher turbidities and thereby severely impairs the depth of penetration of incident radiation.[27] Additionally, nanoparticle slurry process requires a supplementary posttreatment solid/liquid separation for catalyst recovery.[19] There is also a human health hazard associated with fugitive emission of nanoparticles during slurry preparation.[3] An approach to minimize these limitations is to immobilize the nanoparticles onto a fixed or fluidized support.

A popular method for immobilizing TiO_2 for photocatalysis is in situ production of nanoparticles by sol–gel technique and subsequent deposition onto a solid support via dip coating.[17] However, a major drawback of this immobilized TiO_2 catalyst system is lower PC rates compared to the discrete nanoparticle slurry. Lower PC rate of immobilized system is related to the loss of surface area caused by particle sintering or aggregation on the support surface during the thermal treatment.[7,19] Sintering results in formation of large particle aggregate or a film on the support surface. This ultimately produces a surface area smaller than that of discrete nanoparticles by a few orders of magnitude.[21] An alternative approach of producing a catalyst with surface area comparable to that of the nanoparticles is to fabricate TiO_2 nanostructures and subsequently immobilize them onto a support.

A technique for fabricating immobilized nanostructures onto a fixed support is electrospinning. In the electrospinning process, a high static voltage is used to produce ultrafine fibers with diameters within the nanometric range.[37] The electrospinning technique has been successfully exploited to generate small diameter fibers and to fabricate large surface area membranes from a broad range of polymers, including engineering plastics, biopolymers, conducting polymers, block copolymers, and polymer blends.[15,43] Recently, electrospinning has also been applied for producing nanofibers of metal oxides and ceramics.[10,41]

Li and Xia[26] demonstrated the coupling of the sol–gel technique of TiO_2 nanoparticle formation with electrospinning process and produced TiO_2 nanofibers in a two-step process. Initially, the nanofibers are fabricated by electrospinning a sol precursor of TiO_2 with a high molecular weight polymer. The purpose of the polymer was to impart rheological stability and act as carrier for the titanium (Ti) salt during nanofiber formation.[26] Later, the composite nanofibers of polymer and TiO_2 are subjected to a calcination treatment to obtain a pure TiO_2 fiber. To date, several attempts have been reported toward developing an immobilized TiO_2 nanofiber catalyst for PC application.[2,13,29] However, none of the earlier reports have been very successful in developing a high surface area immobilized TiO_2 nanofibers catalyst for PC application. Two limitations observed by the earlier researchers are poor stability of the immobilized catalyst system[13,29] and inferior PC performance compared to nanoparticles.[2,29] Accordingly, the intent of the present study is to develop a photocatalyst system by immobilizing TiO_2 nanofibers onto a fixed solid support. Later, compare the surface area and PC performance of immobilized TiO_2 nanofibers with that of nanoparticles slurry.

6.2 MATERIALS AND METHODS

6.2.1 MATERIALS

Titanium tetraisopropoxide (TTIP), an organotitanium sol–gel precursor to TiO_2 (> 99.95 % purity) and polyvinyl acetate (PVAc (average molecular weight (M_w) 50,000 Daltons)), a carrier for the TTIP, was purchased from Alfa Aesar (Ward Hill, MA). Acetic acid (> 99 % purity), a stabilizer for sol–gel conversion of TTIP, was procured from EMD (Gibbstown, NJ). Dimethylformamide (DMF) and tetrahydrofuran (THF), solvents was supplied by Fischer Scientific (Ottawa, ON). TiO_2 (> 99.9 % purity) nanoparticles (5 and 10 nm particle size) used in the experiment were procured from Alfa Aesar. X-ray diffraction (XRD) was used to ensure the anatase type crystal structure of the nanoparticles. Phenol (reagent grade, > 99 % purity) was procured from Sigma Aldrich (Oakville, ON). Ultrapure water (18 M-ohm resistivity) used in this study was generated by a NANOpure Diamond water unit (Barnstead, IA).

6.2.2 ELECTROSPINNING APPARATUS

The electrospinning apparatus (Fig. 6.1) consisted of a pumping system capable of delivering a viscous solution at a constant flow rate to a metallic capillary feed, which was connected to a positive (anode) terminal of a variable high voltage DC power supply (ES 50P–10 W/dam, Gamma High Voltage Research Inc. Ormond Beach, FL). The pumping system consists of a programmable syringe pump (PHD 22/2000, Havard Apparatus Canada, St. Laurent, QC) equipped with a 10 ml Luer-lock plastic syringe (Becton Dickinson, Oakville, ON). The syringe was fitted with a 22 gauge, 1.5 in long stainless steel hypodermic needle with polypropylene hub (Becton Dickinson, Oakville, ON). The syringe delivery system had a flow capacity (infusion rate) of $0.03 \pm 0.001 \mu l/min$. The transformer was capable of providing a potential difference (applied potential) from 0 to 50 kV. The negative or ground terminal (cathode) was attached to a collector surface (conducting solid catalyst support material), where charged nanofibers are deposited. The two electrodes (needle tip to the surface of the solid support) were separated by a distance (32.5 cm), favorable for forming ultrafine nanofibers (unpublished work). The apparatus was maintained in a horizontal orientation to minimize deposition of excess spinning solution during initial instability of electrospinning process onto the collector surface. The charged section of the electrospinning apparatus (capillary needle and solid support collector) was enclosed in a sealed chamber to prevent the movement of nanofibers by surrounding air currents.[34,35]

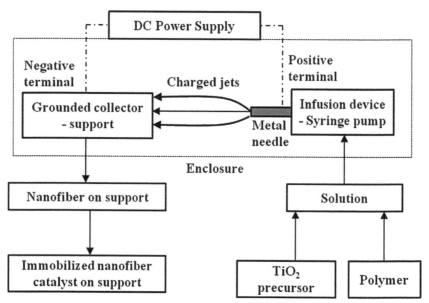

FIGURE 6.1   Schematic layout of the electrospinning apparatus.

6.2.3   CHOICE OF CATALYST SUPPORT MATERIAL

The type of support material used to immobilize TiO_2 nanoparticles can be classified as fixed and fluidized support. Fixed support material include glass plates,[17,27] glass fibres,[33] polymeric fibres,[12] and textile materials.[6] Materials used for fluidized application, include activated charcoal[8] and bentonites.[19] Fluidized materials are not suitable as collector solid support because they are unorganized small particles and in some cases, they are nonconducting. Fixed material, such as glass also presents a problem because it is nonconducting. In comparison, aluminum support is capable of quickly dissipating static charges and, hence, can be used as collector ground. Moreover, previous work reported that aluminum possesses good adhesion property for the TiO_2 nanocatalyst and surface roughness of the support surface improves the adhesion behavior of immobilized TiO_2 nanocatalyst.[32] Accordingly, a newly developed surface etched aluminum foil with the porous surface and well-marked surface roughness was used for supporting the electrospun TiO_2 nanofibers.[24]

6.2.4   PREPARATION OF ELECTROSPINNING SOLUTION

A sol–gel precursor for fabricating TiO_2 is TTIP. TTIP is prepared by stabilizing it with glacial acetic acid in a molar ratio of 1:4 mol TTIP per mol acetic acid under slow stirring conditions (Solution A). The TTIP/acetic acid solution is mixed with a polymer solution to maintain a viscosity within 130–160 cPs.[11] PVAc is reported to have better miscibility with TIP and maintain better homogeneity of the phases during electrospinning[22] and hence, PVAc was chosen for the study. A PVAc solution was prepared by dissolving polymer beads in 3:2 volumetric mixtures of DMF and THF (Solution B). A 45 % (weight per volume) solution of PVAc (Mw 50,000 Da) in 3:2 (v/v) DMF/THF was measured (using cone and plate viscometer (Brookfield CAP 1000 viscometer, Brookfield, Middleboro, MA) to a viscosity of 147.8 ± 0.6 cPs (at shear rate $\geq 10,000s^{-1}$). The electrospinning solution (Solution C) was prepared by mixing the TTIP solution (Solution A) with the PVAc solution (Solution B). The Ti content (by weight) in the electrospinning solution was varied by mixing various proportions of the TTIP solution (Solution A). The different TTIP content (by weight) examined were 11, 22, and 33 %. The lowest TTIP content resulted in a very slow sol-gel conversion and highest TTIP content was restrained by too fast sol-gel conversion in the electrospinning solution.

6.2.5   ELECTROSPINNING AND CATALYST IMMOBILIZATION

A syringe containing the electrospinning solution (Solution C) was placed in the syringe pump and the infusion rate of the pump was adjusted to a desired value of 0.6 mlh^{-1}. The stainless steel needle of the syringe was connected to the positive terminal of the high voltage DC power supply. The ground terminal was attached to the surface-treated aluminum support (collector) and positioned at 32.5 cm from the needle tip. The interaction of PVAc with TTIP results in formation of linking bridge, which is known to favor the adhesion of nanofibers on to the support surface.[42] Accordingly, in the present study, the surface-treated aluminum foil applied with a coating of PVAc (45 % (w/v) in 3:2 DMF/THF) by means of a stainless steel doctors blade (blade angle 45°) prior to electrospinning.

Upon applying a potential gradient within 40 kV to the solution at the needle tip a fluid jet is ejected from the capillary tip. After an initial instability period for few minutes, a steady fluid jet is directed toward the grounded support. As the jet accelerates toward the cathode, the solvent evaporates and a charged TiO_2/PVAc composite fiber is deposited on the solid support. TiO_2/PVAc nanofiber was dried under a vacuum of 600 mm Hg at 105°C for 2 h to remove the residual solvent and allow further condensation of the structure.[29,40] The vacuum dried nanofibers was subjected to a stepwise heat treatment (developed through a complete thermal characterization study (unpublished work)) to remove the polymer back bone (PVAc) and obtain immobilized TiO_2 nanofiber catalyst. Initially, TiO_2/PVAc nanofiber on aluminum support (vacuum dried) was slow heated (at rate of 1.5°C/min) in a temperature programmable oven to 300°C; thereafter, it was calcined in a muffle furnace (Thermolyne 1300, Thermo Fisher Scientific Inc., Newington, NH) at the final calcination temperature (400–500°C) for additional 2 h. The anatase is the most photo-catalytically active crystal form.[4] The calcination temperatures between 400°C and 500°C, was reported to fabricate the anatase TiO_2 photocatalyst.[2,9,23,47] The temperature above 400°C has been reported to induce phase transformation of TiO_2 from anatase to rutile.[44] Calcination temperatures of 450°C[13] and 500°C[2] have also been reported in literature for immobilization of TiO_2 nanofiber catalyst. Accordingly, in the present study, three calcination temperatures (400°C, 450°C, and 500°C) was evaluated for their effect on the morphology and specific surface area of the photocatalyst. The immobilized nanocatalyst was then cooled to ambient temperature, cleaned with a gentle stream of clean dry air (to strip-off the loose particles attached on the surface of the catalyst) and rinsed in ultrapure water to remove any remaining polymer ash. The nanocatalyst was then dried at 105°C to remove any moisture.

6.2.6   NANOCATALYST CHARACTERIZATION

The crystalline phase of the immobilized TiO_2 nanofibers, scrapped from the support surface, were quantified using a X-ray diffractometer (D8 Discover, Bruker Corporation, Milton, ON) configured with a Cu K$_\alpha$ ($\alpha = 1.54$ Å) source and outfitted with general area detector diffraction system (GADDS). The specimen was scanned from 2θ-angle 17–55° in steps of 0.05°. The crystalline phase were identified by comparing the interplanar spacing and the diffraction peaks against Joint Committee on Powder Diffraction Standards cards (JCPDS, powder diffraction file, Card No. 21-1272 (anatase) and 21-1276 (rutile), Swarthmore, PA). The mass fraction of rutile phase (X_R) was computed using Spurr equation, Eq. 6.1.[39] The term I_A and I_R (Eq. 6.3) are the integrated intensities of the (101) anatase and (110) rutile crystal plane, respectively.

$$\frac{1}{X_R} = 1 + 0.8\left(\frac{I_A}{I_R}\right) \tag{6.1}$$

Images of the nanofibers were obtained using a field emission gun scanning electron microscope (FESEM) (Quanta 200, FEI Company, Hillsboro, OR) using Everhart–Thornley secondary electron detector under high vacuum mode. The maximum resolution capacity of the microscope was 0.8 nm. The SEM energy dispersive x-ray spectroscopy (EDX) and GENESIS material characterization software (EDAX Inc., Mahwah, NJ) was used to analyze the elemental composition of the nanofibers. The diameter of the nanofibers was measured from the SEM images of the nanofibers using SCANDIUM image processing software (Olympus Soft Imaging Solutions Corp, Lakewood, CO). The surface details of the nanofibers were imaged using multimode scanning probe atomic force microscope (AFM) (Nanoscope IV, Veeco Instruments Inc., Plainview, NY) fitted with TESP probe in tapping mode. The minimum scanning area of the AFM was 0.16 μm². The AFM images were analyzed using Nanoscope software, version 6.13 (Veeco Instruments Inc., Plainview, NY).

The TiO_2 nanocatalysts were optically characterized for Eg by measuring the transmittance of an incident light with wavelength between 200 and 400 nm using a UV–visible spectrophotometer (Cary 50, Varian Inc, Palo Alto, CA). The specific surface area (m²/g) of the TiO_2 nanocatalyst was determined from physisorption of nitrogen gas (BOC, Windsor, ON) under relative pressure (P/P$_o$) of 0–0.3 at 77.34 K in a surface area analyzer (NOVA 1200e, Quantachrome Instruments, Boynton Beach, FL) using Brunauer–Emmett–Teller (BET) principle.

6.2.7 PHOTOCATALYTIC EXPERIMENTAL SETUP

PC experiments were performed in PC reaction tubes (25 mm ID × 250 mm length), which were fabricated from GE-214 clear fused quartz silica

(Technical Glass Products Inc., Painesvile, Ohio). The model pollutant (phenol) in aqueous solution and TiO_2 nanocatalyst (immobilized or slurry) were placed in reaction tubes, which were purged with oxygen and sealed with aluminum crimp cap (Cobert Associates, St Louis, MO) and PTFE®-silicone rubber septa (Cobert Associates, St Louis, MO). The sealed reaction tubes were then placed in a modified Rayonet RPR-100 UV PC chamber (Southern New England Ultraviolet Co., Connecticut). The custom built chamber was equipped with 16 phosphor-coated low-pressure mercury lamps on the outer perimeter and a centrally located rotating inner carousel (Fig. 6.2). Three or six quartz reaction tubes were placed on the inner rotating carousel and irradiated with 300 nm mono-chromatic UV light at an average irradiance of 9 mW/cm² (measured using a UV-X radiometer (UV Process Supply Inc., Chicago, IL). Over the duration of each experiment, a fixed amount of aqueous solution was withdrawn at specific time intervals and stored in screw capped culture tubes (13 mm ID×100 mm length) (VWR International, Mississauga, ON) wrapped in aluminum foil for further quantitative analysis.[34,35,36]

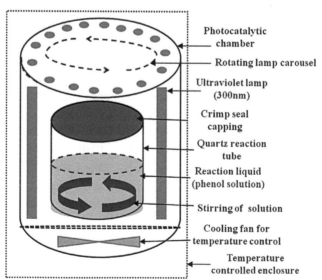

FIGURE 6.2   Schematic diagram of photocatalytic reactor and the experimental setup.

Phenol is a classified carcinogen, teratogen, mutagen, and endocrine disruptor. Notice that the phenol is a basic structural entity of many other ecotoxins and endocrine disrupting chemicals. Phenol and phenol derivatives are routinely used in the manufacture of resins, insulation panels, herbicides and pesticides paints, and lubricants.[44] Moreover, phenol has an annual global production of approximately 3 million tonnes and annual discharge of 500 tonnes into the Canadian environment[14] and hence was chosen as the model pollutant (substrate) for the PC experiment in this study.

6.2.8 ANALYSIS

Degradation of the substrate (phenol) was monitored using a high-performance liquid chromatograph (Dionex Ultimate 3000, Sunnyvale, CA). The instrument was equipped with a UV–visible photodiode array (PDA) detector set at 215 nm and configured with an Acclaim C18-3 µm-2.1 mm (ID) × 100 mm (length) column (Dionex, Sunnyvale, CA). The analysis was conducted isothermally with the oven temperature set at 45°C and with an eluent (acetonitrile–water mixture (1:4)) (Fisher Scientific, Ottawa, ON) flow rate set at 0.4 ml/min. The detection limit for phenol was 5 µg/l.

6.3   RESULTS AND DISCUSSIONS

6.3.1   EFFECT OF VARYING TTIP CONTENT ON THE IMMOBILIZED NANOFIBERS

The diameter of the TiO_2 nanofibers immobilized on support surface was measured to determine the effect of varying TTIP content on the nanofiber dimension. Histograms of the TiO_2 nanofiber diameters produced from different TTIP content were presented in Figure 6.3 (A–C). Smaller diameters were recorded for the nanofibers generated from electrospinning solution with lower TTIP content. Higher variability in nanofiber diameters was observed for increased TTIP content. A smallest fiber diameter of 19 nm (with range of 19–49 nm) was measured for 11 % TTIP content. TTIP gel on hydrolysis converts into TiO_2.

Accordingly, TTIP rich electrospinning solution results in thicker nanofibers due to higher TiO_2 content after thermal stabilization at 400°C for 2 h. Increased TTIP content in the electrospinning solution results in faster gelation tendency. Gelation of TTIP changes the surface tension and the viscosity property of the solution during electrospinning, inducing higher variability in the fiber formation. The gelation tendency of a solution with TTIP content greater than 33 % results in discontinuity of fiber formation in the electro-spinning process. A maximum specific surface area of 259 ± 23 $m^2 \cdot g^{-1}$ was recorded for TiO_2 nanofibers produced from electrospinning solution with 11 % TTIP. The specific surface area of TiO_2 nanofibers electrospun from 22 % TTIP to 33 % TTIP solution were 108 ± 23 and 90 ± 11 $m^2 \cdot g^{-1}$, respectively. Decreasing specific surface area with increasing TTIP content in the electrospinning solution is directly related to the loss of the surface area due to increased fiber diameter at higher TTIP content.

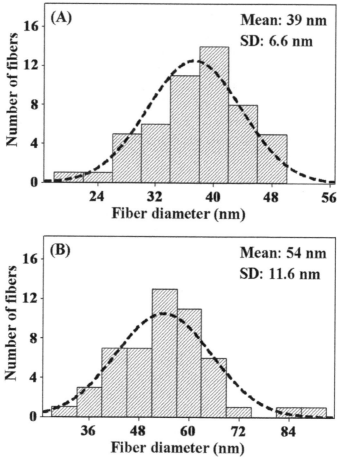

FIGURE 6.3   Histograms of the nanofibers—effect of TTIP content (A) 11 % (B) 22 % (C) 33 %.

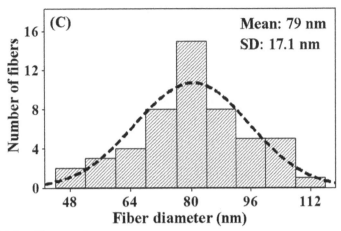

FIGURE 6.3 *(Continued)*

6.3.2 EFFECT OF CALCINATION TEMPERATURE ON THE IMMOBILIZED NANOFIBERS

Earlier studies have reported 400°C as the temperature for phase trans-formation of TiO_2 from anatase to rutile.[44] Calcination temperatures of 450°C[13] and 500°C[2] have also been reported in literature for immo-bilization of TiO_2 nanofiber catalyst. Accordingly, in the present study, the effect of three different calcination temperatures, 400°C, 450°C, and 500°C on the properties of TiO_2 nanofibers were studied. The diameter of TiO_2 nanofibers, electrospun from solution containing 22 % TTIP, after calcination at 400, 450 and 500°C were 54 ± 11.6 nm (A), 50 ± 14.3 nm (B), and 49 ± 15.1 nm (C), respectively. The fiber diameters were statisti-cally examined to conclude on the effect of calcination temperature. The results of *t*-test were 1.55 (t_{A-B}), 0.34 (t_{B-C}), and 1.88 (t_{A-C}), respectively. The calculated *t*-test values were less than tabulated t-value of 2.02. Thus, increasing calcination temperature from 400°C to 500°C does not result in any significant change on the diameter of TiO_2 nanofibers.

The specific surface area of the TiO_2 nanofibers calcined at 400°C, 450°C, and 500°C was measured. The results are tabulated in Table 6.1. The specific surface area of the TiO_2 nanofibers was considerably reduced (from 108 ± 23 to 54 ± 9) on increasing the calcination temperature from 400°C to 450°C. The decrease in specific surface area on further increase in calcination temperature from 450°C to 500°C is much less (from 54±9 to 39±11). Examination of the TiO$_2$ nanofibers calcined at 400°C, 450°C, and 500°C under AFM and FESEM revealed the cause of the decrease in surface area (Fig. 6.4 (A–F)). Notice the decrease in surface roughness in AFM images and appearance of distinct cracks due to aggregations in FESEM images with increase in calcination temperatures. The sintering of the pores and loss of surface texture of the nanofiber with increase in calcination temperatures result in a decrease in specific surface area values. Accordingly, a temperature of 400°C was chosen as the calcination temperature for the TiO$_2$ nanofibers.

TABLE 6.1   Effect of Calcination Temperature on the Diameter and Specific Surface Area of TiO$_2$ Nanofibers.

Calcination temperature (°C)	Fiber diameter (nm)	Specific surface area (m$^2 \cdot$g^{-1})
400	54±11.6	108±23
450	50±14.3	54±9
500	49±15.1	39±11

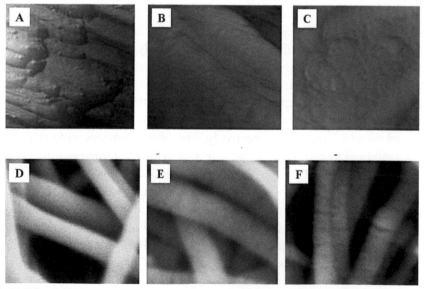

FIGURE 6.4   Effect calcination temperature on the surface texture of TiO$_2$ nanofibers (A) AFM image, 400°C, (B) AFM image, 450°C (C) AFM image, 500°C, (D) FESEM image, 400°C (E) FESEM image, 450°C (F) FESEM image, 500°C.

6.3.3 THE CRYSTALLINE PHASE AND THE BANDGAP ENERGY OF THE IMMOBILIZED NANOFIBERS

The TiO_2 nanofibers calcined at three different temperatures (400°C, 450°C, and 500°C) were analyzed for the crystalline phase and the E_g. XRD studies were conducted to determine the crystalline phase of the nanofibers. From the d-spacing and the 2θ XRD angle, the crystal planes were identified by comparing with the d-spacing values reported for pure crystalline phases. Anatase is the only crystal phase identified in the TiO_2 nanofibers calcined at 400°C. XRD peaks for both anatase and rutile TiO_2 crystal phases were observed in the nanofibers calcined at 450°C and 500°C. The integrated intensities of the (101) anatase crystal plane (101) at 3.51 Å and rutile crystal plane (110) at 3.24 Å (JCPDS, PDF, Card No. 21-1272 (anatase) and 21-1276 (rutile)) were calculated. With the integrated intensities of anatase (I_A) and rutile (I_R), the mass fraction of rutile phase (X_R) was computed using Eq. 6.1. The values are tabulated in Table 6.2. Increasing calcination temperature was observed to increase the mass fraction of rutile phase in the TiO_2 nanofibers.

TABLE 6.2 Effect of Calcination Temperature on Crystal Phase and Bandgap Energy of TiO_2 Nanofibers.

Calcination temperature (°C)	Mass fraction of crystal phase (%)		Bandgap energy (eV)
	Anatase	Rutile	
400	100	0	3.24
450	96	4	3.13
500	73	27	3.03

The bandgap E_g of the TiO_2 nanofibers was computed from the measured transmittance of ultraviolet radiation using Plank–Einstein equation, Eq. 6.2.

$$E_g = hc/\lambda_{min} \tag{6.2}$$

where λ_{min} is the wavelength of incident radiation with minimum transmittance, h is Plank's constant and c is the speed of light (constant). The computed E_g for the TiO_2 nanofibers calcined at 400°C, 450°C, and 500°C were tabulated in Table 6.2. The highest E_g was recorded for the

TiO_2 nanofibers calcined at 400°C. The E_g was observed to decrease with increase in calcination temperature. Note that increase in calcination temperature from 400°C to 500°C increase the rutile mass fraction in the TiO_2 nanofibers. The E_g of rutile phase (3.0 eV) being lower than that of the anatase crystal phase (3.2 eV)[4] progressively lower E_g was observed for TiO_2 nanofibers calcined at 450°C and 500°C.

6.3.4   EFFECT OF NANOFIBER LOADING ON THE SPECIFIC SURFACE AREA OF THE IMMOBILIZED CATALYST

Electrospinning and subsequent immobilization result in layer-by-layer deposition of TiO_2 nanofibers on the surface of the support. Increase in number of layers of nanofiber deposition is expected to affect the specific surface area. Accordingly, the electrospinning deposition and immobilization process was repeated to vary the mass of TiO_2 deposited per unit area of the support. The specific surface area of immobilized catalyst with different mass of nanofibers was determined. Increase in nanofiber loading was observed to decrease the specific surface area (Fig. 6.5A). Maximum specific surface area for TiO_2 nanofiber after loading of 0.9 $g \cdot m^{-2}$ was recorded. Decrease in specific surface area tends to level beyond 1.4 $g \cdot m^{-2}$ of TiO_2 nanofiber loading. The reason is well understood from the schematic diagram presented in Figure 6.5B. The surface to surface contacts of nanofibers in the layerwise buildup cause loss of available surface area at contact portions. Increase in number of nanofiber layers increase the loss due to surface contacts. Add to the fact that the nanofibers are randomly oriented in the electrospinning deposition process. Thus, higher deposition of TiO_2 nanofibers per unit area of support lessen, the available surface area for monolayer adsorption of adsorbate gas molecules (nitrogen) resulting in lowered specific surface area values.

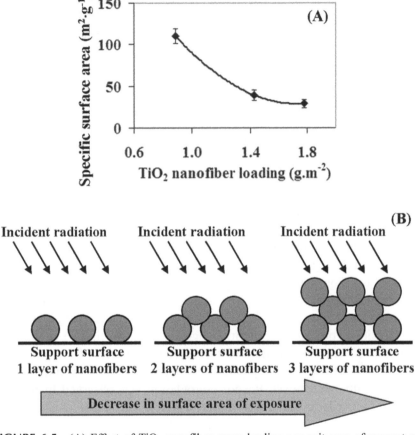

FIGURE 6.5 (A) Effect of TiO_2 nanofiber mass loading per unit area of support on specific surface area. (B) Schematic diagram relating layer-by-layer buildup of nanofibers with loss of surface area.

6.3.5 PHOTOCATALYTIC PERFORMANCE OF IMMOBILIZED TIO$_2$ NANOFIBER CATALYST

The impingement of light on TiO_2 surface with photon energy greater than the bandgap potential generates an electron–hole pair.[25] The charge carriers, that is, electrons in conduction band or hole in valence band either recombine with the bulk of the material or migrate to the particle surface.[28] In aqueous medium, this electron–hole pair initiates an oxidation–reduction reaction at the TiO_2 surface to produce hydroxyl radicals (˙OH).[18] For that reason, a factor controlling the PC performance of TiO_2 is the E_g, which is favorable for formation of hydroxyl radical (˙OH) and subsequent degradation of organic molecules.[4] The specific surface area is another important factor, which controls the diffusion path of the charge carrier and reaction sites on the TiO_2 surface.[7] Accordingly, the chosen immobilized TiO_2 nanocatalyst for PC experiments (11 % TTIP; calcined at 400°C) had minimum fiber (39±6.6 nm), maximum specific surface area (259±23 $m^2 \cdot g^{-1}$), and highest E_g (3.24 eV) among other alternatives, manufactured from 22 % to 33 % TTIP content and calcined at higher temperatures (450°C or 500°C).

The experimental condition for phenol photocatalysis were adopted from the literature.[36] The phenol concentration of 40 mgl^{-1}, TiO_2 concentration of 0.5 gl^{-1}, and reaction temperature of 37±2°C was chosen for PC experiment. The dissolved oxygen (DO) level was maintained at 7.8 mgl^{-1}. About 25 mg of 39±6.6 nm diameter TiO_2 nanofibers (calculated on 50 ml reaction volume at 0.5 gl^{-1} TiO_2) supported on surface-treated aluminium foil (marked as NF) was taken for the PC study. Phenol degradation in the presence and absence of TiO_2 catalyst was assessed by monitoring residual phenol concentration against reaction time (Fig. 6.6A). Around 5 % phenol degradation was observed in absence of TiO_2 catalyst (control). About 60±1 % of phenol was degraded within 60 min in PC reactions with NF catalyst. Phenol degradation was observed to follow apparent first order kinetics according to Eq. (6.3).

$$-(dC/dt) = kC \quad \text{or,} \quad -\left[\ln\left(\frac{C}{C_o}\right)\right] = kt \qquad (6.3)$$

where k is the reaction rate constant, referred hereafter as apparent degradation rate constant (min^{-1}), C is the phenol concentration ($mg \cdot l^{-1}$), and $(-dC/dt)$ is the first order degradation rate. $-\ln(C/C_O)$ was plotted against the reaction time (t) to determine the apparent degradation rate constant (Fig. 6.6B). The PC degradation rate with NF was recorded as 6.5 times faster than the control (photolytic rate).

The apparent degradation rate of phenol with NF was compared with TiO_2 nanoparticles of comparable specific surface area. TiO_2 nanoparticles with particle size of 5 nm, specific surface area of 275±15 $m^2 \cdot g^{-1}$ and E_g

of 3.23 eV (>99 % anatase crystal phase) was chosen for comparison with NF in PC performance. The PC rates of NF and 5 nm nanoparticles are tabulated in Table 6.3. The quantum yield (ε) was determined using Eq. (6.4).[25]

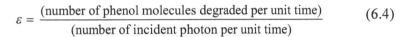

$$\varepsilon = \frac{\text{(number of phenol molecules degraded per unit time)}}{\text{(number of incident photon per unit time)}} \qquad (6.4)$$

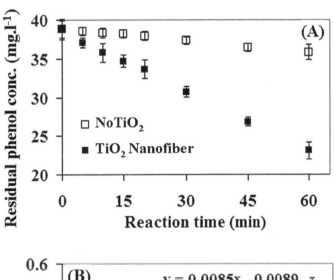

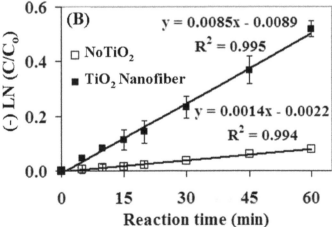

FIGURE 6.6 Degradation profiles for photocatalysis of phenol in presence and in absence of TiO$_2$ nanofiber catalyst (A) residual phenol concentration (B) apparent degradation rate.

TABLE 6.3   Comparative Photocatalytic Degradation Rate for Phenol with Different Catalyst.

Type	Specific surface area $(m^2 \cdot g^{-1})$	Nominal size of nanoparticles (nm)	Mean diameter of nanofibers (nm)	Apparent degradation rate (min^{-1})	Degradation rate $(\mu mol \cdot l^{-1} \cdot min^{-1})$	Quantum yield
Nanoparticle	(275 ± 15)[a]	5		(0.0034 ± 0.0005)[a]	(3.5 ± 0.47)[a]	(0.19 ± 0.025)[a]
Nanofibers	(259 ± 23)[a]		(39 ± 6.6)[b]	(0.0085 ± 0.0001)[a]	(7.4 ± 0.35)[a]	(0.40 ± 0.019)[a]
Control (No TiO$_2$)				(0.0014 ± 0.0002)[a]	(1.2 ± 0.15)[a]	(0.03 ± 0.004)[a]

[a]Average and standard deviation for triplicate samples.
[b]Average and standard deviation for 50 fibers.

The quantum yield of control experiments (without TiO_2) was 10 times lower than the PC experiments with TiO_2 (nanofibers or nanoparticles). Higher degradation rate and quantum yield in PC experiments over control (photolysis) were attributed to the presence of TiO_2. Presence of TiO_2 facilitates higher conversion of photo-generated electrons to hydroxyl radicals onto the catalyst surface for mediating the PC degradation reactions.[4,18] The quantum yield as well as PC degradation rate of NF was double of that observed for 5 nm TiO_2 nanoparticles (of comparable specific surface area). The PC result clearly sets the immobilized NF catalyst ahead of the nanoparticles in terms of PC performance. Lower PC rates and quantum yield of the nanoparticles compared to NF can be accounted to the intrinsic aggregation tendency and loss of surface area of nanoparticles in suspension.

The PC performance of NF generated in this study was compared with literature values.[29] The PC activity of electrospun TiO_2 nanofibers for phenol degradation was studied and the specific surface area, approximate fiber diameter, and PC degradation rate was reported. The observed PC degradation rate for TiO_2 nanofibers (diameter < 100 nm) with specific surface area 32 $m^2 \cdot g^{-1}$ was 1.9 ± 0.16 $\mu mol \cdot l^{-1} \cdot min^{-1}$.[29] The PC rate observed for NF in the present study is 3.9 times (7.4 ± 0.35 $\mu mol \cdot l^{-1} \cdot min^{-1}$) higher than the literature values. Higher surface area of the TiO_2 nanofibers (259 ± 23 $m^2 \cdot g^{-1}$) produced in this study can be accounted for better PC performance of the TiO_2 catalyst reported in the present work.

6.3.6 PERFORMANCE OF IMMOBILIZED TIO_2 NANOFIBER CATALYST ON REPEATED USE

A health hazard associated with the use of nanoparticle in suspension is release of remnant nanocatalyst particle into the environment through treated effluent. Similarly, the loss of catalyst particles is uneconomical. Thus, recycling efficiency of the immobilized TiO_2 nanofiber catalyst is an important characteristic from commercial standpoint. Accordingly, the NF was subjected to repeated PC experimental cycle to evaluate the reusability of the nanocatalyst.

TABLE 6.4   Photocatalytic Degradation Rate for Phenol with TiO_2 Nanofiber Catalyst on Multiple Use.

Photocatalytic cycle	Degradation rate($\mu mol \cdot l^{-1} \cdot min^{-1}$)	Quantum yield
1	$(7.14 \pm 0.16)^a$	$(0.38 \pm 0.01)^a$
2	$(6.74 \pm 0.32)^a$	$(0.36 \pm 0.02)^a$
3	$(6.47 \pm 0.22)^a$	$(0.35 \pm 0.01)^a$
4	$(6.64 \pm 0.44)^a$	$(0.36 \pm 0.02)^a$
-	Heated at 199°C for 120 min	
5	$(6.77 \pm 0.32)^a$	$(0.36 \pm 0.02)^a$

[a]Average and standard deviation for triplicate samples.

The photocatalysis of phenol was monitored for four consecutive experimental cycles after thoroughly washing the NF photocatalyst in ultrapure distilled water after each experimental cycle. The PC degradation rate ($\mu mol \cdot l^{-1} \cdot min^{-1}$) and quantum yield was computed for each PC experimental cycle from the apparent degradation rate (Eq. 6.3 and 6.4). The observed degradation rate and respective quantum yield values are tabulated in Table 6.4. The PC rate of 1st cycle and 4th cycle was compared using t-test at 95 % level of confidence. The calculated t-value 4.27 ($p=0.02$) was smaller than tabulated t-value 3.18. Thus, no significant change was observed in the PC performance of the NF photocatalyst in four consecutive experimental cycles. After the 4th cycle, the NF photocatalyst was heated at 199°C for 120 min and reevaluated for PC performance. The PC rate of 5th cycle 6.77 ± 0.32 $\mu mol \cdot l^{-1} \cdot min^{-1}$ was in close agreement with that observed for the 4th cycle (6.44 ± 0.44 $\mu mol \cdot l^{-1} \cdot min^{-1}$) confirming the self-cleaning ability of the photocatalyst on repeated use.

6.4 CONCLUSION

TiO_2 nanofiber produced by electrospinning a sol precursor (TTIP) solution was immobilized on a surface etched aluminum foil through controlled calcination. The effect of varying sol precursor content (TTIP content) on the spinning solution and final calcination temperature on the fiber diameter and specific surface area of immobilized nanocatalyst was studied. Lower TTIP content produced fiber with smaller diameter but associated with higher variability. Increasing calcination temperature from 400°C to 500°C resulted in considerable loss of specific surface area without significantly affecting the fiber diameter. Surface aggregation and sintering of pores were accounted for loss of specific surface area with increase in calcination temperature. Decrease in E_g was observed at higher calcination temperature due to increase in the rutile fraction in the crystalline phase. The mass of TiO_2 nanocatalyst immobilized per unit area of the aluminum support was observed to affect the specific surface area of the immobilized catalyst. Increase in layerwise deposition of nanofibers on support surface cause loss of surface area at contact portions and thereby results in lowered specific surface area of the immobilized catalyst. The immobilized nanocatalyst with maximum specific surface area (259 ± 23 $m^2 \cdot g^{-1}$) and highest E_g (3.24 eV) was chosen for PC degradation of phenol. The PC rate of the nanofiber catalyst was approximately 3.9 times higher than the literature value and 2 times higher than that observed with TiO_2 nanoparticle of comparable specific surface area (275 ± 15 $m^2 \cdot g^{-1}$). The immobilized nanocatalyst was subjected to repeated PC cycle. No significant change in PC performance was noted till the end of five cycles studied.

6.5 ACKNOWLEDGEMENTS

Financial support for this work was provided by the Natural Sciences and Engineering Research (NSERC) of Canada and the University of Windsor.

KEYWORDS

- **titanium dioxide**
- **immobilized nanofibers**
- **specific surface area**
- **photocatalytic rate**

REFERENCES

1. Allen, N. S.; Edge, M.; Ortega, A.; Sandoval, G.; Liauw, C. M.; Verran, J.; Stratton, J.; McIntyre, R. B. Degradation and Stabilisation of Polymers and Coatings: Nano Versus Pigmentary Titania Particles. *Polym. Degrad. Stab.* **2004**, *85*, 927–946.

2. Alves, A. K.; Berutti, F. A.; Clemens, F. J.; Graule, T.; Bergmann, C. P. Photocatalytic Activity of Titania Fibers Obtained by Electrospinning. *Mater. Res. Bull.* **2009,** *44,* 312–317.

3. Baan, R.; Straif, K.; Grosse, Y.; Secretan, B.; El Ghissassi, F.; Cogliano, V. Carcinogenicity of Carbon Black, Titanium Dioxide, and Talc. *Lancet Oncol.* **2006,** *7,* 295–296.

4. Bhatkhande, D. S.; Pangarkar, V. G.; Beenackers, A. A. C. M. Photocatalytic Degradation for Environmental Applications—A Review. *J. Chem. Technol. Biotechnol.* **2001,** *77,* 102–116.

5. Blake, D. M. *Bibliography of Work on the Heterogeneous Photocatalytic Removal of Hazardous Compounds from Water and Air;* Technical Report, Update Number 3. NREL/TP-570-26797; National Renewable Energy Laboratory: Golden, CO, 1999; pp. 1–7. http://www.nrel.gov/docs/fy99osti/26797.pdf (accessed Oct, 2009).

6. Bozzi, A.; Yuranova, T.; Guasaquillo, I.; Laub, D.; Kiwi, J. Self-cleaning of Modified Cotton Textiles by TiO_2 at Low Temperatures Under Daylight Irradiation. *J. Photochem. Photobiol. A Chem.* **2005,** *174,* 156–164.

7. Carp, O.; Huisman, C. L.; Reller, A. Photoinduced Reactivity of Titanium Dioxide. *Prog. Solid State Chem.* **2004,** *32,* 33–177.

8. Carpio, E.; Zuniga, P.; Ponce, S.; Solis, J.; Rodriguez, J.; Estrada, W. Photocatalytic Degradation of Phenol Using TiO_2 Nanocrystals Supported on Activated Carbon. *J. Mol. Catal. A Chem.* **2005,** *228,* 293–298.

9. Chandrasekar, R.; Zhang L.; Howe, J. Y.; Hedin, N. E.; Zhang, Y.; Fong, H. Fabrication and Characterization of Electrospun Titania Nanofibers. *J Mater Sci.* **2009,** *44,* 1198–1205.

10. Chronakis, I. S. Novel Nanocomposites and Nanoceramics Based on Polymer Nanofibers Using Electrospinning Process—A Review. *J. Mater. Process. Technol.* **2005,** *167,* 283–293.

11. Cui, X. M.; Nam, Y. S.; Lee, J. Y.; Park, W. H. Fabrication of Zirconium Carbide (ZrC) Ultra-Thin Fibers by Electrospinning. *Mater. Lett.* **2008,** *62,* 1961–1964.

12. Ding, B.; Kim, J.; Kimura, E.; Shiratori, S. Layer-by-Layer Structured Films of TiO_2 Nanoparticles and Poly(acrylic acid) on Electrospun Nanofibers. *Nanotechnology* **2004,** *15,* 913–917.

13. Doh, S. J.; Kim, C.; Lee, S. G.; Lee, S. J.; Kim, H. Development of Photocatalytic TiO_2 Nanofibers by Electrospinning and its Application to Degradation of Dye Pollutants. *J. Hazard. Mater.* **2008,** *154,* 118–127.

14. Environment Canada. National Pollutant Release Inventory (NPRI) database. http://www.ec.gc.ca/pdb/querysite/results_e.cfm? (accessed Nov, 2009).

15. Frenot, A.; Chronakis, I. Polymer Nanofibers Assembled by Electrospinning. *Curr. Opin. Colloid Interface Sci.* **2003,** *8,* 64–75.

16. Gogate, P. R.; Pandit, A. B. A Review of Imperative Technologies for Wastewater Treatment I: Oxidation Technologies at Ambient Conditions. *Adv. Environ. Res.* **2004,** *8,* 501–551.

17. Hamid, M. A.; Rahman, I. A. Preparation of Titanium Dioxide (TiO_2) Thin Films by Sol Gel Dip Coating Method. *Malays. J. Chem.* **2003,** *5*(1), 86–91.

18. Herrmann, J. M. Heterogeneous Photocatalysis: State of the Art and Present Applications. *Top. Catal.* **2005**, *34*, 49–65.
19. Houari, M.; Saidi, M.; Tabet, D.; Pichat, P.; Khalaf, H. The Removal of 4-chlorophenol and Dichloroacetic Acid in Water Using Ti-, Zr- and Ti/Zr-Pillared Bentonites as Photocatalyst. *Am. J. Appl. Sci.* **2005**, *2*, 1136–1140.
20. Hurum, D. C.; Agrios, A. G.; Crist, S. E.; Gray, K. A.; Rajh, T.; Thurnauer, M. C. Probing Reaction Mechanisms in Mixed Phase TiO_2 by EPR. *J. Electron Spectrosc. Relat. Phenom.* **2006**, *150*, 155–163.
21. Ibañez, P. F.; Malato, S.; Enea, O. Photoelectrochemical Reactors for the Solar Decontamination of Water. *Catal. Today* **1999**, *54*, 329–339.
22. Jo, S. M.; Song, M. Y.; Ahn, Y. R.; Park, C. R.; Kim, D. Y. Nanofibril Formation of Electrospun TiO_2 Fibers and its Application to Dye-Sensitized Solar Cells. *J. Macromol. Sci. Pure Appl. Chem.* **2005**, *42*, 1529–1540.
23. Kumar, A.; Jose, R.; Fujihara, K.; Wang, J.; Ramakrishna, S. Structural and Optical Properties of Electrospun TiO_2 Nanofibers. *Chem. Mater.* **2007**, *19*, 6536–6542.
24. Lalman, J. A.; Ray, S. Method of Surface Treatment of Aluminum Foil and its Alloy and Method of Producing Immobilized Nanocatalyst of Transition Metal Oxides and Their Alloys. United States Provisional Patent Application 61/272,518, 2009.
25. Lee, S. K.; Mills, A. Detoxification of Water by Semiconductor Photocatalysis. *J. Ind. Eng. Chem.* **2004**, *10*, 173–187.
26. Li, D.; Xia, Y. Fabrication of Titania Nanofibers by Electrospinning. *Nano Lett.* **2003**, *3*, 555–560.
27. Ling, C. M.; Mohamed, A. R.; Bhatia, S. Performance of Photocatalytic Reactors Using Immobilized TiO_2 Film for the Degradation of Phenol and Methylene Blue Dye Present in Water Stream. *Chemosphere* **2004**, *57*, 547–554.
28. Linsebigler, L.; Lu, G.; Yates Jr., J.T. Photocatalysis on TiO_2 Surfaces: Principles, Mechanisms and Selected Results, *Chem. Rev.* **1995**, *95*, 735–758.
29. Madhugiri, S.; Sun, B.; Smirniotis, P. G.; Ferraris, J. P.; Balkus, K. J., Jr. Electrospun Mesoporous Titanium Dioxide Fibers. *Microporous Mesoporous Mater.* **2004**, *69*, 77–83.
30. Matthews, R. W. Photocatalytic Oxidation of Organic Contaminants in Water: An Aid to Environmental Preservation. *Pure Appl. Chem.* **1992**, *64* (1992), 1285–1290.
31. Ollis, D. F.; Pelezzetti, E.; Serpone, N. Photocatalyzed Destruction of Water Contaminants. *Environ. Sci. Technol.* **1991**, *25*, 1522–1529.
32. Peiró, A. M.; Brillas, E.; Peral, J.; Domènech, X.; Ayllón, J. A. Electrochemically Assisted Deposition of Titanium Dioxide on Aluminium Cathodes. *J. Mater. Chem.* **2002**, *12*, 2769–2773.
33. Pozzo, R. L.; Baltanfis, M. A.; Cassano, A. E. Supported Titanium Oxide as Photocatalyst in Water Decontamination: State of the Art. *Catal. Today* **1997**, *39*, 219–231.
34. Ray, S.; Lalman, J. A. Using the Box–Benkhen Design (BBD) to Minimize the Diameter of Electrospun Titanium Dioxide Nanofibers. *Chem. Eng. J.* **2011**, *169*, 116–125.
35. Ray, S.; Lalman, J. A. Fabrication and Characterization of an Immobilized Titanium Dioxide (TiO_2) Nanofiber Photocatalyst. *Mater. Today Proc.* **2016**, *3*, 1582–1591.

36. Ray, S.; Lalman, J. A.; Biswas, N. Using the Box-Benkhen Technique to Statistically Model Phenol Photocatalytic Degradation by Titanium Dioxide Nanoparticles. *Chem. Eng. J.* **2009,** *150*(1), 15–24.

37. Reneker, D. H.; Chun, I. Nanometer Diameter Fibers of Polymer, Produced by Electrospinning. *Nanotechnology* **1996,** *7*, 216–223.

38. Sayilkan, F.; AsiltTurk, M.; Sayilkan, H.; Onal, Y.; Akarsu, M.; Arpae, E. Characterization of TiO_2 Synthesized in Alcohol by a Sol-Gel Process: The Effects of Annealing Temperature and Acid Catalyst. *Turk. J. Chem.* **2005,** *29*, 697–706.

39. Scotti, R.; D'Arienzo, M.; Morazzoni, F.; Bellobono, I. R. Immobilization of Hydrothermally Produced TiO2 with Different Phase Composition for Photocatalytic Degradation of Phenol. *Appl. Catal. B Environ.* **2009,** *88*, 323–330.

40. Sheikh, F. A.; Barakat, N. A. M.; Kanjwal, M. A.; Chaudhuri, A. A.; Jung, I-H.; Lee, J. H.; Kim, H. Y. Electrospun Antimicrobial Polyurethane Nanofibers Containing Silver Nanoparticles for Biotechnological Applications. *Macromol. Res.* **2009,** *17*, 688–696.

41. Sigmund, W.; Yuh, V.; Park, H.; Maneeratana, V.; Pyrgiotakis, G.; Daga, A.; Taylor, J.; Nino, J. C. Processing and Structure Relationships in Electrospinning of Ceramic Fiber Systems. *J. Am. Ceram. Soc.* **2006,** *89*, 395–407.

42. Song, M. Y.; Kim, D. K.; Ihn, K. J.; Jo, S. M.; Kim, D. Y. Electrospun TiO_2 Electrodes for Dye-Sensitized Solar Cells. Nanotechnology, **2004,** *15*, 1861–1865.

43. Subbiah, T.; Bhat, G. S.; Tock, R. W.; Parameswaran, S.; Ramkumar, S. S. Electrospinning of Nanofibers. *J. Appl. Polym. Sci.* **2005,** *96*, 557–569.

44. Teleki, A.; Wengeler, R.; Wengeler, L.; Nirschl, H.; Pratsinis, S. E. Distinguishing Between Aggregates and Agglomerates of Flame-Made TiO_2 by High-Pressure Dispersion. *Powder Technol.* **2008,** *181*, 292–300.

45. World Health Organization. Environmental Health Criteria (EHC) No. 161. Phenol. 1994, http://www.inchem.org/documents/ehc/ehc/ehc161.htm (accessed Nov, 2009).

46. Zhang, H.; Banfield, J. F. Thermodynamic Analysis of Phase Stability of Nanocrystalline Titania. *J. Mater. Chem.* **1998,** *8*, 2073–2076.

47. Zhang, X.; Xu, S.; Han, G.; Fabrication and Photocatalytic Activity of TiO_2 Nanofiber Membrane. *Mater. Lett.* **2009,** *63*, 1761–1763.

CHAPTER 7

ELECTROCHEMICAL PROFILE AND ANTIOXIDANT POTENTIAL OF GALLIC ACID IN PRESENCE OF ASCORBIC ACID

DULCE A. FLORES-MALTOS[1], CRISTOBAL N. AGUILAR[1],
RUTH E. BELMARES[1], RAÚL RODRÍGUEZ[1],
L. V. RODRÍGUEZ-DURAN[1], EDITH M. COLUNGA-URBINA[2]
and JOSÉ SANDOVAL-CORTÉS[2,*]

[1]*Food Research Department, School of Chemistry, Universidad Autónoma de Coahuila, Blvd. V. Carranza and González Lobo s/n, ZIP 25280. Saltillo, Coahuila, México*

[2]*Analytical Chemistry Department, School of Chemistry, Universidad Autónoma de Coahuila, Blv. V. Carranza and González Lobo s/n, ZIP 25280. Saltillo, Coahuila, México*

Corresponding author. E-mail: josesandoval@uadec.edu.mx

CONTENTS

ABSTRACT

Electroanalytical techniques have great perspectives for its application in quality control in the food industry. The determination of the anodic potential of two or more substances in a single sample is a fast, convenient, and low-cost alternative to traditional techniques. Even more can be an identification parameter to be used to determine total antioxidant potential in foodstuff samples. The developed system basically consist of a platinum electrode1 for electrochemical identification of gallic acid in the presence of ascorbic acid at different pH values.

7.1   INTRODUCTION

Polyphenols are a large group of chemical substances and are considered as secondary plant metabolites. Polyphenols include more than 8000 compounds with different chemical structures and biological activities.[1] Chemically, polyphenols are compounds that have an aromatic ring with one or more hydroxyl substituents, including functional derivatives (esters, methyl esters, glycosides, etc.).[2] Their chemical structure is good enough to scavenge free radicals, due to the capacity of the proton in the aromatic hydroxyl group to be donated to the radical species and the stability for the resulting quinone that support a disappeared electron.[3] The nature of polyphenols varies from simple molecules like phenolic acids to highly polymerized compounds. In the plants, these compounds are present in a conjugated form with one or more glycosidic moieties bound by hydroxyl groups. Furthermore, in some cases, a sugar moiety can be directly bound to an aromatic carbon. Thus, the most common form of polyphenols in nature is in the form of glycosides, such as tannins. These compounds are soluble in water and organic solvents and have a large number of hydroxyl groups, among other functional groups. Therefore, they are able to bind to proteins and other macromolecules.[4]

To be considered as an antioxidant, a phenolic compound must meet two basic conditions. First, when present in a low concentration relative to the substrate to be oxidized, antioxidant must delay or prevent autoxidation or oxidation mediated by free radical. Second, the radical formed after the scavenging must be stable and unable to act in subsequent oxidation reactions.[5] Polyphenolic compounds with high antioxidant activity include phenolic acids, flavonoids, anthocyanins, and tannins. These compounds and other natural antioxidants such as ascorbic acid (AA) are abundant in plants.[6]

Analytical techniques used to evaluate the antioxidant capacity are classified into three major groups: biological analysis (xanthine oxidase, lipid peroxidation), spectrophotometric analysis (2,2-diphenyl-1-picrylhy-drazyl (DPPH), ABTS), and electrochemical assays (cyclic voltammetry, differential pulse voltammetry (DPV)). Electrochemical analyses correlate oxidation potentials, electric current, or other electrochemical parameters to the antioxidant capacity. This kind of techniques is more selective and more sensitive than spectrophotometric methods for the evaluation of anti-oxidant power and are also more reproducible than biological analysis.[7] In the present study, we report the electrochemical analysis of the antioxidant potential of gallic acid (GA) in the presence of AA at different pH values.

7.2   EXPERIMENTAL

7.2.1   CHEMICALS

AA, GA, DPPH, acetic acid, sodium acetate, potassium phosphate mono-basic, and potassium phosphate dibasic were purchased from Sigma (USA). All other chemicals used were analytical grade and used without further purification.

7.2.2   CHEMICAL ASSAY: DPPH FREE RADICAL SCAVENGING

AA and GA were added at different concentrations to a methanolic solution of the radical DPPH (6×10^{-5} M). The solutions were mixed and incubated for 30 min in darkness, until a stable absorbance value at $\lambda = 517$ nm was obtained. The reduction of the DPPH radical was calculated as a discoloration percentage using the following equation:

$$\% \, I = \left(\frac{A_{Control} - A_{Sample}}{A_{Control}} \right) \times 100 \qquad (7.1)$$

where A_{Sample} is the sample absorbance at 517 nm and $A_{Control}$ is the absorbance of the control.

7.2.3   ELECTROCHEMICAL ASSAY: CYCLIC VOLTAMMETRY

The cyclic and DPV were achieved with a potentiostat BAS Epsilon controlled with BAS Epsilon EC software (Bioanalytical Systems, USA). Potentiostat was connected to a typical three electrode cell, which used platinum microelectrode as a working electrode, platinum wire as a counter electrode, and the Ag/AgCl electrode as a reference electrode. Always before the analysis of the samples, the electrochemical cell was tested using the redox system Fe^{3+}/Fe^{2+}.

7.2.4   PROCEDURE

The antioxidant potential of AA and GA was studied at several concentrations and pH values. Standards were prepared at different concentrations (1–10 mM) in acetate buffer (0.2 M) to adjust the pH at 4 and 5, and in phosphate buffer (0.2 M) for pH 7. All solutions were freshly prepared and used immediately. To evaluate the antioxidant power of organic acids, the DPV was used between −50 and 900 mV.

During the test, the electrodes were submerged in the buffer solution and increasing amounts of antioxidant were added. For voltammetric measurements, an Epsilon potentiostat was used for controlling the potential scanning between the reference electrode and the working electrode. At the same time, the electrical current generated between the working electrode and the auxiliary electrode, due to the movement of electrical charges in the electrode–solution interface, was measured. Potentiostat was connected to a computer and controlled by the software provided by the manufacturer. Several measurement protocols were employed.

7.2.5   RESULTS AND DISCUSSION

Using DPV, it was possible to obtain the values for the maximal oxidation potentials of AA and GA. Figure 7.1 shows the voltammograms for AA and GA at different pH values. Notable differences can be found between the oxidation processes of both compounds. For GA, two oxidative processes can be observed at pH 7, this could be related to its chemical structure. Figure 7.1b shows that only two of the three hydroxyl groups (enclosed in circles) are involved in oxidative processes. In addition, it appears that these functional groups are susceptible to change according to the pH of the medium. This figure also shows that at pH 7 the oxidation of GA occurs in two processes, whereas pH 7 appears only as a process. On the other hand, it can be observed that regardless of pH, AA oxidation is carried out in a single process. The process is well-defined at pH 5, better than the others at pH 4 and 7, with the highest current and the finest shape.

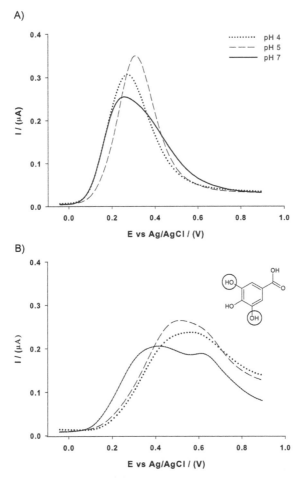

FIGURE 7.1   Differential pulse voltammetry of AA (A) and GA (B) at pH 4, 5, and 7.

Figure 7.2 shows the differential pulse voltammograms of AA, GA, and the mixture of both compounds at 10 mM and pH 5 and 7. When we analyze the solutions at pH 5, we can observe a well-defined shapes for each one of the organic acids separately and together with EpA=0.35 for AA, EpA=0.51 for GA, whereas the peak potentials in the mixed solution were shifted to more positive values, 0.422 and 0.722 mV, respectively; this shift could be due to an interaction between them. At pH 7, we can observe a bigger overlapping of the oxidation processes compared with a lower pH and separately we can observe three oxidation processes, whereas in the mixed solution we can observe only two oxidation processes, due to this the pH 5 was selected to work.

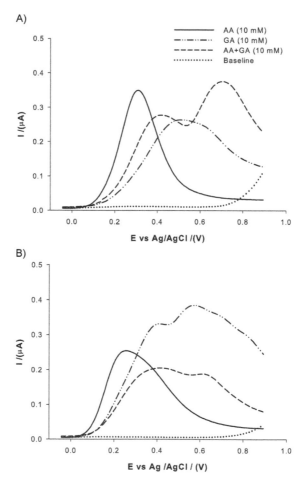

FIGURE 7.2　Differential pulse voltammetry of AA and GA at pH 5 (A) and 7 (B).

To verify that both analytes (AA and GA) can be determined simultaneously, it was carried out in the deconvolution of differential pulse voltammograms of the mixture of AA-AG. Figure 7.3 shows that the magnitude of the current recorded during the oxidation of AA at a concentration of 10 mM does not generate any current at the potential value of the maximum current for GA at a concentration of 10 mM, and vice versa. The difference of potential between the two processes is 180 mV, this is large enough to carry out the simultaneous determination of both acids independently and without overlapping of signals.

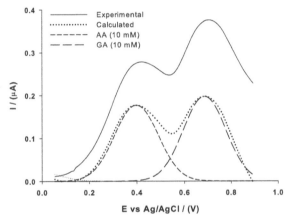

FIGURE 7.3   Deconvolution of the differential pulse voltammogram of a mixture of AA (10 mM) and GA (10 mM).

Figure 7.4 shows differential pulse voltammograms of the mixture of AA and GA at pH 5. This figure shows that the oxidation processes of AA and GA appear as two separate signals and can be determined independently of each other. It was observed that a fixed concentration of GA (1 mM) and varying the concentration of AA from 1 to 10 mM, the current increase is correlated linearly with respect to the concentration of AA ($R^2 = 0.9965$) and the assay has a sensitivity of 2.7×10^{-2} μ A·mM.

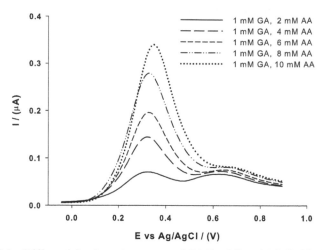

FIGURE 7.4   Differential pulse voltammetry of GA (1 mM) and AA (1–10 mM) at pH 5.

Similarly, when in a solution with a fixed concentration of AA (1 mM), the concentration of AG is increased from 1 to 10 mM, the current increases proportionally and linearly with the concentration of GA ($R^2 = 0.9959$) with a sensitivity of $3.25 10^{-2}$ μ A·mM (Fig. 7.5).

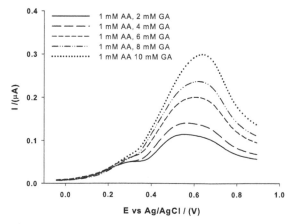

FIGURE 7.5   Differential pulse voltammetry of AA (1 mM) and GA (1–10 mM) at pH 5.

These results show that using a platinum electrode and adjusting the pH of the sample is possible to simultaneously determine the AA and GA present in a solution.

On the other hand, the oxidation potentials suggest the compound with higher antioxidant potential AA, because it has a lower oxidation potential. To confirm this observation, a chemical assay was carried out to evaluate the DPPH free radical scavenging potential of GA and AA. Table 7.1 shows the free radical scavenging activity for both organic acids as well as the oxidation potential at different pH values. It was found that the AA (10 mM) inhibited 71.21% of the free DPPH free radical, whereas GA (10 mM) inhibited 68.68 of free radical. This confirmed the oxidation potentials at both pH 5 and pH 7, where the AA showed a lower oxidation potential.

TABLE 7.1   Relationship Between Oxidation Potential and Antioxidant Activity by DPPH Assay.

Compound	E_{Ox-pH5} (V)	E_{Ox-pH7} (V)	% Inhibition
Ascorbic acid	0.310	0.254	71.21
Gallic acid	0.518	0.414	68.68

7.3   CONCLUSIONS

Through the pH manipulation and using a platinum microelectrode without any special treatment, the determination of GA in the presence of AA and vice versa can be achieved. This allows us to propose this method for the analysis of complex samples that contain these two organic acids very popular today, such as grapes or berries.

7.4   ACKNOWLEDGMENTS

Dulce A. Flores Maltos thanks the National Council for Science and Technology of Mexico (CONACYT) for the financial support provided for their postgraduate studies in the Food Science and Technology Program, Universidad Autónoma de Coahuila, Mexico.

KEYWORDS

- **electroanalysis**
- **antioxidants**
- **gallic acid**

REFERENCES

1. Martínez-Valverde, I.; Periago, M. J.; Ros, G. Nutritional Significance of Dietary Phenolic Compounds (*In Spanish*). *Arch. Latinoam. Nutr.* **2000**, *50*, 5–18.
2. Lattanzio, V.; Lattanzio, V. M. T.; Cardinali, A. Role of Phenolics in the Resistance Mechanisms of Plants Against Fungal Pathogens and Insects. In *Phytochemistry: Advances in Research;* Imperato, F. Ed.; Research Signpost: Kerala, 2006; pp 23–67.
3. Londoño, J.; Montoya, G.; Guerrero, K.; Aristizabal, L.; Arango, G. J. Citrus Juice Inhibits Low Density Lipoprotein Oxidation: Relationship Between Free Radical Scavenger Activity and Electrophoretic Mobility. *Rev. Chil. Nutr.* **2006**, *33*, 544–551.
4. Sanchez, V.; Sandoval, C.; Franco, C. An Evaluation of Polyphenol Release from Cosmetic Formulations. *Ars. Pharm.* **2008**, *49*, 309–320.
5. Eklund, P. C.; Langvik, O. K.; Warna, J. P.; Salmi, T. O.; Willfor, S. M.; Sjoholm, R. E. Chemical Studies on Antioxidant Mechanisms and Free Radical Scavenging Properties of Lignans. *Org. Biomol. Chem.* **2005**, *3*, 3336–3347.
6. Muanda, F.; Kone, D.; Dicko, A.; Soulimani, R.; Younos, C. Phytochemical Composition and Antioxidant Capacity of Three Malian Medicinal Plant Parts. *Evidence-Based Complementary Altern. Med.* **2009**, *6*, 1–8.
7. Bara, M. T. F.; Serrano, S. H. P.; Asquieri, E. R.; Lúcio, T. C.; Gil, E. S. Measurement of Solid-State Anodic Potential: A Tool for Determining the Antioxidant Potential of Phytotherapeutics (*In Spanish*). *Lat. Am. J. Pharm.* **2008**, *27*, 89–92.

CHAPTER 8

EFFICIENT SYNTHESIS OF OXYGEN-STUDDED GRAPHENE NANOLAYERS POSSESSING TUNABLE PHOTOLUMINESCENCE FROM HEARTHSIDE WASTE

ANU N. MOHAN[1,2,*] and MANOJ B.[1]

[1]Material Sciences Research Laboratory, Department of Physics, Christ University, Bengaluru, Karnataka 560029, India

[2]Department of Physics, School of Graduate Studies, Jain University, J C Road, Bengaluru, Karnataka 560027, India

*Corresponding author. E-mail: anunmohan@gmail.com

CONTENTS

ABSTRACT

A facile one-pot synthesis route to Graphene Nanolayers (GNL) from the hearthside waste is reported herein. Nanomaterials with excitation wavelength governing emissions are considered to be highly desirable because of their potential applications in the field of sensors, imaging, and other optical devices. The synthesized GNL exhibits tunable photoluminescence properties and thereby makes it an ideal candidate to cater for today's needs.

8.1 INTRODUCTION

Graphene and its derivatives had gained significant popularity due to their excellent electronic, thermal, and optical properties in the recent years. Graphene, an assembly of carbon atoms with a hexagonal crystal lattice pattern in a single layer, has been used in a long trail of applications due to the considerable electronic and thermal properties it possesses compared to the other 2D materials. Even though graphene was leading in the fields of electronic and thermal applications, its optical applications were very limited because of the material's nonexistent bandgap. This hurdle was overcome by modern researchers by decorating the basal planes of carbon with several oxygen functionalities. The method adopted for the chemical modification of carbon layers was originally put forward by Brodie in 1859, which was later improved by Staudenmaier.[1–3] Later, in 1958, Hummers and Offeman came up with a time-saving and simplified version of the chemical oxidation method for the synthesis of graphite oxide, which can then be exfoliated to obtain reduced graphene oxide (rGO).[4–6]

rGO corresponds to a single or few layers of graphene intercalated with traces of various oxygen functional groups along the basal planes and the edges. The incorporation of the oxygen functionalities considerably increased the solubility of the graphene system and it also put an end to the long wait for the opening up of an optical band gap in the wonder material. rGO and other carbon derivatives such as carbon dots (CDs), graphene quantum dots (GQDs), carbon nano-diamonds (CNDs), etc. possess similar photoluminescence (PL) characteristics owing to the various synthesis method depending on band gap formation. Majority of them exhibit an excitation dependent PL behavior, which is a very enticing property, as it enables one to tune the PL emission wavelengths just by changing the excitation wavelength and thereby eliminating the troubles of any chemical alterations in the composition or particle size of the material. In the present study, we report a facile chemical synthesis route, which is a modification of the existing Hummers' method, to obtain excitation wavelength dependent photoluminescent Graphene Nanolayers (GNL).[7–12]

8.2 EXPERIMENTAL

The burnt wood waste from the hearthside (HS) was washed repeatedly and was subjected to chemical oxidative treatment. The protocol that followed involved a modified Hummers' method. 2 g of HS was mixed with sulfuric acid and sodium nitrate. The mixture was stirred for 15 min and potassium permanganate was then added with constant stirring. The oxidative reaction was allowed to continue for next 48 h with constant agitation with the help of a magnetic stirrer. The reaction was terminated with the addition of hydrogen peroxide and cold water. The mixture was subjected to repetitive washing with ethanol and distilled water and later on, was dialyzed till the pH turned neutral. It was then exfoliated and dried to get GNL.

HS and GNL were spectroscopically and morphologically characterized using Raman spectroscopy, X-ray Diffraction (XRD), Fourier Transform Infrared (FTIR) spectroscopy, PL spectroscopy, and Transmission Electron Microscopy (TEM). Raman analysis was carried out using a Horiba LabRAM HR spectrometer at 514.5 nm. XRD analysis of the samples was performed using a Bruker AXS D8 Advance X-ray diffractometer. Fourier-transform infrared spectra (FTIR) were obtained using a Shimadzu FT-IR-8400 spectrometer and a Horiba LabRAM HR spectrometer was used to obtain the PL spectra of the sample. Morphological analysis of the samples was performed by a JEM-2100 (JOEL) model system.

8.3 RESULTS AND DISCUSSION

Raman spectra of HS and GNL are given in Figure 8.1. The characteristic D and G peaks of rGO were clearly evident in the spectrum of GNL at 1349 and 1587 cm^{-1}, respectively. D peak represents the in-plane vibrations of the disordered carbon of the crystal lattice and G peak is a representation of the E_{2g} mode of the graphitic domains. GNL spectrum also depicts a 2D region at ~2800 cm^{-1}. I_D/I_G ratio of HS and GNL was calculated to be 0.68 and 0.81 indicating the increase in quality of the nanolayers formed. The increase in the D and G peak intensity ratio indicates the reduction in size of the sp[2] clusters in the lattice structure.[13–14]

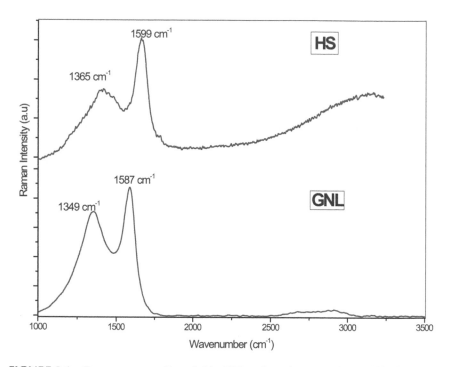

FIGURE 8.1   Raman spectra of hearthside (HS) and graphene nanolayers (GNL).

Figure 8.2 shows the XRD profile of HS and GNL. X-ray diffractogram of HS shows a number of impurity peaks coupled with those arising from the amorphous like carbon. GNL profile shows the elimination of all the impurity peaks and exhibits a prominent peak at $\sim 20°$. Observation of this intense single peak indicates the formation of rGO with ordered nature. It also points out the efficiency of the oxidative treatment protocols followed during the chemical treatment.

FTIR spectra of HS and GNL are shown in Figure 8.3. The comparison of both the spectra indicates the enhancement of oxygen functionalities after the chemical treatment. Peak at ~ 1600 cm^{-1} indicates restoration of the graphene network in GNL.[15] This result also corroborates well with the XRD and Raman analyses.

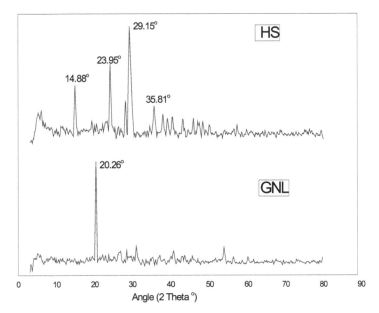

FIGURE 8.2 X-ray diffractogram (XRD) profile of HS and GNL.

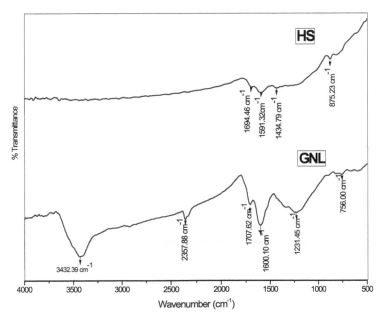

FIGURE 8.3 Fourier-transform infrared (FTIR) spectra of HS and GNL.

Photoluminescence spectrum of GNL (Fig. 8.4) shows an excitation-dependent emission behavior. Graphene oxide sheets are rarely reported to exhibit PL. GNL exhibits a peculiar pattern different from the general cases in which emission intensity decreases with increase in the excitation wavelengths. In the case of GNL, the emission wavelengths increase at first and reach a peak and then decrease with the increase in the excitation wavelengths. The reason can be attributed to the presence of nano-sized aromatic clusters in the GNL. GO is known to give fixed peak positions whereas rGO peaks redshifts with an increase in excitation wavelengths. It is observed in the spectrum of GNL that PL peaks are redshifted at higher excitation wavelengths clearly indicating the reduction of GO to rGO. Excitation dependent PL characteristics of GNL allow one to tune the emission characteristics, thereby opening the windows for many applications.[16]

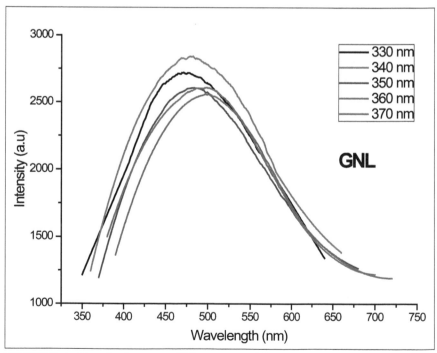

FIGURE 8.4 Photoluminescence (PL) spectrum of GNL.

To deduce the microstructure of the samples, Transmission electron microscopy (TEM) analysis was done. TEM images of HS (Fig. 8.5) show a cluttered morphology with no ordered arrangement. SAED pattern also supports this observed nature.

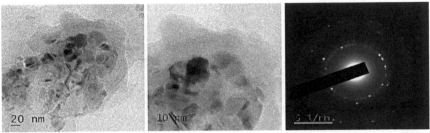

FIGURE 8.5 Transmission electron microscopy (TEM) image and selected area electron diffraction (SAED) pattern of HS.

TEM images of GNL show a layered structure of the sample. From TEM images and SAED pattern (Fig. 8.6), it can be deduced that the GNL formed consists of crumbled multilayers. This was, in turn, supportive of the other spectroscopic analyses.

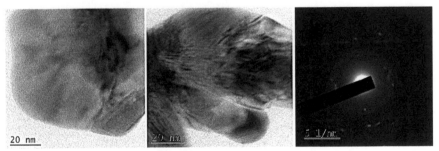

FIGURE 8.6 TEM image and SAED pattern of GNL.

8.4 CONCLUSIONS

An efficient and one-pot synthesis of rGO from the hearthside wood waste is reported herein. Various spectroscopic and morphological characterization of the samples before and after the chemical treatment show the effectiveness of the protocol followed. This was in direct corroboration with the XRD analysis of GLN, depicting a single sharp peak of rGO, and also its FTIR studies that had representations from various oxygen functional groups and the graphitic domain. The increase in the intensity ratio of the D and G peaks of Raman spectrum of the chemically oxidized sample, also supported by the observations from its PL spectrum, points to the reduction of the size of the sp[2] clusters. The opening up of a band gap in the treated sample and the excitation wavelength dependency showcased by GLN is an intriguing at the same time beneficial property, which makes it a potential candidate for many optical applications including bio-tracers and imaging.

8.5 ACKNOWLEDGMENT

The authors are thankful to Center for Research, Christ University, Bengaluru for providing laboratory facilities for the successful completion of this work. We also acknowledge IISc, Bengaluru; IUCNN, M G University, Kottayam; and SAIF, CUSAT, Cochin for the help and facilities provided for the characterization of the samples.

KEYWORDS

- **graphene nanolayers**
- **modified Hummers' method**
- **photoluminescence**
- **tunable PL behavior**

REFERENCES

1. Brodie, B. C. On the Atomic Weight of Graphite. *Philos. Trans. R. Soc. London* **1859,** *149,* 249–259.
2. Staudenmaier, L. Verfahren zur Darstellung der Graphitsäure. *Ber. Dtsch. Chem. Ges.* **1898,** *31,* 1481–1487.
3. Mohan, A. N.; Manoj, B. Synthesis and Characterization of Carbon Nanospheres From Hydrocarbon Soot. *Int. J. Electrochem. Sci.* **2012,** *7,* 9537–9549.

4. Hummers, W. S.; Offeman, R. E. Preparation of Graphitic Oxide. *J. Am. Chem. Soc.* **1958,** *80,* 1339.

5. Pan, S.; Aksay, I. A. Factors Controlling the Size of Graphene Oxide Sheets Produced via the Graphite Oxide Route. *ACS Nano* **2011,** *5,* 4073–4083.

6. Mohan, A. N.; Ramya, A. V.; Manoj, B. Synthesis and Characterization of sp^2-sp^3 Bonded Disordered Graphene Like Nanocarbon From Coconut Shell. Adv. Sci. Eng. Med. **2016,** *8*(2), 112–116.

7. Zhixing, G.; Hao, X.; Yanling, H. Mechanism for Excitation-Dependent Photoluminescence From Graphene Quantum Dots and Other Graphene Oxide Derivates: Consensus, Debates and Challenges. *Nanoscale* **2016,** *8,* 7794–7807.

8. Dong, Y.; Shao, J.; Chen, C.; Li, H.; Wang, R.; Chi, Y.; Lin, X.; Chen, G. Blue Luminescent Graphene Quantum Dots and Graphene Oxide Prepared by Tuning the Carbonization Degree of Citric Acid. *Carbon* **2012,** *50*(12), 4738–4743.

9. Lin, L.; Rong, M.; Luo, F.; Chen, D.; Wang, Y.; Chen, X. Luminescent Graphene Quantum Dots as New Fluorescent Materials for Environmental and Biological Applications. *TrAC Trends Anal. Chem.* **2014,** *54,* 83–102.

10. Shen, J.; Zhu, Y.; Yang, X.; Li, C. Graphene Quantum Dots: Emergent Nanolights for Bioimaging, Sensors, Catalysis and Photovoltaic Devices. *Chem. Commun.* **2012,** *48,* 3686–3699.

11. Sun, H.; Wu, L.; Wei, W.; Qu, X. Recent Advances in Graphene Quantum Dots for Sensing. *Mater. Today* **2013,** *16*(11), 433–442.

12. Mohan, A. N.; Manoj, B.; John, J.; Ramya, A. V. Structural Characterization of Paraffin Wax Soot and Carbon Black by XRD. *Asian J. Chem.* **2013,** *25* (Supplementary Issue), S76–78.

12. Fei, Y.; Zhao, B.; Ran, R.; Shao, X. Facile Mechanochemical Synthesis of Nano SnO2/ Graphene Composite from Coarse Metallic Sn and Graphite Oxide: An Outstanding Anode Material for Lithium-Ion Batteries. *Chem. Eur. J.* **2014,** *20,* 4055–4063.

13. Mohan, A. N.; Ramya, A. V.; Manoj, B. Probing the Nature of Defects of Graphene Like Nano-Carbon From Amorphous Materials by Raman Spectroscopy. *Asian J. Chem.* **2016,** *28*(7), 1501–1504.

14. Manoj, B.; Sreelaksmi, S.; Mohan, A. N.; Kunjomana, A. G. Characterization of Diesel Soot from the Combustion in Engine by X-ray and Spectroscopic Techniques. *Int. J. Electrochem. Sci.* **2012,** *7,* 3215–3221.

15. Gan, Z. X.; Xiong, S J.; Wu, X. L.; Tao Xu, Xiaobin Zhu, Xiao Gan, Junhong Guo, Jiancang Shen, Litao Sun, Paul K. Chu. Mechanism of Photoluminescence From Chemically Derived Graphene Oxide: Role of Chemical Reduction. *Adv. Opt. Mater.* **2013,** *1*(12), 926–932.

CHAPTER 9

INTERACTION OF TERTIARY AMINE WITH ARYL AND ALKYL ETHERS: EXPERIMENTAL AND THEORETICAL APPROACH

ZUBIN R. MASTER, ZUBER S. VAID and NAVED I. MALEK*

Applied Chemistry Department, S. V. National Institute of Technology, Surat 395007, India

Corresponding author. E-mail: navedmalek@chem.svnit.ac.in
navedmalek@yahoo.co.in

CONTENTS

ABSTRACT

In this chapter, densities, ρ, speeds of sound, u, and refractive indices, n_D of the binary mixtures of N,N-diethylaniline (DEA) with anisole (ANS) and tert-butyl methyl ether (MTBE) were determined at 0.1 MPa pressure as a function of composition and temperature from 293.15 to 323.15 K at 5 K interval. Excess molar volume (V_m^E), excess molar isentropic compressibilities ($K_{s,m}^E$), and the deviation in refractive index (Δn_D) were calculated and fitted to the four-parameter Redlich–Kister polynomial equation. V_m^E and $K_{s,m}^E$ were negative, whereas Δn_D was positive for the studied mixtures (except for DEA+ANS, $K_{s,m}^E$ was found positive in the DEA rich region) for the entire range of composition and at all studied temperatures. Several semiempirical equations were used to predict the refractive index of the mixtures. V_m^E results have been discussed in terms of Prigogine–Flory–Patterson statistical theory.

9.1   INTRODUCTION

We have been engaged in a systematic study of thermodynamics, acoustic, optical, and transport properties of the binary liquid mixtures containing amines and ethers. We have reported excess molar volume, excess molar isentropic compressibilities, Rao's molar sound functions, deviation in viscosity, excess viscosity, excess free energy of activation of viscous flow, deviation in refractive index and the deviation in molar refraction for alkyl amines with nonelectrolyte solvents, cyclohexane with benzene and benzaldehyde, cyclohexylamine with cyclohexane and benzene, chloroanilines with diisopropyl ether and oxolane, and ionic liquids with alkyl amines and cyclic ethers at various temperatures.[1–6] Amines are industrially important bases and are used in the preparation of various dyes,[7] whereas ethers have found applications in various fields, such as in the synthesis of organic compounds, fragrances, and pharmaceuticals, used as a solvent and heat transfer medium to name a few.[8]

We had reported the transport, acoustic, and refractive properties for the mixtures containing N-ethylaniline (NEA) with anisole (ANS) and tert-butyl methyl ether (MTBE) recently.[9] In this chapter, we have reported the density (ρ), speeds of sound (u), and refractive index (n_D) of the binary mixtures of N,N-diethylaniline (DEA) with ANS and MTBE in the temperature range 293.15–323.15 K at 5 K intervals and at atmospheric pressure. Various thermodynamic properties along with the optical properties such as Rao's molar sound functions (R), excess molar volume (V_m^E), excess molar isentropic compressibilities ($V_{s,m}^E$), and deviation in refractive index (Δn_D) were derived from the experimental data.

9.2 EXPERIMENTAL

9.2.1 MATERIALS

N,N-diethylaniline, ANS, and MTBE were purchased from Acros Chemicals Ltd., Belgium and were stored over activated 4 Å molecular sieves (Merck) to reduce water content. A specific assembly was set up consisting of two vertical columns; the first column was filled with raschig rings and 4 Å molecular sieves mounted by a vigreux column. First column was used to reduce the impurity and moisture content from the DEA and the vigreux column was used to remove low boiling impurities from the DEA. Care was taken to avoid the degradation of the amine and the purity was checked with gas chromatography (GC) comprising capillary column with a flame ionization detector employed. The purity of the sample was more than 0.998 on mass fraction basis. The details of the chemicals used in the present work with their purity and method used for purification are given in Table 9.1. The experimental ρ, u, and n_D are compared in Table 9.2 with the literature data.[10–25]

Analytical balance (B 204-S, Mettler Toledo, Switzerland), operated in the dry box to prevent the exposure of the sample from atmospheric moisture with an uncertainty of ± 0.0001 g was used for the preparation of the sample by mass in the current investigation. The estimated uncertainty in the mole fraction of the mixtures was less than ± 0.0001. Care was taken to prevent evaporation of the samples after preparation.

TABLE 9.1 CAS Number, Supplier and Purity of Components at T = 298.15 K.

Component	CAS Number	Supplier	Initial Purity in mass fraction	Final	Purification Method
N,N-Diethyl Aniline	91-66-7	Acros	0.990	0.998	CD[a]
Anisole	100-66-3	Acros	0.990		None
MTBE	1634-04-4	Acros	0.990		None

[a]CD column distillation, MTBE tert-butyl methyl ether.

TABLE 9.2 Comparison of Experimental Densities (ρ), Speeds of Sound (u), and Refractive Index (n_D), at Temperatures, T, from 293.15 to 323.15 K and Atmospheric Pressure for Pure Liquids.

T (K)	ρ ($kg \cdot m^{-3}$)		u ($m \cdot s^{-1}$)		n_D	
	Exp	Lit	Exp	Lit	Exp	Lit
N,N-Diethylaniline						
293.15	933.680	—	1473.71		1.54192	—
298.15	929.668	929.9[10] 929.92[11] 930.7[12]	1453.55		1.53944	—
303.15	925.653	926.1[13] 925.9[10] 925.29[11] 926.0[14] 926.1[12]	1433.52	1411[11] 1434[13]	1.53697	—
308.15	921.629	921.9[10] 921.26[11] 922.2[12]	1413.64	1406[11]	1.53450	—
313.15	917.597	918.0[10,11] 917.5[13] 917.7[14] 918.2[12]	1393.93	1396[13]	1.53200	—
318.15	913.556	913.9[10]	1374.35		1.52951	—
323.15	909.505		1354.92	1358[10]	1.52700	—

TABLE 9.2 *(Continued)*

T (K)	ρ (kg·m⁻³)		u (m·s⁻¹)		n_D	
	Exp	Lit	Exp	Lit	Exp	Lit
Anisole						
293.15	993.844	994.0[15]	1428.04		1.51719	1.5175[15]
298.15	989.133	989.32[16]	1407.42	1410[17]	1.51478	1.5148[17]
		988.9[17]				1.5153[18]
		989.30[18]				
303.15	984.418	984.1[17]	1386.97		1.51239	1.5124[17]
		984.3[19]				
308.15	979.690	979.4[17]	1366.67		1.50993	1.5092[17]
		979.71[18]				1.5095[18]
313.15	974.945	974.9[19]	1346.5		1.50747	
318.15	970.183		1326.43		1.50499	
323.15	965.406	963.5[19]	1306.5		1.50253	
Tert-Butyl Methyl Ether						
293.15	740.757	740.585[20]	1059.23	1059.49[20]	1.36900	1.3678[22]
		740.910[22]	742.072[21]		1063.43[21]	
		740.62[23]				
298.15	735.507	735.337[20]	1035.98	1036.25[20]	1.36637	1.36628[24]
			736.826[21]		1040.35[21]	

TABLE 9.2 *(Continued)*

T (K)	ρ $(kg \cdot m^{-3})$ Exp	ρ Lit	u $(m \cdot s^{-1})$ Exp	u Lit	n_D Exp	n_D Lit
303.15	730.222	735.686[22]	1012.85	1013.17[20]	1.36371	1.3633[22]
		735.41[23]		1017.42[21]		
		735.56[24]				
		735.38[25]				
		730.042[20]				
		730.395[22]				
		730.11[23]				
		731.532[21]				
308.15	724.891	724.693[20]	990.04	990.25[20]	1.36112	
		726.185[21]				
		725.051[22]				
		724.77[23]				
		724.72[25]				
313.15	719.511	719.293[20]	967.22	967.35[20]	1.35851	1.3581[22]
		719.649[22]				
318.15	714.051	713.85[25]	944.43		1.35618	
323.15	708.511		921.80		1.35254	

Standard uncertainties u are: $u(\rho)=0.2$ kg·m⁻³, $u(u)=0.5$ m·s⁻¹, $u(n_D)=0.004$, and $u(T)=0.05$ K. All the experiments were carried out at 100.7 kPa pressure.

9.2.2 DENSITY AND SPEED OF SOUND MEASUREMENTS

Anton Paar DSA 5000 digital vibrating tube densimeter with inbuilt solid state thermostat controlling the temperature to ± 0.001 K was used to measure the density and speeds of sound simultaneously. The instrument was calibrated by ultrapure water and dry air prior to each measurement. In a previous publication,[4] we have reported the test system cyclohexane + benzene to check the performance of the system, the same system was investigated in the current study as well. The estimated uncertainty for the density and speeds of sound is lower than ± 0.2 kg·m^{-3} and ± 0.5 m·s^{-1}, respectively.

9.2.3 REFRACTIVE INDEX MEASUREMENTS

Measurement of n_D was carried out using Abbemat 300 automatic refractometer (Anton Paar GmbH) with an inbuilt temperature controller with ± 0.05 K accuracy. The calibration was performed by measuring the n_D of Millipore water at 298.15 K temperature. The calibration was performed at 298.15 K temperature, prior to the experiment. The estimated uncertainty was found to be less than ± 0.004.

9.2.4 PREDICTION OF REFRACTIVE INDEX

The n_D of the binary mixtures was predicted through the pure component n_D by employing several mixing rules, such as Gladstone–Dale (G-D),[26] Arago–Biot (A-B),[27] Heller (H),[28] Weiner (W),[29] Oster (Os),[30] Newton (N),[31] Lorentz–Lorenz (L-L),[32] and Eykman (EK).[33]

9.3 RESULTS AND DISCUSSION

In Table 9.2, we had compared our experimental ρ, u, and n_D of the pure DEA, ANS, and MTBE with literature values at all the studied temperatures. Experimental ρ, u, and n_D data for both the mixtures have been reported in Tables 9.3–9.5 at all the studied temperatures.

TABLE 9.3 Experimental Densities (ρ) of N,N-diethylaniline (DEA) with Anisole (ANS) and Tert-Butyl Methyl Ether (MTBE).

X_1 (g)	Temperature (K)						
	293.15	298.15	303.15	308.15	313.15	318.15	323.15
	Densities (ρ)/kg·m^{-3}						
N,N-diethylaniline (1) + Anisole (2)							
0.0000	993.844	989.133	984.418	979.690	974.945	970.183	965.406
0.1000	985.728	981.091	976.455	971.805	967.121	962.453	957.743
0.1994	978.241	973.707	969.156	964.601	960.033	955.451	950.842
0.2974	971.440	966.984	962.526	958.057	953.566	949.064	944.527
0.3991	964.825	960.440	956.060	951.668	947.262	942.845	938.414
0.4886	959.376	955.065	950.743	946.411	942.070	937.714	933.348
0.5882	953.693	949.440	945.183	940.916	936.639	932.354	928.055
0.6974	947.852	943.671	939.493	935.291	931.089	926.864	922.625
0.7980	942.841	938.716	934.576	930.442	926.295	922.138	917.969
0.8995	938.150	934.071	929.981	925.891	921.803	917.704	913.575
1.0000	933.680	929.668	925.653	921.629	917.597	913.556	909.505
N,N-diethylaniline (1) + Tert-butyl methyl ether (2)							
0.0000	740.757	735.507	730.222	724.891	719.511	714.051	708.511
0.1005	768.015	763.551	758.752	753.867	748.739	743.854	739.001
0.2015	793.214	789.203	784.766	780.237	775.612	770.885	766.286
0.3011	816.345	812.374	807.940	803.584	798.972	794.478	789.895
0.4015	837.583	833.555	829.245	824.896	820.505	816.111	811.749
0.5017	857.139	853.022	848.821	844.624	840.399	836.113	831.910
0.6025	875.254	871.389	867.244	863.114	859.097	854.919	850.899
0.7008	891.252	887.430	883.598	879.751	875.791	871.791	867.934
0.7988	906.011	902.406	898.567	894.575	891.033	887.277	883.479
0.8992	919.739	915.938	912.251	908.574	904.744	900.961	896.979
1.0000	933.680	929.668	925.653	921.629	917.597	913.556	909.505

Standard uncertainties $u(\rho)=0.2$ kg·m^{-3} and $u(T)=0.05$ K. All the experiments were carried out at 100.7 kPa pressure.

TABLE 9.4 Experimental Speed of Sound (u) of N,N-Diethylaniline (DEA) with Anisole (ANS) and Tert-Butyl Methyl Ether (MTBE).

X_1 (g)	Temperature (K)						
	293.15	298.15	303.15	308.15	313.15	318.15	323.15
	Speeds of Sound, u(m·s^{-1})						
N,N-diethylaniline (1) + Anisole (2)							
0.0000	1428.04	1407.42	1386.97	1366.67	1346.50	1326.43	1306.50
0.1000	1434.76	1414.14	1393.65	1373.28	1353.08	1333.02	1313.07
0.1994	1440.55	1419.95	1399.47	1379.13	1358.97	1338.93	1319.02
0.2974	1445.67	1425.10	1404.65	1384.36	1364.24	1344.24	1324.37
0.3991	1450.61	1430.08	1409.68	1389.45	1369.37	1349.41	1329.58
0.4886	1454.54	1434.06	1413.71	1393.51	1373.46	1353.55	1333.80
0.5882	1458.67	1438.24	1417.97	1397.83	1377.83	1358.00	1338.31
0.6974	1462.83	1442.47	1422.26	1402.18	1382.26	1362.51	1342.88
0.7980	1466.49	1446.17	1426.03	1406.03	1386.16	1366.48	1346.92
0.8995	1469.90	1449.64	1429.56	1409.61	1389.83	1370.20	1350.69
1.0000	1473.71	1453.55	1433.52	1413.64	1393.93	1374.35	1354.92
N,N-diethylaniline (1) + Tert-butyl methyl ether (2)							
0.0000	1059.23	1035.98	1012.85	990.04	967.22	944.43	921.80
0.1005	1114.16	1091.45	1068.89	1046.61	1024.36	1002.30	980.43
0.2015	1167.50	1145.34	1123.26	1101.34	1079.67	1058.08	1036.71
0.3011	1212.53	1190.39	1168.71	1147.15	1125.81	1104.72	1083.77
0.4015	1258.47	1237.03	1215.71	1194.52	1173.48	1152.58	1131.80
0.5017	1298.98	1277.81	1256.74	1235.86	1215.17	1194.65	1174.31
0.6025	1336.50	1319.79	1299.02	1278.40	1257.93	1237.63	1217.54
0.7008	1375.39	1354.70	1334.13	1313.71	1293.46	1273.35	1253.41
0.7988	1410.85	1390.34	1369.98	1349.76	1329.71	1309.80	1290.06
0.8992	1442.72	1422.39	1402.18	1382.12	1362.25	1342.52	1322.93
1.0000	1473.71	1453.55	1433.52	1413.64	1393.93	1374.35	1354.92

Standard uncertainties $u(u)$=0.5 m·s^{-1} and $u(T)$ =0.05 K. All the experiments were carried out at 100.7 kPa pressure.

TABLE 9.5 Experimental Refractive Index (n_D) of N,N-Diethylaniline (DEA) with Anisole (ANS) and Tert-Butyl Methyl Ether (MTBE).

X_1 (g)	Temperature (K)						
	293.15	298.15	303.15	308.15	313.15	318.15	323.15
	Refractive Index (n_D)						
N,N-diethylaniline (1) + Anisole (2)							
0.0000	1.51719	1.51478	1.51239	1.50993	1.50747	1.50499	1.50253
0.1000	1.52065	1.51798	1.51539	1.51281	1.51022	1.50762	1.50509
0.1994	1.52394	1.52132	1.51875	1.51613	1.51351	1.51082	1.50815
0.2974	1.52685	1.52424	1.52171	1.51911	1.51648	1.51389	1.51128
0.3991	1.52955	1.52698	1.52445	1.52188	1.51929	1.51666	1.51409
0.4886	1.53166	1.52903	1.52647	1.52388	1.52132	1.51868	1.51612
0.5882	1.53378	1.53108	1.52852	1.52592	1.52331	1.52066	1.51802
0.6974	1.53591	1.53324	1.53061	1.52798	1.52535	1.52276	1.52016
0.7980	1.53789	1.53524	1.53264	1.53007	1.52745	1.52486	1.52225
0.8995	1.53992	1.53733	1.53478	1.53222	1.52969	1.52717	1.52462
1.0000	1.54192	1.53944	1.53697	1.53450	1.53200	1.52951	1.52700
N,N-diethylaniline (1) + Tert-butyl methyl ether (2)							
0.0000	1.36900	1.36637	1.36371	1.36112	1.35851	1.35618	1.35254
0.1005	1.39441	1.39324	1.39234	1.39123	1.38962	1.38759	1.38468
0.2015	1.41982	1.41929	1.41863	1.41706	1.41554	1.41499	1.41251
0.3011	1.44226	1.44141	1.44067	1.43971	1.43808	1.43697	1.43506
0.4015	1.46086	1.45999	1.45942	1.45872	1.45727	1.45598	1.45443
0.5017	1.47659	1.47568	1.47561	1.47473	1.47385	1.47252	1.47182
0.6025	1.49096	1.49032	1.49012	1.48963	1.48901	1.48799	1.48729
0.7008	1.50421	1.50358	1.50262	1.50216	1.50211	1.50147	1.50073
0.7988	1.51678	1.51578	1.51468	1.51372	1.51311	1.51294	1.51226
0.8992	1.52922	1.52781	1.52641	1.52477	1.52355	1.52283	1.52106
1.0000	1.54192	1.53944	1.53697	1.53450	1.53200	1.52951	1.52700

Standard uncertainties $u(n_D) = 0.004$ and $u(T) = 0.05$ K. All the experiments were carried out at 100.7 kPa pressure.

Excess molar volumes V_m^E for both of the systems over the entire range of composition were calculated from the measured density results at $T = (293.15–323.15)$ K at 5 K interval and at atmospheric pressure using the equation:

$$V_m^E = \sum_{i=1}^{2} x_i M_i \left(\rho^{-1} - \rho_i^{-1} \right) \tag{9.1}$$

where ρ and ρ_i are the density of the pure and mixture component, respectively; x_i and M_i represent the mole fraction and molar mass of component i, respectively.

Isentropic compressibility κ_s, was calculated using Newton–Laplace equation[34] by:

$$\kappa_s = -V_m^{-1} \left(\frac{\partial V_m}{\partial P} \right)_s = \left(\rho u^2 \right)^{-1} = V_m \left(M u^2 \right)^{-1} \tag{9.2}$$

where u is the experimental speeds of sound and V_m is the molar volume of the mixture.

Molar isentropic compressibility $K_{s,m}$ [34,35] and excess molar isentropic compressibility $K_{s,m}^E$ were calculated according to the Equations 9.3 and 9.4, respectively.

$$K_{S,m} = -(\partial V_m / \partial P)_S = V_m \kappa_S = M_m / (\rho u)^2 \tag{9.3}$$

$$K_{S,m}^E = K_{S,m} - K_{S,m}^{id} \tag{9.4}$$

where $K_{s,m}^{id}$ is the molar isentropic compressibility of ideal solution that can be calculated as:

$$K_{S,m}^{id} = \sum_{i=1}^{2} x_i \left[K_{S,i}^* + T(E_{p,i}^{*2} / C_{p,i}^*) \right] - T \left[\sum x_i E_{p,i}^* \right)^2 / \sum x_i C_{p,i}^* \right] \tag{9.5}$$

where $E_{p,i}^*$ (expansibility), $C_{p,i}^*$ (isobaric molar heat capacity), and $K_{s,m}^*$ (molar isentropic compressibility) are variable parameters of the pure liquid component i, respectively.

Rao's molar sound function[36] R, with an estimated uncertainty of 0.2%, was obtained from following relation:

$$R = u^{1/3} V_m \tag{9.6}$$

Experimental refractive index of the pure components of the mixtures, $n_{D,i}$ and their binary mixtures, n_D, were used to calculate the deviation in refractive index Δn_D by:

$$\Delta n_D = n_D - \sum x_i n_{D,i} \qquad (9.7)$$

where x_i is the mole fraction of the component i.

Excess thermodynamic properties were correlated by Redlich–Kister polynomial equation:

$$Y^E = x_1 \left(1 - x_1\right) \sum_{i=1}^{n} B_i \left(1 - 2x_1\right)^{i-1} \qquad (9.8)$$

The coefficient B_i of Equation 9.8 at different temperatures for both mixtures are given in Table 9.6.

TABLE 9.6 Temperature Dependence of B_i of Eq. (9.8) for Excess Molar Volume V_m^E(m³/mol), Excess Molar Isentropic Compressibilities $K_{S,m}^E$(dm³/TPa·mol), and Deviation in Refractive Index Δn_D Along with Their Standard Deviation (σ).

T (K)	B_1	B_2	B_3	B_4	σ
N,N-diethylaniline + Anisole					
$V_m^E (\times 10^6$ m³/mol)					
293.15	−0.3595	−0.1230	-0.0490	0.1753	0.0034
298.15	−0.3553	−0.1232	-0.0129	0.1740	0.0025
303.15	−0.3514	−0.1164	0.0354	0.1427	0.0022
308.15	−0.3457	−0.1192	0.0665	0.1464	0.0016
313.15	−0.3407	−0.1301	0.1029	0.2010	0.0015
318.15	−0.3313	−0.1334	0.1088	0.2039	0.0012
323.15	−0.3250	−0.1218	0.1705	0.1840	0.0008
$K_{S,m}^E$ (dm³/TPa·mol)					
293.15	−0.3173	−0.3095	0.1761	−0.4865	0.0039
298.15	−0.2816	−0.3124	0.2366	−0.5570	0.0043
303.15	−0.2368	−0.2874	0.2815	−0.5951	0.0048
308.15	−0.1891	−0.2886	0.3641	−0.5715	0.0066
313.15	−0.1326	−0.3271	0.4239	−0.5001	0.0072
318.15	−0.0802	−0.3031	0.4306	−0.5504	0.0081
323.15	−0.0247	−0.2801	0.5330	−0.6070	0.0095

TABLE 9.6 *(Continued)*

T (K)	B_1	B_2	B_3	B_4	σ
Δn_D					
293.15	0.0094	0.0056	−0.0019	−0.0033	0.00002
298.15	0.0087	0.0065	−0.0039	−0.0061	0.00003
303.15	0.0083	0.0072	−0.0056	−0.0083	0.00003
308.15	0.0078	0.0072	−0.0066	−0.0087	0.00004
313.15	0.0073	0.0075	−0.0073	−0.0101	0.00003
318.15	0.0067	0.0075	−0.0078	−0.0111	0.00001
323.15	0.0062	0.0072	−0.0082	−0.0111	0.00005
N,N-diethylaniline + Tert-butyl methyl ether					
$V_m^E(int)$ ($\times 10^6$ m³/mol)					
293.15	−3.6570	−0.1439	1.3868	−1.6630	0.0196
298.15	−4.1579	−0.3912	0.5522	−1.8674	0.0330
303.15	−4.5083	−0.5527	−0.2029	−1.5186	0.0280
308.15	−4.8859	−0.8691	−0.8676	−0.8344	0.0268
313.15	−5.3382	−0.7607	−1.1555	−0.6446	0.0385
318.15	−5.7302	−0.7723	−1.9527	−0.7028	0.0352
323.15	−6.2493	−0.5418	−2.5191	−1.7331	0.0389
$K_{S,m}^E$ (dm³/TPa·mol)					
293.15	−58.0168	−24.2652	−10.1974	−1.4607	0.1833
298.15	−64.6744	−25.8537	−11.3038	−5.0238	0.2010
303.15	−71.3751	−29.1237	−13.5224	−5.7544	0.2177
308.15	−78.7000	−32.6962	−15.9263	−6.5820	0.2276
313.15	−87.0510	−36.8374	−18.2972	−7.1694	0.2630
318.15	−96.3760	−41.5174	−21.9751	−9.0708	0.2646
323.15	−106.8748	−46.5981	−26.2469	−12.3698	0.2797
Δn_D					
293.15	0.0857	0.0477	−0.0218	−0.0391	0.00037
298.15	0.0927	0.0473	−0.0105	−0.0340	0.00039
303.15	0.1006	0.0471	−0.0001	−0.0264	0.00015
308.15	0.1076	0.0404	0.0075	−0.0099	0.00021
313.15	0.1139	0.0308	0.0172	0.0023	
318.15	0.1194	0.0321	0.0291	−0.0144	0.00030
323.15	0.1280	0.0246	0.0287	−0.0058	0.00028

The standard deviations for the studied parameters m and with N experimental points were calculated by:

$$\sigma = \left[\sum_{i=1}^{M} \left(X_{calc} - X_{exp} \right)^2 / (N-m) \right]^{0.5}$$ (9.9)

Here, we had reported the excess molar volume (V_m^E), excess molar isentropic compressibilities ($K_{s,m}^E$), Rao's molar sound functions (R), and deviation in refractive index (Δn_D) for both of the systems over the entire range of composition and at all the temperatures studied.

Graphical representations of V_m^E against the mole fraction of DEA for both of the studied mixtures are presented in Figures 9.1 and 9.2. For both of the mixtures, V_m^E were negative at all the temperatures and over the entire range of compositions. For the mixture containing ANS, V_m^E decreased negatively with temperature, whereas for the MTBE, the V_m^E increased negatively with increasing temperature from 293.15 K to 323.15 K. The maximum V_m^E were found to be -0.0912×10^{-6} and -1.0067×10^{-6} m$^3 \cdot$mol^{-1} for the mixtures containing ANS and MTBE, respectively, near 0.4 mole fraction of the DEA at 298.15 K.

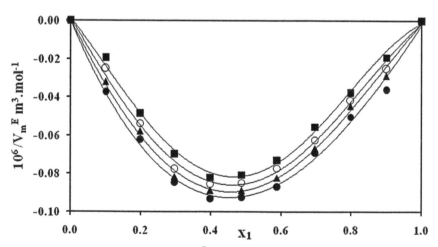

FIGURE 9.1 Excess molar volumes (V_m^E) for N,N-Diethyl aniline + Anisole at 293.15 K (•), 303.15 K (▲), 313.15 K (○), and 323.15 K (■). Solid lines have been drawn from Equation 9.8 using the coefficients given in Table 9.6.

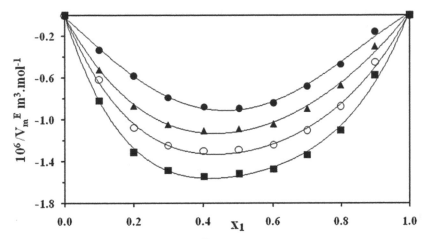

FIGURE 9.2   Excess molar volumes (V_m^E) for N,N-Diethyl aniline + Tert-butyl methyl ether at 293.15 K (●), 303.15 K (▲), 313.15 K (○), and 323.15 K (■). Solid lines have been drawn from Equation 9.8 using the coefficients given in Table 9.6.

Manukonda[14] reported negative V_m^E in the mixtures of aliphatic ketones as well as for the lower alkyl chain length (C_1–C_4) ketones with DEA. In the current investigation, maximum V_m^E was found to be the lowest (-0.0912×10^{-6} $m^3 \cdot mol^{-1}$) negative for ANS as compared to the ketones and alcohols.[37] The order of the magnitude of V_m^E in the mixture of DEA with organic solvents were found as: propanoic acid < Di-isopropyl Ether (DIPE) < acetone < MTBE < methyl propyl ketone < diethyl ketone < methyl isobutyl ketone at 303.15 K.[13,14]

Comparative graph for V_m^E of DEA + ANS and MTBE with diethylketone, 2-propanone, acetone, and DIPE is represented in Figure 9.3. The observed negative V_m^E between the DEA and ethers may be due to the dipole–dipole interaction between the component organic mixtures, structural effect, and formation of charge transfer complex in DEA.[38–43] The lone pairs of electron on the N atom of the DEA resulted in the specific interaction with the ether.[36] The much lower V_m^E of MTBE than that of ANS may be due to higher dipole moment of MTBE (1.32 D) as compared to the ANS (1.24 D). Structural effect such as the interstitial accommodation of the comparatively smaller ANS ($V_m = 118.14 \times 10^{-6}$ $m^3 \cdot mol^{-1}$) than that of MTBE ($V_m = 119.15 \times 10^{-6}$ $m^3 \cdot mol^{-1}$) in DEA contribute to the negative V_m^E, but this effect is reasonably lower than that of other specific interaction and dipole–dipole interaction between the mixture of amines and ethers. Similar observations were made in the system of MTBE with alcohols[44] and aromatic hydrocarbons.[15]

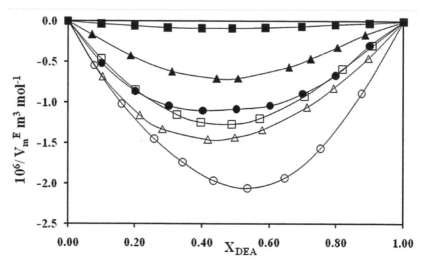

FIGURE 9.3   Comparison of excess molar volume (V_m^E) for N,N-diethyl aniline + ANS (■), + diethylketone (▲), + MTBE (●), + 2-propanone (□), + acetone (△), and + DIPE (○) at 303.15 K.

At fixed temperature, speeds of sound for both the systems increases as the composition of the DEA increases (Table 9.4), which indicate more close packing as the concentration of the DEA increases. At fix composition of the mixture, speeds of sound decrease with increasing temperature in all the studied mixtures. This may be due to the fact that as the temperature increases, more spaces are available for the smaller molecules (MTBE and ANS) to get accommodated in the DEA. The observation was supported by the negative V_m^E data, which also increases as the temperature increases. Figures 9.4 and 9.5 represent the $K_{s,m}^E$ with respect to the composition of the mixtures. $K_{s,m}^E$ for the ANS decreases with temperature and for the MTBE, $K_{s,m}^E$ increases with temperature from 293.15 to 323.15 K. For the mixture containing ANS, the curve of $K_{s,m}^E$ was found to be sigmoid (positive in the DEA rich region). R, calculated from the experimental ρ and u, increases as the concentration of the DEA increases and remains unchanged with temperature for the fixed composition. Further, slight negative deviations from the mole fraction additivity were observed in R.

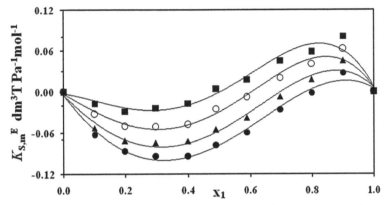

FIGURE 9.4   Excess molar isentropic compressibilities ($K_{s,m}^E$) for N,N-Diethyl aniline + Anisole at 293.15 K (●), 303.15 K (▲), 313.15 K (○), and 323.15 K (■). Solid lines have been drawn from Equation 9.8 using the coefficients given in Table 9.6.

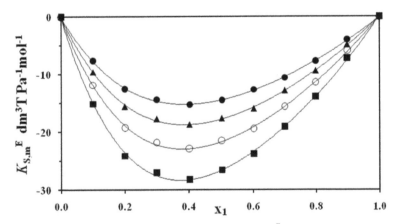

FIGURE 9.5   Excess molar isentropic compressibilities ($K_{s,m}^E$) for N,N-Diethyl aniline + Tert-butyl methyl ether at 293.15 K (●), 303.15 K (▲), 313.15 K (○), and 323.15 K (■). Solid lines have been drawn from Equation 9.8 using the coefficients given in Table 9.6.

As reported in Table 9.5, n_D for both the mixtures decreases with increasing temperature at the fixed composition of the mixtures. n_D also increases as the concentration of the DEA increases in the mixtures at all the studied temperatures. As the general observations, Δn_D was found to be positive if V_m^E was negative.[45–49] Current study fit perfectly for such observations. Δn_D was found to be positive for both of the systems in the entire range of composition and represented graphically in Figures 9.6 and 9.7.

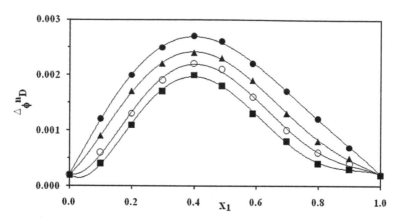

FIGURE 9.6   Deviation in Refractive index (Δn_D) in N,N-Diethyl aniline + Anisole at 293.15 K (●), 303.15 K (▲), 313.15 K (○), and 323.15 K (■). Solid lines have been drawn from Equation 9.8 using the coefficients given in Table 9.6.

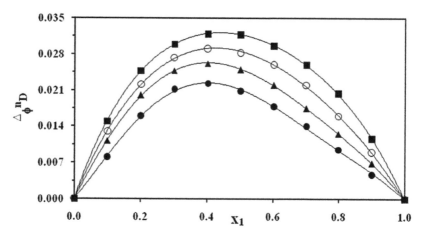

FIGURE 9.7   Deviation in Refractive index (Δn_D) in N,N-Diethyl aniline + Tert-butyl methyl ether at 293.15 K (●), 303.15 K (▲), 313.15 K (○), and 323.15 K (■). Solid lines have been drawn from Equation 9.8 using the coefficients given in Table 9.6.

Among the several mixing rules proposed to estimate the refractive index of the mixtures from the pure components, L-L relation have been the best fit with the experimental refractive index. Predicted refractive indices follow the sequence L-L > H > W > G-D > A-B > Os > N > EK as far as the agreement concerned.

9.4 THE PRIGOGINE–FLORY–PATTERSON (PFP) THEORY

The Prigogine–Flory–Patterson (PFP) statistical theory of nonelectrolyte liquid mixtures has been commonly and successfully employed to calculate the V_m^E of the liquid mixtures.[50–62] According to PFP theory, V_m^E is divided into three contributional terms: (i) interactional contribution, V_m^E (int), (ii) a free volume contribution, V_m^E (fv), and (iii) P* contribution, V_m^E (P*). According to PFP theory, a molecule is made up of equal portions having contact sites interacting with the neighboring sites in numbers r.

$$\frac{V_m^E}{\sum_{i=1}^{2} x_i V_i^*} = \frac{(\tilde{V}^{1/3} - 1)\tilde{V}^{2/3}\psi_1\theta_2\chi_{12}}{\left[(4/3)\tilde{V}^{-1/3} - 1\right]P_1^*} \left(\text{Interactional Contribution}\right)$$

$$-\frac{(\tilde{V}_1 - \tilde{V}_2)^2\left[(14/9)\tilde{V}^{-1/3} - 1\right]\psi_1\psi_2}{\left[(4/3)\tilde{V}^{-1/3} - 1\right]\tilde{V}} \left(\begin{array}{c}\text{Free Volume}\\\text{Contribution}\end{array}\right)$$

$$+\frac{(\tilde{V}_1 - \tilde{V}_2)(P_1^* - P_2^*)\psi_1\psi_2}{P_2^*\psi_1 + P_1^*\psi_2} \left(P^*\text{Contribution}\right) \qquad (9.10)$$

The values of Flory's parameters, reduced volume of the pure components ($\tilde{V}$), molecular contact energy fraction of components (ψ_i), characteristic volume (V_i^*), characteristic pressure (P_i^*), hard-core volume fractions of pure components (ϕ_i), molecular surface fraction (θ_2), and the molecular surface to volume ratio (S) used in the theoretical calculations are defined elsewhere[3] and reported in Table 9.7. In all these calculations, the required contact interaction parameter χ_{12} is considered the only adjustable parameter, which can be obtained from the experimental H_m^E or V_m^E. In the current investigation, we had used the experimental V_m^E to obtain the χ_{12} and were negative for DEA + ANS and positive at lower temperatures and then became negative at the higher temperatures for DEA + MTBE. As reported in Table 9.8, χ_{12} increases as the temperature increases for DEA + ANS, whereas it decreases as the temperature increases for DEA + MTBE binary mixtures. Such kind of behavior in both of the mixtures are very well correlated with the experimental results, as the temperature increases, V_m^E for DEA + ANS increases from -0.0930×10^{-6} to -0.0817×10^{-6} m^3·mol^{-1}, whereas V_m^E decreases from -0.8908×10^{-6} to -1.5375×10^{-6} m^3·mol^{-1} as the temperature increases from 293.15 K to 323.15 K. The compatible values of the contact interaction parameter, three contributional terms

TABLE 9.7 Pure Component Thermal Expansion Coefficient, α, and Molar Heat Capacity, C_p, Along with the Flory's Interaction Parameters Such as: Isothermal Compressibility k_T, Characteristic Volume, V^*, Reduce Volume, $\tilde{V}$, Pressure, P^*, and Molecular Surface to Volume Ratio S at Temperature Range from 293.15 to 323.15 K.

Component	T/K	$10^4 \alpha$ (K^{-1})	10^4 kT (M/Pa)	10^6 V* (m³/mol)	$\tilde{V}$	P*	C_p	S^a (nm^{-1})
DEA	293.15	8.630	6.152	131.47	159.84	607.88	286.0[b]	12.84
	298.15	8.667	6.337	131.61	160.53	606.63	288.5[b]	12.84
	303.15	8.705	6.530	131.76	161.23	605.10	291.0[10]	12.84
	308.15	8.743	6.729	131.91	161.23	603.34	293.5[b]	12.84
	313.15	8.781	6.935	132.06	161.93	601.35	296.0[10]	12.84
	318.15	8.820	7.150	132.22	163.36	599.10	298.5[b]	12.84
	323.15	8.859	7.372	132.39	164.09	596.63	301.0[10]	12.84
Anisole	293.15	9.535	6.494	88.12	108.81	658.84	189.0[b]	12.74
	298.15	9.581	6.700	88.24	109.33	662.57	197.5[b]	12.74
	303.1	9.627	6.912	88.35	109.85	665.52	206.0[26]	12.74
	308.15	9.673	7.133	88.47	109.85	667.75	214.5[b]	12.74
	313.15	9.720	7.362	88.60	110.38	669.26	223.0[b]	12.74
	318.15	9.768	7.600	88.72	111.46	670.07	231.5[b]	12.74
	323.15	9.816	7.848	88.85	112.02	670.25	240.0[b]	12.74
MTBE	293.15	14.497	15.977	89.55	119.00	469.73	185.9[24]	14.29
	298.15	14.601	16.731	89.78	119.85	463.70	187.5[24]	14.29
		14.230[52]	16.906[52]	90.20[52]	119.88[52]	442.90[52]		

TABLE 9.7 *(Continued)*

Component	T/K	$10^4\,\alpha$ (K^{-1})	$10^4\,kT$ (M/Pa)	$10^6\,V^a$ (m^3/mol)	$\tilde{V}$	P^*	C_p	S^a (nm^{-1})
	303.15	14.706	17.534	90.01	120.72	457.34	189.2[24]	14.29
	308.15	14.815	18.384	90.26	121.60	450.77	190.8[24]	14.29
	313.15	14.925	19.295	90.51	122.51	443.78	192.6[b]	14.29
	318.15	15.039	20.274	90.79	123.45	436.39	194.3[b]	14.29
	323.15	15.157	21.322	91.07	124.42	428.71	196.0[b]	14.29

[a]Calculated as per Bondi (Ref. 63).
[b]Calculated as per group additive method from the available literature data.
[c]C_p in Ref 64 is at 304.65 K.

V_m^E (fv), V_m^E (P^*), and V_m^E (int) at equimolar composition and the standard deviation σ (V_m^E) between the experimental V_m^E and the theoretical ($V_{s,m}^E$) at all studied temperatures are recorded in Table 9.8.

TABLE 9.8 Values of Flory Interaction Parameter χ_{12}, Three Contributions V_m^E(int), V_m^E(ip), V_m^E(fv) in Equation (9.18), Theoretical Excess Molar Volume V_{PFP}^E at $x=0.5$, Standard Deviation $\sigma(V_m^E)$ at 293.15 K and 323.15 K.

Temp (K)	χ_{12} (J/cm³)	$10^6 V_m^E$ (int) (m³/mol)	$10^6 V_m^E$ (ip) (m³/mol)	$10^6 V_m^E$ (fv) (m³/mol)	$\sigma(V_m^E)^a$
N,N-diethylaniline + Anisole					
293.15	−8.79	−0.1166	0.0385	−0.0145	0.005
298.15	−8.63	−0.1132	0.0391	−0.0150	0.004
303.15	−8.39	−0.1089	0.0397	−0.0156	0.005
308.15	−8.20	−0.1054	0.0403	−0.0162	0.006
313.15	−7.99	−0.1019	0.0408	−0.0168	0.007
318.15	−7.81	−0.0991	0.0414	−0.0174	0.008
323.15	−7.44	−0.0933	0.0419	−0.0181	0.010
N,N-diethylaniline + Tert-butyl methyl ether					
293.15	17.95	0.3764	−0.7539	−0.4763	0.1361
298.15	12.22	0.2647	−0.8012	0.4937	0.1245
303.15	8.37	0.1874	−0.8515	−0.5116	0.1447
308.15	4.82	0.1114	−0.9040	−0.5299	0.1754
313.15	1.62	0.0316	−0.9606	−0.5486	0.2402
318.15	−1.67	−0.0414	−1.0214	−0.5679	0.2851
323.15	−4.96	−0.1270	−1.0861	−0.5878	0.3278

[a]σ represents the standard deviation between experimental and theoretical   over the whole composition range.

The first term, V_m^E (int) represents interaction between unlike components of the mixtures, is negative for DEA + ANS at all the studied temperatures, whereas it is positive up to 313.15 K after that it became negative for the DEA + MTBE. The second term V_m^E (fv), describing the geometrical accommodation in the binary mixture, is negative for both of the mixtures and is in the order: ANS < MTBE (Table 9.8). V_m^E (fv) is proportional to $(\tilde{V}_1 - \tilde{V}_2)^2$. Here, $\left|\tilde{V}_1 - \tilde{V}_2\right|$ is larger for DEA + MTBE than for DEA + ANS. Therefore, the term V_m^E (fv) is comparatively larger negative for DEA+MTBE than that for DEA + ANS. The third term V_m^E (P^*), depends on the relative cohesive energy of the expanded and less expanded component, is positive for DEA + ANS and negative for DEA + MTBE. As reported in Table 9.8, (V_m^E) between the experimental V_m^E and the theoretical V_{PFP}^E at all the studied temperatures varies from 0.004 to 0.010 for the mixture containing ANS, whereas for MTBE containing binary mixture, it varies from 0.1245 to 0.3278.

9.5 CONCLUSION

The experimental density, speeds of sound, and refractive index of pure and binary mixtures of tertiary amine (N,N-diethylaniline) with aryl (ANS) and alkyl (MTBE) ether have been measured over the entire composition range and at temperatures (293.15–323.15) K. Experimental results were used to calculate various thermodynamic functions and excess functions and correlated using Redlich–Kister type polynomial equation. The results of V_m^E were compared with the theoretical predictions of PFP theory. The signs and magnitude of various quantities have been discussed in terms of dipole–dipole interactions, structural effects, and complex formation between the component molecules. L-L equation for the refractive index was found to be having good agreement with the experimental results.

9.6 ACKNOWLEDGMENT

N.I.M. and Z.S.V acknowledges Department of Science and Technology, New Delhi and Maulana Azad National Fellowship for providing the financial assistance through grants No. SR/FT/CS-014/2010 and F1-17.1/2012-13/MANF-2012-13-MUS-GUJ-10818, respectively to carry out this work. Financial assistance by Council of Scientific and Industrial Research (CSIR), New Delhi through grant No. 01 (2545)/11/EMR-II is also acknowledged. Financial assistance through Institute Research Grants to the Assistant Professors by SVNIT is also acknowledged.

KEYWORDS

- **N, N-diethylaniline**
- **excess molar volume**
- **excess molar isentropic compressibilities**
- **Prigogine–Flory–Patterson theory**

REFERENCES

1. Malek, N. I.; Ijardar, S. P.; Master, Z. R.; Oswal, S. B. Temperature Dependence of Densities, Speeds Of Sound, and Derived Properties of Cyclohexylamine + Cyclohexane or Benzene in the Temperature Range 293.15–323.15 K. *Thermochim. Acta.* **2012,** *547*, 106–119.
2. Oswal, S. L.; Desai, J. S.; Ijardar, S. P.; Malek, N. I. Studies of Viscosities of Dilute Solutions of Alkylamine in Non-electrolyte Solvents. II. Haloalkanes and Other Polar Solvents. *Thermochim. Acta.* **2005,** *427*, 51–60.
3. Ijardar, S. P.; Malek, N. I.; Oswal, S. L. Studies on Volumetric Properties of Triethylamine in Organic Solvents with Varying Polarity. *Indian J. Chem.* **2011,** *50A*, 1709–1718.
4. Malek, N. I.; Ijardar, S. P.; Oswal , S. B. Volumetric and Acoustic Properties of Binary Mixtures of Cyclohexane + Benzene and + Benzaldehyde at (293.15–323.15) K. *Thermochim. Acta.* **2012,** *539*, 71–83.
5. Pandiyan, V.; Oswal, S. L.; Malek, N. I.; Vasantharani, P. Thermodynamic and Acoustic Properties of Binary Mixtures of Ethers. V. Diisopropyl Ether or Oxolane with 2- or 3-Chloroanilines at 303.15, 313.15 and 323.15 K. *Thermochim. Acta.* **2011,** *524*, 140–150.
6. Ijardar, S. P.; Malek, N. I. Experimental and Theoretical Excess Molar Properties of Imidazolium Based Ionic Liquids with Molecular Organic Solvents–I. 1-Hexyl-3-Methylimidazlouim Tetraflouroborate and 1-octyl-3-methylimidazlouim Tetraflouroborate with Cyclic Ethers. *J. Chem. Thermodyn.* **2014,** *71*, 236–248.
7. Nietzki, R.; Collin, A.; Richarson, W. *Chemistry of the Organic dye-Stuffs*; Taylor and Francis: London, 1888.
8. Fiege, H.; Voges, H. W.; Hamamoto, T.; Umemura, S.; Iwata, T.; Miki, H.; Fujita, Y.; Buysch, H. J.; Garbe, D.; Paulus, W. *Phenol Derivatives, Ullmann's Encyclopedia of Industrial Chemistry*; Wiley-VCH: Weinheim, 2002.
9. Master, Z. R.; Vaid, Z. S.; More, U. U.; Malek, N. I. Molecular Interaction Study Through Experimental and Theoretical Volumetric, Transport and Refractive Properties of N-Ethylaniline with Aryl and Alkyl Ethers at Several Temperatures. *Phy. Chem. Liq.* **2015**. DOI: 10.1080/00319104.2015.1074047.

10. Palepu, R.; Oliver, J.; Campbell, D. Thermodynamic and Transport Properties of O-chlorophenol with Aniline and N-alkylanilines. *J. Chem. Eng. Data.* **1985,** *30,* 355–360.

11. Pandiyan, V.; Oswal, S. L.; Vasantharani, P. Thermodynamic and Acoustic Properties of Binary Mixtures of Ethers. IV. Diisopropyl Ether or Oxolane with N,N-dimethylaniline or N,N-diethylaniline at 303.15, 313.15 and 323.15 K. *Thermochim. Acta.* **2011,** *518,* 36–46.

12. Reid, T. M.; Prausnitz, J. M.; Poling, B. E. *The Properties of Gases and Liquids,* 4th ed.; McGraw Hill: New York, 1987.

13. Kondaiah, M.; Sravana Kumar, D.; Sreekanth, K.; Krishna Rao, D. Densities and Viscosities of Binary Mixtures of Propanoic Acid with N,N-Dimethylaniline and N,N-Diethylaniline at T = (303.15, 313.15, and 323.15) K. *J. Chem. Eng. Data.* **2012,** *57,* 352–357.

14. Manukonda, G. S.; Ponneri, V.; Kasibhatta, K. S.; Sakamuri, S. R. B. Thermodynamics of Amine + Ketone Mixtures: Volumetric, Speed of Sound Data and Viscosity at 303.15 K and 308.15 K for the Binary Mixtures of N,N-Diethylaniline + Aliphatic Ketones (C3–C5) + 4-methyl-2-pentanone. *Arab. J. Chem.* DOI: http://dx.doi.org/10.1016/j.arabjc.2013.09.042.

15. Viswanathan, S.; Rao, M. A.; Prasad, D. H. L. Densities and Viscosities of Binary Liquid Mixtures of Anisole or Methyl tert-Butyl Ether with Benzene, Chlorobenzene, Benzonitrile, and Nitrobenzene. *J. Chem. Eng. Data.* **2000,** *45,* 764–770.

16. Joshi, S. S.; Aminabhavi, T. M. Densities and Viscosities of Binary Liquid Mixtures of Anisole with Methanol and Benzene. *J. Chem. Eng. Data.* **1990,** *35,* 187–189.

17. Joshi, S. S.; Aminabhavi, T. M. Densities and Shear Viscosities of Anisole with Nitrobenzene, Chlorobenzene, Carbon Tetrachloride, 1,2-Dichloroethane, and Cyclohexane from 25 to 40°C. *J. Chem. Eng. Data.* **1990,** *35,* 247–253.

18. Baragi, J. G.; Aralaguppi, M. I.; Aminabhavi, T. M.; Kariduraganavar, M. Y.; Kittur, A. S. Density, Viscosity, Refractive Index, and Speed of Sound for Binary Mixtures of Anisole with 2-Chloroethanol, 1,4-Dioxane, Tetrachloroethylene, Tetrachloroethane, DMF, DMSO, and Diethyl Oxalate at (298.15, 303.15, and 308.15) K. *J. Chem. Eng. Data.* **2005,** *50,* 910–916.

19. Weng, W. Viscosities and Densities for Binary Mixtures of Anisole with 1-Butanol, 1-Pentanol, 1-Hexanol, 1-Heptanol, and 1-Octanol. *J. Chem. Eng. Data.* **1999,** *44,* 63–66.

20. Montano, D.; Bolts, R.; Gmehling, J.; Artigas, H.; Lafuente, C. Calorimetric and Acoustic Study of Binary Mixtures Containing an Isomeric Chlorobutane and Butyl Ethyl Ether or Methyl Tert-Butyl Ether. *J. Therm. Anal. Calorim.* In Press. DOI: 10.1007/s10973-015-4797-4.

21. Pal, A.; Kumar, H.; Sharma, S.; Maan, R.; Sharma, H. K. Mixing Properties for Binary Liquid Mixtures of Methyl tert-Butyl Ether with Propylamine and Dipropylamine at Temperatures from (288.15 to 308.15) K. *J. Chem. Eng. Data.* **2010,** *55,* 1424–1429.

22. Li, D.; Qin, X.; Fang, W.; Guo, M.; Wang, H.; Feng, Y. Densities, Viscosities and Refractive Indices of Binary Liquid Mixtures of Methyl Tert-Butyl Ether or Ethyl Tert-Butyl Ether with a Hydrocarbon Fuel. *Exp. Therm. Fluid. Sci.* **2013,** *48,* 163–168.

23. Hoga, H. E.; Torres, R. B. Volumetric and Viscometric Properties of Binary Mixtures of {methyl tert-butyl ether (MTBE) + alcohol} at Several Temperatures and p=0.1 MPa: Experimental Results and Application of the ERAS Model. *J. Chem. Thermodyn.* **2011,** *43,* 1104–1134.

24. Gomez-Marigliano, A. C.; Arce, A.; Rodil, E.; Soto, A. Isobaric Vapor–Liquid Equilibria at 101.32 kPa and Densities, Speeds of Sound, and Refractive Indices at 298.15 K for MTBE or DIPE or TAME + 1-Propanol Binary Systems. *J. Chem. Eng. Data.* **2010,** *55,* 92–97.

25. Domanska, U.; Zolek-Tryznowska, Z. Measurements of the Density and Viscosity of Binary Mixtures of (hyper-branched polymer, B-H2004 + 1-butanol, or 1-hexanol, or 1-octanol, or methyl tert-butyl ether). *J. Chem. Thermodyn.* **2010,** *42,* 651–658.

26. Dale, T. P.; Gladstone, J. H. On the Influence of Temperature on the Refraction of Light. *Phil. Trans. R. Soc. Lond.* **1858,** *148,* 887–894.

27. Arago, D. F.J.; Biot, J. B. *Mem. Acad. Fr.* **1806,** *1806,* 7–11.

28. Heller, W. J. Remarks on Refractive Index Mixture Rules. *J. Phys. Chem.* **1965,** *69,* 1123–1129.

29. Weiner, O. Berichte (Leipzig) **1910,** *62,* 256–262.

30. Oster, G. *Chem. Rev.* **1948,** *43,* 319.

31. Pineiro, A.; Brocos, P.; Amigo, A.; Pintos, M.; Bravo, R. Prediction of Excess Volumes and Excess Surface Tensions From Experimental Refractive Indices. *Phys. Chem. Liq.* **2000,** *38,* 251–260.

32. Lorentz, H. A. *The Theory of Electrons,* 2nd edn.; Teubner: Leipzig, 1916.

33. Eykman, J. F. Rec. *Trav. Chim. Pays-Bas* **1895,** *14,* 887–894.

34. Douheret, G.; Davis, M. I.; Reis, J. C. R.; Blandamer, M. J. Isentropic Compressibilities—Experimental Origin and the Quest for their Rigorous Estimation in Thermodynamically Ideal Liquid Mixtures. *Chem. Phys. Chem.* **2001,** *2,* 148–161.

35. Douheret, G.; Davis, M. I.; Reis, J. C. R.; Fjellanger, I. J.; Vaage, M. B.; Hoiland, H. Aggregative Processes in Aqueous Solutions of Isomeric 2-butoxyethanols at 298.15 K. *Phys. Chem. Chem. Phys.* **2002,** *4,* 6034–6042.

36. Rao, M. R. Velocity of Sound in Liquids and Chemical Constitution. *J. Chem. Phys.* **1941,** *9,* 682–685.

37. Gowrisankar, M.; Venkateswarlu, P.; Siva kumar, K.; Sivarambabu, S. Density, Ultrasonic Velocity, Viscosity and Their Excess Parameters of the Binary Mixtures of N,N- diethyl aniline with 1-Alkanols (C3-C5), + 2-Alkanols (C3-C4) at 303.15 K. *Int. J. Sci. Eng. Res.* **2013,** *4,* 1008–1027.

38. Canosa, J.; Rodrıguez, A.; Tojo, J. Binary Mixture Properties of Diethyl Ether with Alcohols and Alkanes from 288.15 K to 298.15 K. *Fluid Phase Equilib.* **1999,** *156,* 57–71.

39. Rezanova, E. N.; Lichtenthaler, R. N. Excess Properties of Binary Mixtures of an Alkanol or an Alkane with Butyl-Vinyl Ether Oriso-Butyl-Vinyl Ether. *J. Chem. Thermodyn.* **2000,** *32,* 517–528.

40. Letcher, T. M.; Govender, P. U. The Excess Molar Volumes of (an alkanol + a branched chain ether) at the Temperature 298.15 K and the Application of the ERAS Model. *Fluid Phase Equilib.* **1997,** *140,* 207–220.

41. Kammerer, K.; Oswald, G.; Rezanova, E.; Silkenbaumer, D.; Lichtenthaler, R. N. Thermodynamic Excess Properties and Vapor–Liquid Equilibria of Binary and Ternary Mixtures Containing Methanol, Tert-Amyl Methyl Ether and an Alkane. *Fluid Phase Equilib.* **2000,** *167,* 223–241.

42. Roy, M. N.; Sinha, A.; Sinha, B. Excess Molar Volumes, Viscosity Deviations and Isentropic Compressibility of Binary Mixtures Containing 1,3-Dioxolane and Mono-alcohols at 303.15 K. *J. Solution Chem.* **2005,** *34,* 1311–1325.

43. Bernazzani, L.; Ceccanti, N.; Conti, G.; Gianni, P.; Mollica, V.; Tine, M. R.; Lepori, L.; Matteoli, E.; Spanedda, A. Volumetric Properties of (an organic compound + di-n-butyl ether) at T = 298.15 K. *J. Chem. Thermodyn.* **2001,** *33,* 629–641.

44. Pal, A.; Dass, G. Excess Molar Volumes and Viscosities for Binary Liquid Mixtures of Methyl tert-Butyl Ether and of tert-Amyl Methyl Ether with Methanol, 1-Propanol, and 1-Pentanol at 298.15 K. *J. Chem. Eng. Data.* **1999,** *44,* 1325–1329.

45. Ali, A.; Nain, A. K.; Kamil, M. Physico-Chemical Studies of Non-Aqueous Binary Liquid Mixtures at Various Temperatures. *Thermochim. Acta.* **1996,** *274,* 209–221.

46. Nakata, M.; Sakurai, M. Refractive Index and Excess Volume for Binary Liquid Mixtures. Part 1. Analyses of New and Old Data for Binary Mixtures. *J. Chem. Faraday Trans.* **1987,** *83,* 2449–2487.

47. Orge, B.; Marino, G.; Iglesias, M.; Tojo, J.; Pineiro, M. M. Thermodynamics of (anisole + benzene, or toluene, orn-hexane, or cyclohexane, or 1-butanol, or 1-pentanol) at T = 298.15 K. *J. Chem. Thermodyn.* **2000,** *32,* 617–629.

48. Rodriguez, A.; Canosa, J.; Tojo, J. Binary Mixture Properties of Methyl tert-Butyl Ether with Hexane or Heptane or Octane or Nonane from 288.15 K to 298.15 K. *J. Chem. Eng. Data.* **1999,** *44,* 666-671.

49. Munoz, R.; Burguet, M. C.; Martinez-Soria,V.; Nogueira de Araujo, R. Densities, Refractive Indices, and Derived Excess Properties of Tert-Butyl Alcohol, Methyl Tert-Butyl Ether and 2-Methylpentane Binary and Ternary Systems at 303.15 K. *Fluid Phase Equilib.* **2000,** *167,* 99–111.

50. Prigogine, I. Molecular Theory of Solution; North-Holland: Amsterdam, 1957.

51. Flory, P. J. *J. Am. Chem. Soc.* **1965,** *87,* 1833–1838.

52. Flory, P. J. Statistical Thermodynamics of Liquid Mixtures. *J. Am. Chem. Soc.* **1965,** *87,* 1833–1838.

53. Kermanpour, F.; Sharifi, T. Thermodynamic Study of Binary Mixture of x1[C$_6$mim] [BF$_4$] + x21-propanol: Measurements and Molecular Modeling. *Thermochim. Acta* **2012,** *527,* 211–218.

54. Qi, F.; Wang, H. Application of Prigogine–Flory–Patterson theory to Excess Molar Volume of Mixtures of 1-butyl-3-methylimidazolium Ionic Liquids with N-methyl-2-Pyrrolidinone. *J. Chem. Thermodyn.* **2009,** *41,* 265–272.

55. Iloukhani, H.; Khanlarzadeh, K. Volumetric Properties for Binary and Ternary Systems Consist of 1-chlorobutane, n-butylamine and Isobutanol at 298.15 K with Application of the Prigogine–Flory–Patterson Theory and ERAS-Model. *Thermochim. Acta.* **2010,** *502,* 77–84.

56. Kermanpour, F.; Niakan, H. Z. Volumetric Properties for Binary and Ternary Systems Consist of 1-chlorobutane, n-butylamine and Isobutanol at 298.15 K with Application

of the Prigogine–Flory–Patterson theory and ERAS-Model. *J. Chem. Thermodyn.* **2012,** *54*, 10–19.

57. Kumar, A.; Singh, T.; Gardas, R. L.; Coutinho, J. A. P. Non-Ideal Behaviour of a Room Temperature Ionic Liquid in an Alkoxyethanol or Poly Ethers at T=(298.15 to 318.15) K. *J. Chem. Thermodyn.* **2008,** *40*, 32–39.

58. Domanska, U.; Pobudkowska, A.; Wisniewska, A. Solubility and Excess Molar Properties of 1,3-Dimethylimidazolium Methylsulfate, or 1-Butyl-3-Methylimidazolium Methylsulfate, or 1-Butyl-3-Methylimidazolium Octylsulfate Ionic Liquids with n-Alkanes and Alcohols: Analysis in Terms of the PFP and FBT Models[1]. *J. Soln. Chem.* **2006,** *35*, 311–334.

59. Torres, R. B.; Ortolan, M. I.; Volpe, P. L. O. Volumetric Properties of Binary Mixtures of Ethers and Acetonitrile: Experimental Results and Application of the Prigogine–Flory–Patterson theory. *J. Chem. Thermodyn.* **2008,** *40*, 442–459.

60. Pal, A.; Bhardwaj, R. K. Excess Molar Volumes and Viscosities of Binary Mixtures of 1,2-diethoxyethane with Chloroalkanes at 298×15 K. *Proc. Indian Acad. Sci. Chem. Sci.* **2001,** *113*, 215–225.

61. Taghi, M.; Moattar, Z.; Shekaari, H. Application of Prigogine–Flory–Patterson Theory to Excess Molar Volume and Speed of Sound of 1-n-butyl-3-methylimidazolium Hexafluorophosphate or 1-n-butyl-3-methylimidazolium Tetrafluoroborate in Methanol and Acetonitrile. *J. Chem. Thermodyn.* **2006,** *38*, 1377–1384.

62. Santosh, M. S.; Bhat, D.K. Application of Prigogine–Flory–Patterson Theory to Volumetric, Ultrasonic, and Compressibility Parameters of (glycylglycine + CuCl$_2$) in Aqueous Ethanol Mixtures. *J. Chem. Thermodyn.* **2011,** *43*, 1336–1341.

63. Bondi, J. Van der Waals Volumes and Radii. *J. Phys. Chem.* **1964,** *68*, 441–443.

64. Riddick, J. A.; Bunger, W. B.; Sakano, T. K. *Organic Solvents: Physical Properties and Method of Purifications*, 4th edn.; Wiley-Interscience: New York, 1986.

PART II
Biophysical Chemistry from a Different Angle

CHAPTER 10

MOLECULAR CLASSIFICATION OF 2-PHENYLINDOLE-3-CARBALDEHYDES AS POTENTIAL ANTIMITOTIC AGENTS IN HUMAN BREAST CANCER CELLS

FRANCISCO TORRENS[1,*] and GLORIA CASTELLANO[2]

[1]Institut Universitari de Ciència Molecular, Universitat de València, Edifici d'Instituts de Paterna, P. O. Box 22085, E-46071 València,Spain

[2]Departamento de Ciencias Experimentales y Matemáticas, Facultad de Veterinaria y Ciencias Experimentales, Universidad Católica de Valencia San Vicente Mártir, Guillem de Castro-94, E-46001 València, Spain

*Corresponding author. E-mail: torrens@uv.es

CONTENTS

ABSTRACT

Algorithms are proposed for classification and taxonomy, based on criteria as *information entropy* and its production. The 32 2-phenylindole-3-carbaldehydes (PICs) present inhibition of breast cancer cells MDA-MB231 and MCF-7. On the basis of PIC structure–activity relationship (SAR) new derivatives are designed. The PICs are classified using five characteristic chemical properties of different moieties. Many classification algorithms are based on information entropy. When applying procedures to sets of moderate size, an excessive number of results appear compatible with data and suffer a combinatorial explosion. However, after *equipartition conjecture* one has a selection criterion among different variants, resulting from classification between hierarchical trees. Information entropy permits classifying compounds and agrees with principal component analysis. Features denote positions R_{1-2} on indole, R_{3-4} on phenyl and R_5 on carbaldehyde. A periodic table of MB231/MCF-7 inhibitors is obtained. Inhibitors in the same group and period are suggested to present maximum similarity; the ones with the same group will present important resemblance. Indoles are attractive as inhibitors of tubulin polymerization. A number of PICs, with lipophilic substituents in both aromatic rings, were synthesized and evaluated for MB231/MCF-7 antitumor activity. Some 5-alkylindoles, with a 4-methoxy group in 2-phenyl ring, strongly inhibit MB231/MCF-7 growth with 50% inhibitory concentration (IC_{50}) 5–20 nm. The action can be rationalized by the cell cycle arrest in phase G_2/M, because of tubulin polymerization inhibition. Quantitative SAR (QSAR) was done on PICs to find out structural requirements, for more active antimitotic agents.

10.1   INTRODUCTION

The colchicine (COL) is a natural product obtained from *Colchicum autumnale*. It is a bioactive alkaloid used in the treatment of a wide variety of diseases.[1] It received attention in cancer study by its capacity for interrupting *mitosis*, ending it in metaphase.[2] It acts as a tubulin polymerization inhibitor.[3] It was used as a probe to understand *microtubule* role in cells because of its affinity to tubulin, whose structure presents a binding site called COL *domain*.[4,5] Mitosis is a cell cycle part where chromosomes are divided into separate cell fractions.[6,7] Microtubules are responsible for chromosome capturing/aligning in metaphase and separating to daughter cells in anaphase.[8] They are targets for antimitotic agents, for example, vinca alkaloids, taxanes, etc., which are used for cancer treatments. However, adverse effects, difficulty in synthesis, and high cost limit their use.[9] In order to find out structural requirements for more active antimitotic agents, quantitative structure–activity relationship (QSAR) was performed on 2-phenylindole-3-carbaldehyde (PIC) (cf. Fig. 10.1).[10] The concentration for 50% inhibition (IC_{50}) of PIC was collected on breast cancer cells MDA-MB231.[11] Microtubule system is essential for cellular functions, for example, mitosis/cell replication, cell shape maintenance, cellular transport, and motility. Microtubules are hollow fibers formed by α/β-tubulin heterodimer polymerizations. Their formation/depolymerization is a dynamic process, which can be interrupted by their stabilization and polymerization inhibition. Many natural products shift the dynamic equilibrium of microtubule system to one/other side and abrogate microtubule biofunctions. Some natural products, for example, taxanes and epothilones, stabilize microtubule structures whereas others, for example, colchicine, CA4, and vinca alkaloids inhibit α/β-tubulin dimer polymerization.[12] Some natural products present complex chemical structures, which make synthesis and chemical modifications difficult. Others, for example, CA4, show simple scaffolds that can easily be modified.[13] Microtubules' biological importance makes them an interesting target for anticancer drugs. For studies on antimitotic agent use in cancer therapy, molecules with simple structures allow extensive chemical modifications, for example, stilbenes, aryl-substituted heterocycles,[14] anthracenones,[15] benzophenones[16] and analogues,[17] indoles,[18–21] and aryl-substituted ones,[22–27] and so forth. Three of the last carry a trimethoxyphenyl ring, which is considered as important for COL-site binding on tubulin. Comparative molecular field analysis of anti-tubulin agents with indole binding at COL binding site was performed.[28] The antivascular effect is interesting in CA4 and related agent applications in cancer chemotherapy. [29] Since cytoskeleton microtubules play a major role in maintaining cell shape, the elongated endothelial cells of tumor neovasculature are sensitive to drugs, which depolymerize microtubules and degrade cytoskeleton. In contrast to drugs that target tumor angiogenesis, CA4 phosphate disrupts tumor vasculature.[30] Methoxy-substituted PICs inhibit growth of human breast cancer cells.[31] Microtubules are their primary target. With bovine tubulin a marked inhibition on its polymerization was observed. Indole derivatives inhibited COL binding to tubulin. Since 2-phenylindoles lack structural features typical for tubulin polymerization inhibitors, for example,

3, 4, 5-trimethoxyphenyl, which is characteristic for colchicine, CA4, and podophyllotoxin, structural requirements for activity had to be elaborated by a substituent systematic variation in both aromatic rings. Since substituents should be lipophilic, alkyl groups of variable length and halogens/CF_3 were introduced. Five-membered ring 1-position was kept unsubstituted because indole N–H is essential for activity. Derivatives were tested for cytostatic activity. Since interaction with tubulin system results in cell cycle arrest in G_2/M phase, most potent compounds were submitted to a fluorescence-activated cell sorting (FACS) to record cell-cycle distribution. Some derivatives were studied for inhibitory effects on tubulin polymerization. A computerized algorithm is proposed, useful for establishing a relationship between chemical structures.[32,33] The starting point is the entropy of information theory for pattern recognition, which is formulated based on *similarity matrix* between biochemicals. As it is weakly discriminating for classification, more powerful concepts of *entropy making hypothesis of equipartition* are introduced.[34] In earlier publications, the periodic classifications of local anesthetics,[35–37] human immunodeficiency virus inhibitors,[38–43] cancer substances and (anti-) cancer agents[44–47] were analyzed. The aim of the present chapter is to develop code learning potentialities to study general approaches to structured information processing since molecules are naturally described via a varying size-structured representation. The second goal is to present a 2-phenylindole-3-carbaldehyde periodic table (PIC PT), and its validation with an external property of anticancer activity, not used in PT development. The next section presents the computational method. Section 10.3 illustrates and discusses the calculation results. The last section summarizes the final remarks.

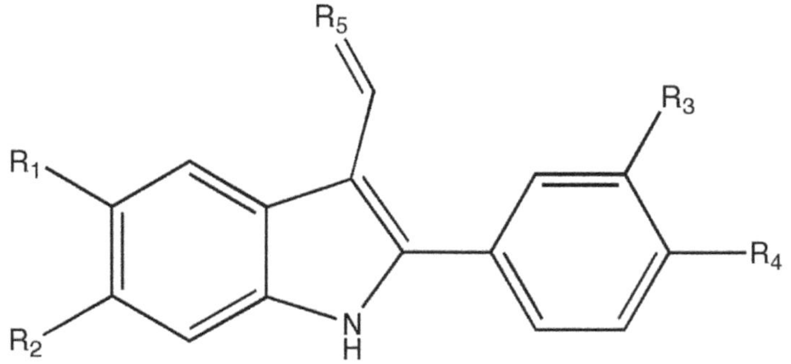

FIGURE 10.1   The general structure of 2-phenylindole-3-carbaldehyde (PIC) compounds.

10.2 COMPUTATIONAL METHOD

The main question in categorization is to define *similarity indices* if several comparison criteria exist. The first step, for PIC compounds, is to list the most important moieties. *The vector of properties* $\overline{i} = <i_1, i_2, \ldots i_k, \ldots>$ is hierarchically associated; their components relate to different groups in PIC. If *mth* part of PIC is more significant for antimitotic potency than *kth* one, then $m < k$. Components i_k are 1/0, along with an equal portion of rank k is present/absent in PIC i, compared to reference PIC. The examination takes in five parts of structural variation in PIC compounds: positions R_1 and R_2 on the indole cycle, R_3 and R_4 on the phenyl ring, and R_5 on the carbaldehyde group. The PICs are inhibitory to breast cancer cells MB231 and MCF-7. Consider that the *structural elements* of a PIC compound are *ranked*, along with their input to MB231/MCF-7 inhibition, in the following order: $R_3 > R_2 > R_4 > R_1 > R_5$. Index $i_1 = 1$ explains $R_3 = H$ ($i_1 = 0$, otherwise), $i_2 = 1$ stands for $R_2 = H$, $i_3 = 1$ means $R_4 = OMe$, $i_4 = 1$ signifies $R_1 = n$-Pent and $i_5 = 1$ explains $R_5 = O$. In PIC 13, $R_3 = R_2 = H$, $R_4 = OMe$, $R_1 = n$-Pent, and $R_5 = O$; clearly its corresponding vector is <11111>. In this work, PIC 13 was taken as *reference* owing to its greatest MB231/MCF-7 inhibition. Table 10.1 lists the vectors corresponding to 33 PICs with antimitotic potencies. Vector <11101> corresponds to PIC 1 as $R_3 = R_2 = H$, $R_4 = R_1 = OMe$ and $R_5 = O$.

TABLE 10.1 Vector Properties of 2-phenylindole-3-carbaldehydes (PICs) as Potential Antimitotic Agents (R_3, R_2, R_4, R_1, R_5).

1. –H–H–OMe–OMe=O <11101>

2. –H–OMe–OMe–H=O <10101>

3. –H–F–OMe–H=O <10101>

4. –H–H–OMe–F=O <11101>

5. –H–Cl–OMe–H=O <10101>

6. –H–Cl–OMe–Me=O <10101>

7. –H–H–OMe–Me=O <11101>

8. –H–H–OMe–n-Pr=O <11101>

9. –H–H–OMe–i-Pr=O <11101>

10. –H–H–OMe–n–But=O <11101>

11. –H–H–OMe–i-But=O <11101>

12. –H–H–OMe–t-But=O <11101>

TABLE 10.1 *(Continued)*

---

13. –H–H–OMe–*n*–Pent=O <11111>

14. –H–H–OMe–*n*–Hex=O <11101>

15. –OMe–OMe–H–H=O <00001>

16. –OMe–OMe–OMe–H=O <00101>

17. –OH–OMe–OMe–H=O <00101>

18. –H–OMe–Me–H=O <10001>

19. –H–Cl–Me–H=O <10001>

20. –H–H–Me–Me=O <11001>

21. –H–H–Me–*n*–But=O <11001>

22. –H–H–Et–*n*–But=O <11001>

23. –H–H–*n*–But–Et=O <11001>

24. –H–H–F–*n*–But=O <11001>

25. –H–H–CF$_3$–*n*–But=O <11001>

26. –H–H–CF$_3$–*n*–Pent=O <11011>

27. –H–H–CF$_3$–*n*–Hex=O <11001>

28. –H–OMe–OMe–H=NCH$_3$ <10100>

29. –H–H–OMe–*n*–But=NCH$_3$ <11100>

30. –H–H–OMe–*n*–Pent=NCH$_3$ <11110>

31. –H–H–CF$_3$–*n*–But=NCH$_3$ <11000>

32. –H–H–OMe–*n*–But=NOH <11100>

33. –H–H–CF$_3$–*n*–But=NOH <11000>

The initial step in quantifying the concept of similarity for chemical species in a mixture is to list the most important structural elements or properties of such species. To every species can be associated a vector, the components of which take only two values, "1" or "0," where "1" means the presence of a given structural element or property and "0" means its absence; for example, "1" may correspond to the presence of an H atom at position R_3 on the phenyl ring, whereas "0" corresponds to its absence. Binary bit string representations of molecular structure and properties, usually called fingerprints, are standard tools to analyze chemical similarity. Vectors associated with the chemicals are denoted by $i = <i_1, i_2 \ldots i_k \ldots>$, where i_k is either "1" or "0." Binary characterization, according to the presence ("1") or the absence ("0") of a given property, was used initially. The use of multivalued digits or the real properties instead of Boolean ones was also tested. A hierarchy of the structural elements or properties is required; for example, it is considered that the property indexed by i_1 is more significant than the property indexed by i_2, this is more significant than i_3, and so forth, in order of the coordinates in the associated vectors. For any set of chemicals, a similarity matrix is associated and to this an entropy of information theory. On this basis, the components of the mixture may be selected. Indicated by r_{ij} $(0 \leq r_{ij} \leq 1)$ the descriptor of similarity of two PICs, corresponding to vectors $\bar{i}$ and $\bar{j}$, respectively. The similarity relationship is characterized by a *similarity matrix* $R = [r_{ij}]$. The descriptor of similarity between two PICs $\bar{i} = <i_1,i_2,...i_k...>$ and $\bar{j} = <j_1,j_2,...j_k...>$ is described by:

$$r_{ij} = \sum_k t_k (a_k)^k \quad (k = 1,2,...) \tag{10.1}$$

Here, $0 \leq a_k \leq 1$ and $t_k = 1$ if $i_k = j_k$ but $t_k = 0$ if $i_k \neq j_k$. This designation allocates a weight $(a_k)^k$ to any feature implicated in the explanation of compound i or j. The hierarchical order of the 5 structural features is expressed in their corresponding weights. The upper bound for the similarity index is one; for example, for only five parameters, for all $a_k = 0.5$ these weights are: 0.5, 0.25, 0.125, 0.0625, 0.03125 and the upper bound for the similarity index is $0.5 + 0.25 + 0.125 + 0.0625 + 0.03125 = 0.96875$. The MB231/MCF-7 antimitotic potency data by Halder et al. were used for the present classification study. *Grouping algorithm* uses *stabilized* similarity matrix, obtained *via max–min composition rule o*:

$$(R \circ S)_{ij} = \max_k \left[\min_k (r_{ik}, s_{kj}) \right] \tag{10.2}$$

Where, $R = [r_{ij}]$ and $S = [s_{ij}]$ are similarity matrices and $(R \circ S)_{ij}$, element (i,j) of matrix $R \circ S$.[48–51] *Grouping rule*: i and j are assigned to the same class if $r_{ij}(n) \geq b$. The matrix of classes is:

$$\hat{R}(n) = \left[\hat{r}_{ij} \right] = \max_{s,t} (r_{st}) \quad (s \in \hat{i}, t \in \hat{j}) \tag{10.3}$$

where s/t stands for any index of a species belonging to class $\hat{i}/\hat{j}$. The *entropy of information theory h* measures the surprise that the source emitting sequences can give.[52,53] The entropy of information theory associated with the matrix of similarity **R** is:

$$h(\mathbf{R}) = -\sum_{i,j} r_{ij} \ln r_{ij} - \sum_{i,j} (1 - r_{ij}) \ln (1 - r_{ij})$$

(10.4)

Equipartition conjecture implies a constant entropy production along b scale; *equipartition line* is:

$$h_{\text{eqp}} = h_{\text{max}} b$$

(10.5)

The best variant is chosen to be the one minimizing the sum of squares of the deviations:

$$SS = \sum_{b_i} (h - h_{\text{eqp}})^2$$

(10.6)

Learning procedures similar to the ones encountered in *stochastic methods* are implemented.[54] The distance between the partitions into classes characterized by **R** and **S** is given by:

$$D = -\sum_{ij} (1 - r_{ij}) \ln \frac{1 - r_{ij}}{1 - s_{ij}} - \sum_{ij} r_{ij} \ln \frac{r_{ij}}{s_{ij}} \qquad \forall 0 \le r_{ij}, s_{ij} \le 1$$

(10.7)

which was suggested by that introduced to measure that between two probability distributions.[55]

The procedure was used in the synthesis of complex dendrograms *via* the entropy of information theory.[56,57] Our code MolClas is efficient and fast for molecular classification, based on the Equations 10.1–10.7.[58–66]

10.3   CALCULATION RESULTS AND DISCUSSION

The antiproliferative information, reported by Halder et al. for substituted PICs, was utilized as the model data collection. The Pearson correlation coefficient matrix was calculated between the pairs of vector properties $<i_1, i_2, i_3, i_4, i_5>$, for 33 PICs. Pearson's correlations can be shown in partial correlation diagram (PCD) that includes high ($r \ge 0.75$), medium

$(0.50 \leq r < 0.75)$, low $(0.25 \leq r < 0.50)$, and *zero* $(r < 0.25)$ partial intercorrelations. Couples of inhibitors with high partial correlations present an alike vector feature. Notwithstanding, the outcomes should be considered with attention, owing to the PIC with constant vector $<11111>$ (Entry 13) presents zero standard deviation, producing the greatest partial intercorrelations of one with any PIC, which results in an artifact. Pearson's correlation coefficient assumes bivariate normal data and, hence is not appropriate for the binary vector properties. Pearson's correlation coefficient r between two vector properties, for example, $<10101>$ and $<11111>$ corresponding to Entries 2 and 13, respectively, in Table 10.1 is defined as:

$$r = \frac{\sum_{i=1}^{n}(x_i - \bar{x})(y_i - \bar{y})}{n\sigma_x\sigma_y} \qquad (10.8)$$

Where, $x = \{1,0,1,0,1\}$, $\bar{x}$, the mean of x $(\bar{x} = 3/5 = 0.6)$, $y = \{1,1,1,1,1\}$, $\bar{y}$, the mean of y $(\bar{y} = 1)$, n, the number of points $(n=5)$, σ_x the standard deviation of x $\left(\sigma_x = \left(\sum_{i=1}^{n} x_i^2 / n - \bar{x}^2\right)^{1/2} = 0.48990\right)$ and σ_y, the standard deviation of y $\left(\sigma_y = \left(\sum_{i=1}^{n} y_i^2 / n - \bar{y}^2\right)^{1/2} = 0\right)$. Notice that as $\sigma_y = 0$, r should be maximum $(r=1)$, which is counterintuitive. In contrast, our method corrects it: $r = 0.5 + 0.125 + 0.03125 = 0.65625$. With our method, the associations result shown in PCD that includes 277 high (cf. Fig. 10.2, *red lines, greyscale*), 161 medium (*orange, greyscale*), 21 low (*yellow, greyscale*), and 69 *zero* (*black, greyscale*) partial intercorrelations. Observe that 10 out of the 32 high partial correlations of Entry 13 were fixed; for example, its intercorrelations with Entries 2, 3, 5, 6, 18, 19, and 28 are medium, and its interrelations with Entries 15–17 are 0 partial intercorrelations.

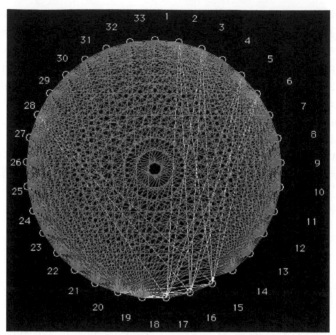

FIGURE 10.2 Partial correlation diagram: High (*red*), medium (*orange*), low (*yellow*) correlations of PICs.

The classifying law in the situation with the same weights $a_k = 0.5$ for $0.91 \leq b_1 \leq 0.93$ presents the groupings:

$$C - b_1 = (1,4,7-12,14,29,32)(2,3,5,6,28)(13,30)$$
$$(15)(16,17)(18,19)(20-25,27,31,33)(26)$$

The eight groupings result with linked entropy: $h-R-b_1 = 29.32$. The binary tree corresponding to $<i_1,i_2,i_3,i_4,i_5>$ and $C-b_1$ is computed (cf. Fig. 10.3);[67–69] it gives a dual classification that divides equal eight groupings: from top to down, the data split into groupings 1, 3, 8, 7, 2, 6, 4 and 5 with 11, 2, 1, 9, 5, 2, 1 and 2 PICs, correspondingly.[70] Chiefly, PICs 13 and 30 with the highest antiproliferative potency are classed into equal grouping. The PICs fitting in equal grouping result greatly associated with PCD. At stage b_2 with $0.85 \leq b_2 \leq 0.87$, the collection of groupings that results is:

$$C - b_2 = (1,4,7-14,29,30,32)(2,3,5,6,28)(15)$$
$$(16,17)(18,19)(20-27,31,33)$$

Six groupings appear in this situation and the entropy decays to h–R–$b_2 = 17.20$. The binary tree corresponding with $<i_1, i_2, i_3, i_4, i_5>$ and C–b_2 splits equal six groupings: 1, 6, 2, 5, 3, and 4 with 13, 10, 5, 2, 1 and 2 PICs. One more time, PICs 13, 30, etc. with the highest antiproliferative potency are classed into equal grouping. The PICs fitting in equal grouping result greatly associated with PCD and binary tree, in concordance with earlier outcomes. An analysis of the set containing 1–33 classes resulted in concordance with earlier outcomes.

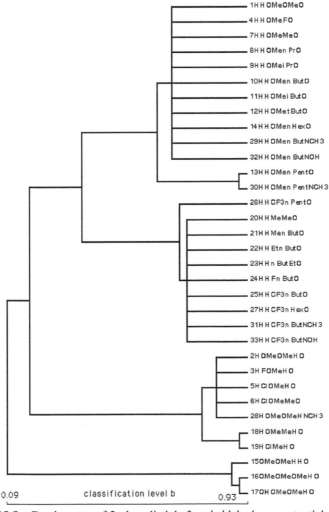

FIGURE 10.3 Dendrogram of 2-phenylindole-3-carbaldehydes as potential antimitotic agents at level b_1.

In view of the earlier PCD and binary trees, we propose to divide the information into four groupings (1,4,7–14,29,30,32)(20–27,31,33) (2,3,5,6,18,19,28)(15–17) with 13, 10, 7 and 3 PICs, respectively. The binary tree is displayed (cf. Fig. 10.4). The figure is calculated varying the classification level b from 1 (every PIC in its own class of 33 classes) to 0 (all PICs in the same class of 33 units). Once more, PICs 13, 30, *etc.* are grouped into the same class.

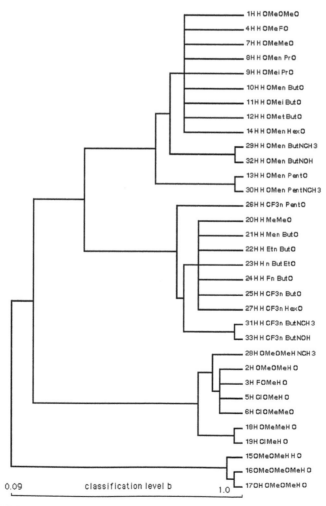

FIGURE 10.4   Dendrogram of 2-phenylindole-3-carbaldehydes as potential antimitotic agents.

Code SplitsTree allows examining cluster analysis (CA) information.[71] Founded on the technique of *split decomposition*, it inputs a *distance matrix* or a collection of CA information and outputs an SG, which stands for the relations among classes. For perfect information, SG is a tree, while less perfect information will cause a tree-like net, which is interpreted as probable proof for dissimilar and contradictory information. Moreover, as SG decomposition does not try to compel information onto a tree, it gives a high-quality sign of how *tree*-like provided information is. The SG for PICs (cf. Fig. 10.5) shows no contradictory relation among PICs. The majority of collections collapse: (1,4,7–12,14,29,32)(2,3,5,6,28)(13,30) (16,17)(18,19)(20–25,27,31,33). The SG is in concordance with PCD, binary trees, and earlier outcomes.

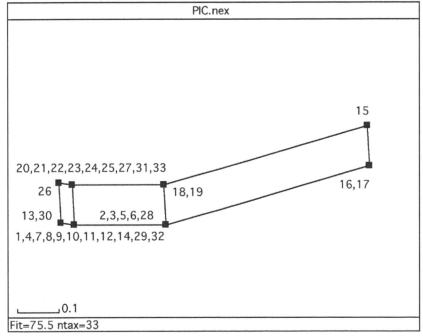

FIGURE 10.5   Split graph for the vector properties corresponding to PICs.

Principal components analysis is a helpful method to *sum up* informa-tion in **X** matrix.[72–77] It functions decomposing **X** matrix as a product of two smaller ones, **P** and **T**. *Loading matrix* **P**, with information on the variables, includes some vectors (PCs), which are gotten as linear combinations of the first X-variables. *Score matrix* **T**, with information on the items, results such that each item results are expressed in terms of the projections onto PCs, instead of the first variables: $\mathbf{X} = \mathbf{TP'} + \mathbf{E}$, where "'" indicates the transpose matrix. Information not included in the matrices stays as *unexplained* X-*variance* in a *residual matrix* **E**. Each PC$_i$ is a novel coordinate described as a linear combination of the first characteristics x_j: PC$_i = \Sigma_j b_{ij} x_j$. The novel coordinates PC$_i$ are named *scores* (*factors*), whereas coefficients b_{ij} are named *loadings*. Scores are sorted consistent with the information matter, according to the total variation between the objects. A PCA was performed for PICs. The significance of PCA PCs F_{1-5} for $\{i_1, i_2, i_3, i_4, i_5\}$ was computed. Chiefly, the utilization of merely the first PC F_1 justifies 33% of the variation (67% error), the joint application of the first two PCs $F_{1/2}$ accounts for 55% of variation (45% error), the utilization of the first three PCs F_{1-3} rationalizes 73% of variation (27% error), and so forth. The PCA PC loadings were calculated. The PCA F_{1-5} outlines for the vector feature was computed. Chiefly, for PCs F_1 and F_5, variable i_2 shows the highest weight in the outline; notwithstanding, F_1 cannot be decreased to two variables $\{i_1, i_2\}$ devoid of a 24% error. For PC F_2, variable i_3 presents the highest weight; nevertheless, F_2 cannot be decreased to 2 variables $\{i_3, i_5\}$ devoid of a 20% error. For PC F_3, variable i_4 assigns the highest weight; however, F_3 cannot be decreased to two variables $\{i_1, i_4\}$ devoid of an 18% error. For PC F_4, variable i_5 consigns the greatest weight; however, F_4 cannot be reduced to 2 variables $\{i_3, i_5\}$ without a 13% error. For PC F_5, variable i_2 represents the greatest weight; notwithstanding, F_5 cannot be reduced to two variables $\{i_1, i_2\}$ without a 6% error. The PCs F_{1-5} can be regarded as linear mixtures of $\{i_1, i_2\}$, $\{i_3, i_5\}$, $\{i_1, i_4\}$, $\{i_3, i_5\}$ and $\{i_1, i_2\}$, correspondingly, with 24, 20, 18, 13, and 6% errors. In the PCA $F_2 - F_1$ *scores plot* (cf. Fig. 10.6), PICs with equal vector feature collapse. Four groupings of PICs are differentiated: cluster 1 with 13 molecules $(F_2 > F_1 > 0, top)$, grouping 2 with 10 compounds $(F_1 > F_2, bottom)$, cluster 3 with 7 substances $(F_1 < F_2, center)$ and grouping 4 with 3 organics $(F_1 \ll F_2, left)$. The categorization agrees with PCD, binary trees, SG, and earlier outcomes.

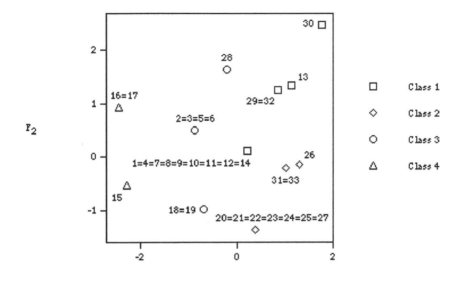

FIGURE 10.6   Principal component analysis F_2–F_1 scores plot for vector properties of PICs.

The PCA PC loadings of PICs F_2–F_1 *loadings plot* (cf. Fig. 10.7) shows the five features. Moreover, as an accompaniment to the scores plot for the loadings, it results corroborated that PICs in cluster 1 located at the top shows an input of R_4=OMe, located in equal place. The PICs in grouping 2 at the bottom show an additional marked input from R_2=H, placed in the same location. The PICs in cluster 3 at the center have an additional marked input from R_3=H, positioned in the same site. The PICs in grouping 4 at the left side present an additional marked input from R_5=O put in the same side. The features are classed into two groupings: cluster 1 (R_{1-3}, $F_1 > F_2$, *right*) and grouping 2 (R_{4-5}, $F_1 < F_2$, *left*).

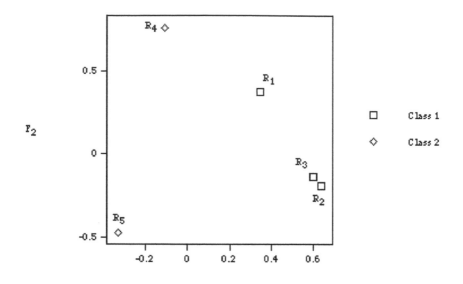

FIGURE 10.7   Principal component analysis F_2-F_1 loadings plot for vector properties of PICs.

As an alternative of 33 PICs in the $\Re^5$ space of five vector features, bear in mind 5 features in the $\Re^{33}$ space of 33 PICs. The binary tree for the vector features (cf. Fig. 10.8) divide features R_3-R_2-R_1 (cluster 1) from R_4 and R_5 (grouping 2) in concordance with PCA loadings plot.

The SG for features (cf. Fig. 10.9) indicates no contradictory relation among vector components. It divides $R_{3/2/1}$ from $R_{4/5}$ in concordance with PCA loadings plot and binary tree.

A PCA was carried out for vector features. The utilization of merely the first PC F_1 justifies 47% of variation (53% error), the joint application of PCs $F_{1/2}$ accounts for 68% of variation (32% error), the utilization of PCs F_{1-3} rationalizes 83% of variation (17% error), and so forth. The PCA F_2–F_1 scores plot (cf. Fig. 10.10) separates properties into 2 groupings: cluster 1 (R_{1-3}, $F_1>F_2$, *bottom*) and grouping 2 (R_{4-5}, $F_1<F_2$, *top*), in concordance with PCA loadings plot, binary tree, and SG.

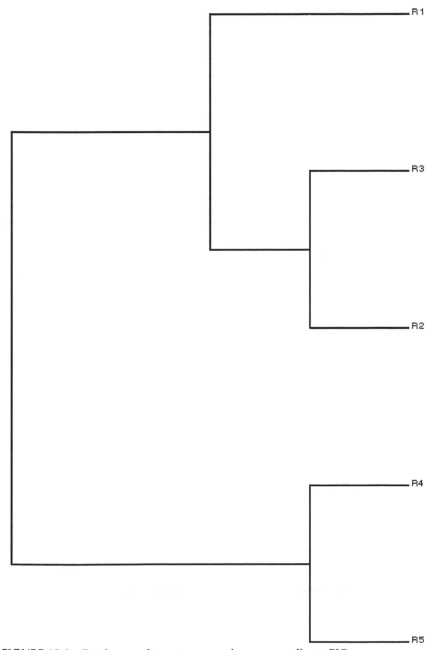

FIGURE 10.8 Dendrogram for vector properties corresponding to PICs.

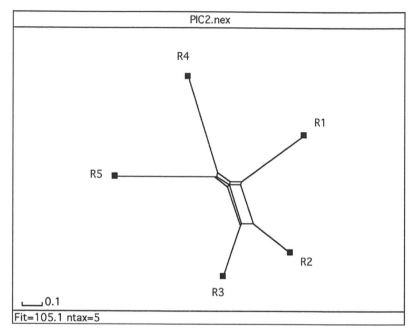

FIGURE 10.9 Split graph for vector properties corresponding to 2-phenylindole-3-carbaldehydes.

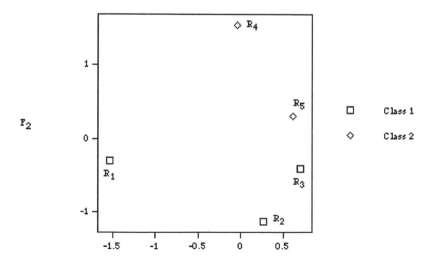

FIGURE 10.10 PCA F_2-F_1 scores plot for PICs corresponding to vector properties.

The suggested arrangement for PIC PT, Table 10.2, shows that the result is categorized first by R_3, then by R_2, R_4, R_1 and, finally, by R_5. However, instead of 2^5 now 6 classes with common bit patterns are of interest. Periods of 6 components are considered; for example, group g000 is for $<i_1,i_2,i_3> = <000>$, viz. $<00001>$ ($R_3 \neq H$, $R_2 \neq H$, $R_4 \neq OMe$, $R_1 \neq nPent$, $R_5 = O$), and so forth. The table shows our results of classification of the studied PIC compounds. Generally, groups of compounds with similar structures follow similar trends. The PICs in equal column result near in PCD, binary tree, SG, PCA scores, and earlier outcomes (Figs. 10.2–10.6).

The change of feature P, inhibition of breast cancer cells MB231/MCF-7 of vector $<i_1,i_2,i_3,i_4,i_5>$ is expressed in the decimal system, $P = 10^4 i_1 + 10^3 i_2 + 10^2 i_3 + 10 i_4 + i_5$, vs. molecular structural design features $\{i_1,i_2,i_3,i_4,i_5\}$ for PICs. Most data appears superimposed. The feature was not utilized in PT progress and works to confirm it. The outcomes correspond to a PT of features, with vertical groups described by $\{i_1,i_2,i_3\}$ and horizontal periods explained by $\{i_4,i_5\}$. The change of feature P of vector $<i_1,i_2,i_3,i_4,i_5>$, in base 10, vs. the figure of the group in PIC PT exposes maxima matching to compounds with $<i_1,i_2,i_3>$ ca. $<111>$ (group g111). Most points come superimposed. Periods p00, p01, p10, and p11 stand for rows 1–4 in PT, respectively. The matching curve $P\,(i_1,i_2,i_3,i_4,i_5)$ indicates a sequence of periodic *waves*, controlled by maxima and minima, which imply a cyclic performance that remembers the shape of a trigonometric curve. For $<i_1,i_2,i_3,i_4,i_5>$, a maximum is presented. The separation in $<i_1,i_2,i_3,i_4,i_5>$ units among every couple of successive maxima is six, which agrees with PIC collections in the consecutive periods. The maxima reside in similar locations in the curve and result in phase. The characteristic positions in phase match with the constituents in the equal group in PT. For $<i_1,i_2,i_3,i_4,i_5>$ maxima, consistency exists among both descriptions; notwithstanding the coherence is not universal. The assessment of the curves shows two dissimilarities: periods 1, 3, and 4 are unfinished and period 2 is staircase-like. The most distinguishing positions of the chart are maxima, which are positioned near group g111. The significance of $<i_1,i_2,i_3,i_4,i_5>$ is done again as periodic law (PL) utters. An experiential curve $P\,(p)$ replicates the dissimilar $<i_1,i_2,i_3,i_4,i_5>$ quantities. A minimum of $P\,(p)$ presents significance merely if it is contrasted to the previous $P\,(p-1)$ and afterwards $P\,(p+1)$ positions, required to satisfy:

TABLE 10.2 Periodic Properties for 2-Phenylindole-3-Carbaldehyde Derivatives

g000	g001	g100	g101	g110	g111
–OMe–OMe–H– H=O	–OMe–OMe–OMe– H=O	–H–OMe–Me–H=O	–H–OMe–OMe–H =NCH$_3$	–H–H–CF$_3$–n-But =NCH$_3$	–H–H–OMe– nBut=NCH$_3$
	–OH–OMe–OMe– H=O	–H–Cl–Me–H=O	–H–OMe–OMe– H=O	–H–H–CF$_3$–n-But =NOH	–H –H –OMe –n-But =NOH
			–H–F–OMe–H=O	–H–H–Me–Me=O	–H–H–OMe– OMe=O
			–H–Cl–OMe–H=O	–H–H–Me–n-But=O	–H–H–OMe–F=O
			–H–Cl–OMe–Me=O	–H–H–Et–n-But=O	–H–H–OMe–Me=O
				–H–H–n-But–Et=O	–H–H–OMe–n-Pr=O
				–H–H–F–n-But=O	–H–H–OMe–i-Pr=O
				–H–H–CF$_3$–n-But=O	–H–H–OMe–n- But=O
				–H–H–CF$_3$ –n- Hex=O	–H–H–OMe–i- But=O
					–H–H–OMe–t- But=O
					–H–H–OMe–n- Hex=O
					–H–H–OMe–n- Pent=NCH$_3$
				–H–H–CF$_3$–n- Pent=O	–H–H–OMe–n- Pent=O

$$P_{min}(p) < P(p-1) \quad P_{min}(p) < P(p+1) \tag{10.9}$$

Sequence relationships (Eq. 10.9) should be done again at certain gaps equivalent to period dimension and are equal to:

$$P_{min}(p) - P(p-1) < 0 \quad P(p+1) - P_{min}(p) > 0 \tag{10.10}$$

As relationships (Equation 10.10) result is suitable merely for minima, universally others are wished for all quantities of p. The $D(p) = P(p+1) - P(p)$ dissimilarities are computed appointing every quantity to PIC p:

$$D(p) = P(p+1) - P(p) \tag{10.11}$$

Instead of $D(p)$, $R(p) = P(p+1)/P(p)$ are allocated to PIC p. If PL was general, the elements in the equal group in vertical positions in dissimilar cyclic curves would convince:

Either $\qquad\qquad\qquad D(p) > 0 \text{ or } D(p) < 0 \tag{10.12}$

Either $\qquad\qquad\qquad R(p) > 1 \text{ or } R(p) < 1 \tag{10.13}$

Notwithstanding, the outcomes present that it is not the situation so that PL is not universal, being certain irregularities; for example, the change of $D(p)$ vs. group figure shows lack of consistency among $<i_1, i_2, i_3, i_4, i_5>$ Cartesian and PT charts. Most results appear superimposed. If coherence was exact, all positions in every period would present equal signs. Usually, a tendency exists in the positions to provide $D(p) > 0$ for the smaller groups but not for the higher ones. Nevertheless, irregularities exist in which PICs for consecutive periods are not at all times in phase. The variation of $R(p)$ vs. group figure corroborates the need for Cartesian/PT reliability. Most data comes superimposed. If evenness was precise, all points in every period would present $R(p)$ as either smaller or higher than one. A tendency exists to provide $R(p) > 1$ for the smaller groups but not for the higher ones. However, corroborated strangeness exists in which PICs for consecutive curves are not at all times in phase.

10.4   FINAL REMARKS

From the discussion of the present results, the following final remarks can be drawn.

1. Some reasons, chosen to decrease the examination to a convenient amount of 33 PICs, relate to the features of molecular architecture connected to sites R_{1-2} on indole, R_{3-4} on phenyl, and R_5 on carbaldehyde. Molecular *structural elements* can be *ranked* according to inhibitory potency as $R_3 > R_2 > R_4 > R_1 > R_5$. In compound 13, $R_3 = R_2 = H$, $R_4 = OMe$, $R_1 = n$-Pent and $R_5 = O$ <11111>, which was selected as a *reference*. The carbaldehydes are inhibitors of breast cancer cells MB231. A lot of categorization procedures are founded on the entropy of information theory. For collections of reasonable dimension, an extreme figure of outcomes result well-matched with information and undergo a sudden combinatorial increase. Nevertheless, following the *hypothesis of equipartition*, one possesses a reason of choice among dissimilar alternatives coming from categorization among hierarchical trees, consistent with which the best arrangement is that in which the entropy making is maximally regularly allocated. This approach keeps difficulty away from others of range variables for the molecule with steady <11111> vector, owing to zero standard deviation producing a Pearson's correlation coefficient of the unit. The classification is in agreement with the principal component analysis.

2. Algorithm MolClas is an easy, consistent, competent, and rapid code for compounds categorization, founded on the hypothesis of equipartition of entropy making. The procedure of MolClas was programmed not only to examine the hypothesis of equipartition of entropy making but also to discover compounds categorization.

3. The PL does not convince the rank of the laws of physics: (a) the inhibitory potencies of PICs do not result finished again, maybe their pharmacological nature; (b) the sequence relationships are done again with exemptions. The examination compels the declaration: The relationships that whichever molecule p presents with its closest $p + 1$ result are roughly replicated, for every period. Periodicity is not universal; notwithstanding, if a usual sequence of molecules is recognized, then the rule ought to be phenomenological.

The antitumor potency was not utilized in the production of the table of periodic properties and works to confirm it. The analysis of other features of PICs in the table of periodic properties would provide a mental picture of its potential generalization.

10.5 ACKNOWLEDGMENT

Francisco Torrens belongs to the Institut Universitari de Ciència Molecular, Universitat de València. Gloria Castellano belongs to the Departamento de Ciencias Experimentales y Matemáticas, Facultad de Veterinaria y Ciencias Experimentales, Universidad Católica de Valencia *San Vicente Mártir*. The authors thank for the support from Generalitat Valenciana (Project No. PROMETEO/2016/094) and Universidad Católica de Valencia *San Vicente Mártir* (Project No. PRUCV/2015/617).

KEYWORDS

- periodic law
- periodic property
- periodic table
- classification
- information entropy
- equipartition conjecture

REFERENCES

1. Santavy, F. Substanzen der herbstzeitlose und ihre derivate. 22. Photochemische produkte des colchicins und einige seiner derivate. *Collect. Czech. Chem. Commun.* **1951,** *16,* 655–675.
2. Andreu, J. M.; Perez-Ramirez, B.; Gorbunoff, M. J.; Ayala, D.; Timasheff, S. N. Role of the Colchicine Ring A and its Methoxy Groups in the Binding to Tubulin and Microtubule Inhibition. *Biochemistry.* **1998,** *37,* 8356–8368.
3. Nunez, J.; Fellous, A.; Francon, J.; Lennon, A. M. Competitive Inhibition of Colchicine Binding to Tubulin by Microtubule-Associated Proteins. *Proc. Natl. Acad. Sci. U. S. A.* **1979,** *76,* 86–90.

4. Lee, R. M.; Gewirtz, D. A. Colchicine Site Inhibitors of Microtubule Integrity as Vascular Disrupting Agents. *Drug Dev. Res.* **2008,** *69,* 352–358.

5. Bhattacharyya, B.; Panda, D.; Gupta, S.; Banerjee, M. Anti-Mitotic Activity of Colchicine and the Structural Basis for its Interaction with Tubulin. *Med. Res. Rev.* **2008,** *28,* 155–183.

6. Lodish, H.; Berk, A.; Matsudaira, P.; Kaiser, C. A.; Krieger, M.; Scott, M. P.; Zipurski, S. L.; Darnell, J. *Molecular Cell Biology*; Freeman: New York, 2004; Chap. 20.

7. Alberts, B.; Bray, D.; Lewis, J.; Raff, M.; Roberts, K.; Watson, J. D. *Molecular Biology of the Cell*; Garland: New York, 1994; Chap. 18.

8. Jordan, M. A.; Wilson, L. Microtubules as a Target for Anticancer Drugs. *Nat. Rev. Cancer.* **2004,** *4,* 253–265.

9. Tripathi, K. D. *Essentials of Medical Pharmacology*; Jaypee: Delhi, India, 2003; Chap. 60.

10. Halder, A. K.; Adhikari, N.; Jha, T. Comparative QSAR Modelling of 2Phenylindole3Carbaldehyde Derivatives as Potential Antimitotic Agents. *Bioorg. Med. Chem. Lett.* **2009,** *19,* 1737–1739.

11. Kaufmann, D.; Pojarová, M.; Vogel, S.; Liebl, R.; Gastpar, R.; Gross, D.; Nishino, T.; Pfaller, T.; von Angerer, E. Antimitotic Activities of 2Phenylindole3Carbaldehydes in Human Breast Cancer Cells. *Bioorg. Med. Chem.* **2007,** *15,* 5122–5136.

12. Von Angerer, E. Tubulin as a Target for Anticancer Drugs. *Curr. Opin. Drug. Discov. Dev.* **2000,** *3,* 575–584.

13. Tron, G. C.; Pirali, T.; Sorba, G.; Pagliai, F.; Busacca, S.; Genazzani, A. A. Medicinal Chemistry of Combretastatin A4: Present and Future. *J. Med. Chem.* **2006,** *49,* 3033–3044.

14. Von Angerer, E. New Inhibitors of Tubulin Polymerisation. *Expert Opin. Ther. Pat.* **1999,** *9,* 1069–1081.

15. Prinz, H.; Ishii, Y.; Hirano, T.; Stoiber, T.; Camacho Gomez, J. A.; Schmidt, P.; Düssmann, H.; Burger, A. M.; Prehn, J. H.; Günther, E. G.; Unger, E.; Umezawa, K. Novel benzylidene-9(10*H*)-anthracenones as highly active antimicrotubule agents. Synthesis, antiproliferative activity, and inhibition of tubulin polymerization. *J. Med. Chem.* **2003,** *46,* 3382–3394.

16. Liou, J. P.; Chang, J. Y.; Chang, C.-W.; Chang, C. Y.; Mahindroo, N.; Kuo, F. M.; Hsieh, H. P. Synthesis and Structure–Activity Relationships of 3-Aminobenzophenones as Antimitotic Agents. *J. Med. Chem.* **2004,** *47,* 2897–2905.

17. Romagnoli, R.; Baraldi, P. G.; Pavani, M. G.; Tabrizi, M. A.; Preti, D.; Fruttarolo, F.; Piccagli, L.; Jung, M. K.; Hamel, E.; Borgatti, M.; Gambari, R. Synthesis and Biological Evaluation of 2-Amino-3-(3′,4′,5′-trimethoxybenzoyl)-5-Aryl Thiophenes as a New Class of Potent Antitubulin Agents. *J. Med. Chem.* **2006,** *49,* 3906–3915.

18. Brancale, A.; Silvestri, R. Indole, a Core Nucleus for Potent Inhibitors of Tubulin Polymerization. *Med. Res. Rev.* **2007,** *27,* 209–238.

19. De Martino, G.; Edler, M. C.; La Regina, G.; Coluccia, A.; Barbera, M. C.; Barrow, D.; Nicholson, R. I.; Chiosis, G.; Brancale, A.; Hamel, E.; Artico, M.; Silvestri, R.; New Arylthioindoles: Potent Inhibitors of Tubulin Polymerization. 2. Structure–Activity Relationships and Molecular Modeling Studies. *J. Med. Chem.* **2006,** *49,* 947–954.

20. Dupeyre, G.; Chabot, G. G.; Thoret, S.; Cachet, X.; Seguin, J.; Guénard, D.; Tillequin, F.; Scherman, D.; Koch, M.; Michel, S. Synthesis and Biological Evaluation of (3,4,5-trimethoxyphenyl)indol-3-ylmethane Derivatives as Potential Antivascular Agents. *Bioorg. Med. Chem.* **2006**, *14*, 4410–4426.

21. Mahboobi, S.; Sellmer, A.; Eichhorn, E.; Beckers, T.; Fiebig, H. H.; Kelter, G. Synthesis and Cytotoxic Activity of 2-Acyl-1*H*-Indole-4,7-Diones on Human Cancer Cell Lines. *Eur. J. Med. Chem.* **2005**, *40*, 85–92.

22. Kuo, C. C.; Hsieh, H. P.; Pan, W. Y.; Chen, C. P.; Liou, J. P.; Lee, S. J.; Chang, Y. L.; Chen, L. T.; Chen, C. T.; Chang, J. Y. BPR0L075, a Novel Synthetic Indole Compound with Antimitotic Activity in Human Cancer Cells, Exerts Effective Antitumoral Activity *in Vivo*. *Cancer Res.* **2004**, *64*, 4621–4628.

23. Liou, J. P.; Chang, Y. L.; Kuo, F. M.; Chang, C. W.; Tseng, H. Y.; Wang, C. C.; Yang, Y. N.; Chang, J. Y.; Lee, S. J.; Hsieh, H. P. Concise Synthesis and Structure–Activity Relationships of Combretastatin A4 Analogues, 1-Aroylindoles and 3-Aroylindoles, as Novel Classes of Potent Antitubulin Agents. *J. Med. Chem.* **2004**, *47*, 4247–4257.

24. Liou, J. P.; Mahindroo, N.; Chang, C. W.; Guo, F. M.; Lee, S. W. H.; Tan, U. K.; Yeh, T. K.; Kuo, C. C.; Chang, Y. W.; Lu, P. H.; Tung, Y. S.; Lin, K. T.; Chang, J. Y.; Hsieh, H. P. Structure-Activity Relationship Studies of 3-Aroylindoles as Potent Antimitotic Agents. *Chem. Med. Chem.* **2006**, *1*, 1106–1118.

25. Mahboobi, S.; Pongratz, H.; Hufsky, H.; Hockemeyer, J.; Frieser, M.; Lyssenko, A.; Paper, D. H.; Bürgermeister, J.; Böhmer, F. D.; Fiebig, H. H.; Burge, A. M.; Baasner, S.; Beckers, T. Synthetic 2-Aroylindole Derivatives as a New Class of Potent Tubulin-Inhibitory, Antimitotic Agents. *J. Med. Chem.* **2001**, *44*, 4535–4553.

26. Wang, L.; Woods, K. W.; Li, Q.; Barr, K. J.; McCroskey, R. W.; Hannick, S. M.; Gherke, L.; Credo, R. B.; Hui, Y.-H.; Marsh, K.; Warner, R.; Lee, J. Y.; Zielinski-Mozng, N.; Frost, D.; Rosenberg, S. H.; Sham, H. L. Potent, Orally Active Heterocycle-Based Combretastatin A4 Analogues: Synthesis, Structure–Activity Relationship, Pharmacokinetics, and in Vivo Antitumor Activity Evaluation. *J. Med. Chem.* **2002**, *45*, 1697–1711.

27. Pandit, B.; Sun, Y.; Chen, P.; Sackett, D. L.; Hu, Z.; Rich, W.; Li, C.; Lewis, A.; Schaefer, K.; Li, P. K. Structure-Activity-Relationship Studies of Conformationally Restricted Analogs of Combretastatin A-4 Derived from SU5416. *Bioorg. Med. Chem.* **2006**, *14*, 6492–6501.

28. Lin, I. H.; Hsu, C. C.; Wang, S. H.; Hsieh, H. P.; Sun, Y. C. Comparative Molecular Field Analysis of Anti-Tubulin Agents with Indole Ring Binding at the Colchicine Binding Site. *J. Theor. Comput. Chem.* **2010**, *9*, 279–291.

29. Thorpe, P. E. Vascular Targeting Agents as Cancer Therapeutics. *Clin. Cancer Res.* **2004**, *10*, 415–427.

30. Chaplin, D. J.; Horsman, M. R.; Siemann, D. W. Current Developments Status of Small-Molecule Vascular Disrupting Agents. *Curr. Opin. Investig. Drugs* **2006**, *7*, 522–528.

31. Gastpar, R.; Goldbrunner, M.; Marko, D.; von Angerer, E. Methoxy-Substituted 3-formyl-2-Phenylindoles Inhibit Tubulin Polymerization. *J. Med. Chem.* **1998**, *41*, 4965–4972.

32. Varmuza, K. *Pattern Recognition in Chemistry*; Springer: New York, 1980.

33. Benzecri, J. P. L'Analyse des Données; Dunod: Paris, 1984; Vol. 1.
34. Tondeur, D.; Kvaalen, E. Equipartition of Entropy Production. An Optimality Criterion for Transfer and Separation Processes. *Ind. Eng. Chem. Res.* **1987,** *26,* 50–56.
35. Torrens, F.; Castellano, G. Periodic Classification of Local Anaesthetics (procaine analogues). *Int. J. Mol. Sci.* **2006,** *7,* 12–34.
36. Castellano-Estornell, G.; Torrens-Zaragozá, F. Local Anaesthetics Classified Using Chemical Structural Indicators. *Nereis* **2009,** *2,* 7–17.
37. Torrens, F.; Castellano, G. Information Entropy and the Table of Periodic Properties of Local Anaesthetics. *Int. J. Chemoinf. Chem. Eng.* **2011,** *1*(2), 15–35.
38. Torrens, F.; Castellano, G. Classification of Complex Molecules. In *Foundations of Computational Intelligence*; Hassanien, A.-E., Abraham, A., Eds.; Springer: Berlin, 2009; Vol. 5, pp 243–315.
39. Torrens, F.; Castellano, G. Table of Periodic Properties of Human Immunodeficiency Virus Inhibitors. *Int. J. Comput. Intell. Bioinf. Syst. Biol.* **2010,** *1,* 246–273.
40. Torrens, F.; Castellano, G. Molecular Classification of Thiocarbamates with Cytoprotection Activity against Human Immunodeficiency Virus. *Int. J. Chem. Model.* **2011,** *3,* 269–296.
41. Torrens, F.; Castellano, G. Structural Classification of Complex Molecules by Artificial Intelligence Techniques. In *Advanced Methods and Applications in Chemoinformatics: Research Methods and New Applications*; Castro, E. A., Haghi, A. K., Eds.; IGI Global: Hershey, PA, 2012; pp 25–91.
42. Torrens, F.; Castellano, G. Structural Classification of Complex Molecules by Information Entropy and Equipartition Conjecture. In *Chemical Information and Computational Challenges in 21st Century*; Putz, M. V., Ed.; Nova: New York, NY, 2012; pp 101–139.
43. Torrens, F.; Castellano, G. Complexity, Emergence and Molecular Diversity *via* Information Theory. In *Complexity Science, Living Systems and Reflexing Interfaces: New Models and Perspectives*; Orsucci, F., Sala, N., Eds.; IGI Global: Hershey, PA, 2013; pp 196–208.
44. Torrens, F.; Castellano, G. Modelling of Complex Multicellular Systems: Tumour–Immune Cells Competition. *Chem. Central J.* **2009,** *3*(Suppl I), 75-1-1.
45. Torrens-Zaragozá, F. Polymer bisphenol-A, the Incorporation of Silica Nanospheres into Epoxy-Amine Materials and Polymer Nanocomposites. *Nereis.* **2011,** *3,* 17–23.
46. Torrens, F.; Castellano, G. Information Theoretic Entropy for Molecular Classification: Oxadiazolamines as Potential Therapeutic Agents. *Curr. Comput.-Aided Drug Des.* **2013,** *9,* 241–253.
47. Torrens, F.; Castellano, G. Molecular Classification of 5-Amino-2-Aroylquinolines and 4-Aroyl-6,7,8-Trimethoxyquinolines as Highly Potent Tubulin Polymerization Inhibitors. *Int. J. Chemoinf. Chem. Eng.* **2013,** *3*(2), 1–26.
48. Kaufmann, A. *Introduction à la Théorie des Sous-ensembles Flous*; Masson: Paris, 1975; Vol. 3.
49. Cox, E. *The Fuzzy Systems Handbook*; Academic: New York, 1994.
50. Kundu, S. The Min-Max Composition Rule and its Superiority over The Usual Max-Min Composition Rule. *Fuzzy Sets Sys.* **1998,** *93,* 319–329.

51. Lambert-Torres, G.; Pereira Pinto, J. O.; Borges da Silva, L. E. Minmax Techniques. In *Wiley Encyclopedia of Electrical and Electronics Engineering*; Wiley: New York, 1999.
52. Shannon, C. E. A Mathematical Theory of Communication: Part I, Discrete Noiseless Systems. *Bell Syst. Tech. J.* **1948,** *27*, 379–423.
53. Shannon, C. E. A Mathematical Theory of Communication: Part II, the Discrete Channel with Noise. *Bell Syst. Tech. J.* **1948,** *27*, 623–656.
54. White, H. Neural Network Learning and Statistics. *AI Expert* **1989,** *4*(12), 48–52.
55. Kullback, S. *Information Theory and Statistics*; Wiley: New York, NY, 1959.
56. Lordache, O.; Corriou, J. P.; Garrido-Sánchez, L.; Fonteix, C.; Tondeur, D. Neural Network Frames. Application to Biochemical Kinetic Diagnosis. *Comput. Chem. Eng.* **1993,** *17*, 1101–1113.
57. Lordache, O. *Modeling Multi-Level Systems*; Springer: Berlin, 2011.
58. MacLane, S. *Categories for the Working Mathematician*; Springer: New York, NY, 1971.
59. Leinster, T. *Higher Operands, Higher Categories*; Cambridge University Press: Cambridge, 2004.
60. Baez, J. An Introduction to n-categories. In *7th Conference on Category Theory and Computer Science*; Moggi, E., Rosolini, G., Eds. Lecture Notes in Computer Science No. 1290; Springer: Heidelberg, 1997; pp 1–33.
61. Gordon, R.; Power, A. J.; Street, R. Coherence for Tricategories. *Memoirs Am. Math Soc.* **1995,** *117*(558), 1–1.
62. Street, R. The Algebra of Oriented Simplexes. *J. Pure Appl. Algebra* **1987,** *49*, 283–335.
63. Street, R. Categorical and Combinatorial Aspects of Descent Theory. *Appl. Categor. Struct.* **2004,** *12*, 537–576.
64. Baez, J.; Dolan, J. Higher Dimensional Algebra and Topological Quantum Field Theory. *J. Math. Phys.* **1995,** *36*, 6073–6105.
65. Leinster, T. *Higher Operands, Higher Categories*; Cambridge University: Cambridge, 2004.
66. Crans, S. On Braidings, Syllepses and Symmetries. *Cahiers Topologie Geom. Differentielle Categ.* **2000,** *41*(1), 2–74.
67. IMSL, Integrated Mathematical Statistical Library (IMSL); IMSL: Houston, 1989.
68. Tryon, R. C. A Multivariate Analysis of the Risk of Coronary Heart Disease in Framingham. *J. Chronic Dis.* **1939,** *20*, 511–524.
69. Jarvis, R. A.; Patrick, E. A. Clustering Using a Similarity Measure Based on Shared Nearest Neighbors. *IEEE Trans. Comput.* **1973,** *C22*, 1025–1034.
70. Page, R. D. M. *Program TreeView*; Universiy of Glasgow: UK, 2000.
71. Huson, D. H. SplitsTree: Analyzing and Visualizing Evolutionary Data. *Bioinformatics.* **1998,** *14*, 68–73.
72. Hotelling, H. Analysis of a Complex of Statistical Variables into Principal Components. *J. Educ. Psychol.* **1933,** *24*, 417–441.
73. Kramer, R. *Chemometric Techniques for Quantitative Analysis*; Marcel Dekker: New York, 1998.

74. Patra, S. K.; Mandal, A. K.; Pal, M. K. State of Aggregation of Bilirubin in Aqueous Solution: Principal Component Analysis Approach. *J. Photochem. Photobiol., A* **1999,** *122*, 23–31.
75. Jolliffe, I.T. *Principal Component Analysis*; Springer: New York, 2002.
76. Xu, J.; Hagler, A. Chemoinformatics and Drug Discovery. *Molecules.* **2002,** *7*, 566–600.
77. Shaw, P. J. A. *Multivariate Statistics for the Environmental Sciences*; Hodder-Arnold: New York, 2003.

CHAPTER 11

APPROACHES FOR IDENTIFICATION OF CHARACTERISTIC LESIONS IN MEDICAL IMAGING

PEDRO FURTADO*

Departamento de Engenharia Informatica, Faculdade de Ciências e tecnologia da Univrsidade de Coimbra, Coimbra, Portugal

Corresponding author. E-mail: pnf@dei.uc.pt

CONTENTS

ABSTRACT

Nowadays, imaging technologies have a very important role in medical procedures. Automated computerized processing helps diagnose diseases and find structures, lesions, and other objects. An automatic procedure may detect or highlight potential cancerous cells, lesions in eye fundus images, or characteristic lesions in skin cancer. One major application area is to use these as aids to help the medical doctor diagnose a disease, automatically indicating areas that may be causing that disease. Another application area is to simply segment structures of the body area appearing in the image. In this chapter, we review the steps and some of the approaches used in each step of medical imaging processing with the objective of finding characteristic features.

11.1 INTRODUCTION

Thanks to imaging technologies, diagnosis of medical conditions have evolved during the last century from a stage where indirect measures would be used to a stage where images of interior parts of the body are used to detect conditions and help diagnosis. One very relevant aspect of dealing with these images is the possibility of processing such images automatically using computerized means, to improve visualization (preprocessing the image), to individualize regions (segment), to identify parts (classify), and to superimpose identified regions for visualization purposes. In this chapter, we review some of the steps and techniques that allow this to happen. In Section 11.2, we summarize these steps; the next sections describe each step in detail. Section 11.3 describes acquisition and preprocessing. Section 11.4 describes segmentation, and Sections 11.5 and 11.6 describe feature extraction issues. Sections 11.7 and 11.8 give details on the classification step. Today, new approaches are still being investigated. Section 11.9 is dedicated to briefly introduce convolution network-based image classification. Finally, Section 11.10 concludes and discusses future work on the issue.

11.2 STEPS INVOLVED IN AUTOMATED MEDICAL IMAGE PROCESSING

Medical image processing goes through a set of steps that are illustrated in Figure 11.1. A source dataset is assumed at the onset. The dataset is usually a large matrix of image pixels (pixels are individual dots in an image with numeric values for color channels or for the gray scale level), but it can also be any type of raw signal. Preprocessing (step 1) is an important step to try to correct image imperfections resulting from bad lighting, noise, and other causes, and to try to enhance some image features to help in further processing. The second, and especially important, step is segmentation (step 2), where the image is divided into regions based on homogeneity or certain other characteristics, or at least some of the regions are identified based on those characteristics. This a crucial step in image processing, both for visualization (step 3), highlighting specific regions and structures, or for further processing in particular for identifying structures using classification algorithms (steps 4, 5, 6). When the objective is to classify lesions or illnesses automatically, then it typically relies on evaluating characteristics of segmented regions. Feature extraction (step 4) is the process of determining characteristics (features) for individual regions (or sometimes for the whole image). A classifier (step 6a) is a mathematical model that tries to identify an object (corresponding to some region in an image) based on its features. The model is built using an algorithm (step 6b) and training cases that identify features for known objects of each of the types. The labeling step (step 5) comprises identifying regions of specific types (called classes) so that a classifier training dataset is built from those. The classifier (6a) is then used to classify new instances of objects (step 6c). In a medical image, the output of segmentation might be an outlining of structures, lesions, parts, or regions in the visualized image, while the output of classification might be the visualization of those elements together with their type (class) that were automatically identified by the classification procedure.

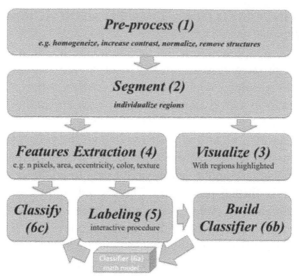

FIGURE 11.1   Steps involved in processing medical images.

11.3   ACQUISITION AND PREPROCESSING

Acquisition refers to technologies that capture and represent measurements of some body part based on sensors. There are a lot of image acquisition technologies in the medical field. For instance, magnetic fields and sensors are used to acquire signals in magnetic resonance imaging (MRI) technologies, X-rays are used in radiography and photosensors are used in photographic imaging. The acquired data may need to be preprocessed to turn it into a "readable image" format. Whatever the preprocessing, the digital output of acquisition and preprocessing is expected to be one or many 2D or 3D matrices containing measurements per pixel. For instance, a digital photography equipment transforms light rays into electrical signals that are captured and are transformed by a sensor chip into individual pixels for each position of the image. The image is an $m \times n$ matrix, where each position is a pixel with a value representing a specific "point" (smallest space region considered) in the targeted body part. A pixel may be represented by a single numerical value in gray scale, or more usually as a set of values that represent different color and intensity channels (e.g., RGB images contain a red, a blue, and a green component per pixel, that together represent a huge number of different perceptual alternatives).

Some preprocessing can be done in the equipment acquiring the data itself, other preprocessing is done as the first computerized treatment of the image after acquisition and transfer to image storage. Depending on the context, the acquisition may have been done in a context of bad illumination, sources of noise, even dirty lenses, or bad positioning. Preprocessing may be done to correct illumination and shadowing problems, remove noise, enhance contrast, or even remove unwanted structures from the image. A typical preprocessing approach is based on the convolution filters consisting of matrices of coefficients that compute sum products for each pixel, based on neighboring pixels. Convolution filters can smooth, enhance edges, remove noise, and so on. More specific operators and algorithms are also applied to remove unwanted structures, to highlight specific structures, or to do any other kind of preprocessing that may be useful in specific scenarios.

11.4 SEGMENTING MEDICAL IMAGES

Segmentation refers to dividing the image into regions or finding specific regions or contours[18] in the image. In general, segmentation algorithms try to find boundaries of regions that are homogeneous in some way and are distinct from the surrounding. Homogeneity might be evaluated, for instance, in terms of a threshold on gray scale intensity, some measure of color homogeneity or texture homogeneity. Locality is also usually present in segmentation, meaning that it is more probable to keep together close by regions in a single segment than distant images. In other terms, segmentation can be based on a distance threshold that is defined based on a subset of spatial distance, color, texture, or other possible attributes. Segmentation might also be template based. In this case, we have a template of some well-known structure and we try to find where that structure can be seen in the image. We discuss some of the approaches generically in the next subsections.

11.4.1 PARTITIONING-BASED CLUSTERING, SUPER-PIXELATION, AND MERGING-BASED CLUSTERING

Partition-based clustering submits a multidimensional dataset (or an image) to a partitioning process that determines a set of regions. The resulting clusters are such that intra-cluster homogeneity and inter-cluster heterogeneity are as large as possible. In K-means clustering,[24] a distance function between two points in the multidimensional space (pixels in the case of an image) is defined based on coordinates. The distance between two pixels with features F, $P_1(x_1, y_1, F_1)$ and $P_2(x_2, y_2, F_2)$, can be defined as $d(P_1, P_2) = \mathrm{sqrt}(w_x(x_2-x_1)^2 + w_y(y_2-y_1)^2 + w_f(F_2-F_1)^2)$, where F_1 and F_2 are the features and w_i is a weight factor. K-means clustering starts by defining k initial cluster centroids (e.g., randomly) and assigning each point to the closest centroid according to the distance metric. At each step, new centroids are computed as the mean of the coordinates of all points belonging to the cluster. Next, every point is reassigned to the closest centroid, according to the distance function. The algorithm stops when there is no modification of centroids.

Superpixelation is the definition of a usually large number of small regions larger than pixels that capture a degree of locality and distance homogeneity. Superpixels can be obtained using an algorithm called Simple Linear Iterative Clustering (SLIC).[1] The algorithm applies K-means with a weighting of color and coordinates distance as described before and adjusts boundaries of clusters iteratively. The visualization of the output is an image with an irregular mesh superimposed which is made of a large number of irregular "tiles" that enclose homogeneous regions, according to a homogeneity threshold.

While partitioning-based clustering is based on space partitioning iterations, region merging,[30] another image segmentation algorithm, takes initial locations all over the image and iteratively merges together neighboring pixels and smaller regions based on homogeneity tests.

11.4.2 DENSITY CLUSTERING

Density-based spatial clustering of applications with noise (DBSCAN)[9] is an example of a density-based clustering algorithm. Given a specific point in the multidimensional space (e.g., a pixel in an image), the algorithm evaluates which points in its neighborhood will belong to the same region (cluster) based on density (i.e., number of neighboring points within a radius). Another point B will belong to the same cluster of point A if its radius r contains point A and a number of points larger or equal to a defined value m, or if it is a part of the cluster of point C using the same rule and point C is part of the cluster of point A using the same rule again (transitivity). Density clustering is able to determine even very irregular and non-convex regions, thanks to transitivity.

11.4.3   OTHER ALGORITHMS

There are myriad of other segmentation algorithms. Some of the most used ones include segmentation based on multi scale J-images (JSEG),[6] OTSU's method,[21,33,43] and Watershed.[36,39] JSEG is a two-step procedure; the first one quantizing colors in every pixel of the image to a chosen number of levels and the second being a clustering over the quantized image. Given a desired number of thresholds, OTSU method determines the best threshold values to quantize the image. The best threshold is the one that minimizes the sum of errors, defined as the sum of the differences between the value and the quantized value for all pixels. Watershed is named after its model of flooding of a terrain whose topographic levels are the pixel intensities. The flooding starts from local minima, and a region merging post-processing step is used to avoid an excessive number of regions.

11.4.4   USE OF SEGMENTATION

OTSU's method is very usual in image segmentation and other image processing tasks targeted at detecting and isolating regions for further processing. Density-based segmentation (DBSCAN adapted for handling images and other density-based variants) and JSEG are also well adapted to image segmentation and typically produce well-defined regions at least partly individualizing objects or parts of objects of interest. On the other hand, DBSCAN and JSEG require heavy computation and for this reason, take more time than simpler approaches. Besides these techniques, there are also other segmentation algorithms that are frequently used to grow regions from specific seed points. In particular, active contours[18] use a mathematical model to iteratively grow region boundaries from an initial specification of either a seed point or a rough region.

Segmentation may be used for visualization, adding a definition of regions superimposed on the medical image. It can also be used together with region properties to identify specific structures and to classify structures, lesions, and other types of objects and regions in images. At the same time, there are other procedures that may use segmentation or simpler threshold-based isolation of regions. For instance, it is common to follow a procedure to isolate a certain type of structure, such as a vascular network or an optic disk in an eye fundus image (EFI). In those cases, gray scale or color channel thresholds can identify the desired structures, or more complex segmentation algorithms can also be used. Figure 11.2 shows two examples of EFI with vascular tree and optic disk removed, replacing those regions with black masks.

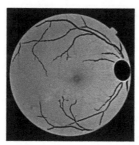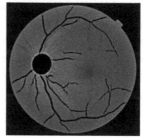

FIGURE11.2   Eye fundus images—removal of optic disk and vascular tree.

11.5   OBTAINING FEATURES OF REGIONS

Segmentation simply finds regions, but further identification and processing of regions require characterization of those regions. Features are characteristics extracted from regions. They usually summarize the details of the region in some way that can be used to assign a specific type (as known as a class) to the region. Typical region features include statistics or histograms on color or gray scale intensities, texture, shape, or contours. Statistical descriptors include mean, max, variance, percentiles, and others. A feature is a single value so that the features extracted from a region are used to build a complete vector of features. The vector of features is expected to describe "well" a region. This means that, given a set of types of regions (classes), the regions of a certain type should have feature vectors that are similar among them and different from feature vectors of regions pertaining to other types. That way we can check the type of the region based on its characteristics. The set of characteristics that is relevant for detecting some structure, lesion, or other types of object is very dependent on the specific object being described.

There are some other specific types of features and feature extraction methods that are worth mentioning. Local binary patterns (LBP)[31,32] based on the texture spectrum model[14,40] can be used for texture classification. For each pixel, it creates a code by traversing neighbors in a specific order and filling each code digit with a 0 or a 1 depending on whether that neighbor has higher or lower pixel value. Then, it creates a histogram of the number of occurrences of each code. Local binary patterns can be combined with another approach, the histogram of oriented gradients (HOG),[5] for improved accuracy. Scale-invariant feature transform (SIFT)[22,23] is another technique to extract features, in this case describing key points in the image or region, and speeded up robust features (SURF),[3] an approach derived from scale-invariant feature transform (SIFT) but which is much faster.

11.6   FIXING FEATURE VECTOR SIZE

Feature extraction with SIFT or SURF results in a variable number of n key points, each having a set of m features associated with it. The bag-of-words approach reduces these $n \times m$ feature values into a feature vector with exactly k positions, k being defined as the dictionary size. In order to do that, a k-means clustering algorithm is applied to the feature vectors of the n key points (m-dimensional space) to find k centroids. Each key point is then represented by the closest centroid. Finally, a feature vector with k positions is created where each position i has the number of key points with centroid i. Parameter k can be adjusted based on evaluating classification accuracy with varied values of k. The bag-of-words approach can be used with other feature extraction algorithms besides SIFT and SURF. In fact, we can concatenate results from multiple feature extraction algorithms and then apply a bag-of-words procedure to find k feature vectors from those.

11.7   MULTIDIMENSIONAL DATASETS (TRAIN AND TEST) AND LABELING

We have seen in the previous section that each feature vector characterizes a region. For classification, we need to create a dataset with multiple cases of well identified regions that will be fed to an algorithm that builds a mathematical model that learns how to classify or distinguish different types of object. The "type of object" is called a class, and labeling is the process of assigning classes to cases. The set of cases (objects together with their classes) is a multidimensional dataset, where each case is a point with coordinates given by the feature vector values. The classifier is some model that is able to map specific points in the multidimensional space to a specific class, such that if a feature vector corresponds to point P, then it belongs to class C. For instance, the model can divide the multi-dimensional space into regions, each with a corresponding class. In order to be able to correctly infer a model for classification, the classifier needs to be fed with a number of cases that is statistically significant for each class that is considered. The test dataset is also a multidimensional dataset, but in that case, the objective is to test how many of those test cases are correctly classified. It is important that the test dataset be distinct from the training dataset and statistically relevant, to avoid overfitting by testing the model with the same data that was used to train the model and to have a significant evaluation of the model. There are many alternatives concerning testing. One alternative is to divide the cases dataset into p% train and $(1-p)$% test cases. Another alternative is cross-validation with f equal-sized folds (e.g., 10 folds). The cases dataset is divided f times such that $f-1$ folds are used to train and 1 fold is used to test.

An issue that is frequent in classification tasks is the need to reduce the number of features. Too many features may lead to overfitting.[13] A simplified definition of overfitting is when the mathematical model captures in its formulas characteristics that are not related to the actual traits that should define the classes that are being modeled, but instead, they are related to other non-related image characteristics that exist by chance in certain images. The more features we have, the larger the dataset needs to be in order to be statistically relevant (dimensionality curse[25]), and the number of cases necessarily grows rapidly as the number of features (size of the feature vector) increases. Among alternative approaches for dimensionality reduction, feature selection by ranking features in order of their correlation to the class or their information gain is a typical way to choose only those features that are assumed to best describe the data. Another approach is the use of principal components analysis,[17] which maps the multidimensional space to another space based on linear combinations of features (principal components), such that each one will be orthogonal to all the previous ones (uncorrelated), and where the components are ordered in order of relevance to the classification. By choosing only the first k principal values (coefficients of the principal components), the size of the feature vector is reduced.

11.8 IDENTIFYING STRUCTURES, LESIONS, OR OTHER OBJECTS

Classification of an image region is the procedure of identifying the object present in the region automatically. The input to classification is the region itself, and the output is a class, the identification of the type of object. In a medical image, the object may be a lesion characteristic of a disease or a structure. As an example, consider detection of diabetic retinopathy lesions based in eye fundus images. Classes include "micro-aneurysm," "exudates," "hemorragy," and other lesions that need to be detected. But besides those classes, there should also be at least a class "normal" = "non-lesion," and there may be classes such as "fundus," "optic disk," "macula," and other classes identifying non-lesion structures that need to be identified in the image as well.

A classifier is a mathematical model that "learns" to classify by adjusting the coefficients of the model. For instance, a linear regression model tries to approximate the distribution of data points by some. It adjusts coefficients based on examples (cases) to fit the data distribution. After training, the linear regression model is able to predict the outcome for new inputs using the equation of the line, with adjusted coefficients (slope and y axis value at the origin). Logistic regression is a type of regression model targeted at categorical (class-based) prediction. Figure 11.3 shows the process of building a classifier, based on a training dataset that includes the class of each training case. The training dataset is a set of feature vectors known as the training dataset. The model adjusts its coefficients to reflect the training cases so that after adjusting the model it will be able to identify the class of the training dataset as well as possible.

The test dataset also shown in Figure 11.3 should be an independent dataset with the class of each case included. This test dataset is fed to the classifier and the fraction of correct classifications of the test dataset is used as a measure of accuracy. Other measures of accuracy are also output in this testing procedure.

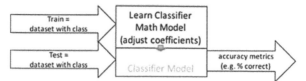

FIGURE 11.3 Building a classifier: train and test.

Figure 11.4 illustrates the use of a classifier. Given an observation (a feature vector representing a region), the classifier uses its mathematical model to identify (classify) the object (class).

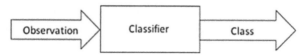

FIGURE 11.4 Using a classifier.

There are many classifier models in the literature.[12,26,41] We briefly introduce some of the most commonly used ones.

K-nn: K-nearest neighbors[2] is based on the proximity of the feature vector to other observations in the training dataset (the model is the training dataset itself in k-nn). Given a new observation (region) to be classified, the Euclidean distance of that new observation to each of the model (training) cases is evaluated, and the shortest k distances are selected. The class of the new observation is then the class given by a majority vote on the classes of the k-nearest neighbors.

Decision trees: Figure 11.5 exemplifies a decision tree.[34] In this example, the green channel is analyzed first. If its value is below 0.1 (normalized values), and the maximum value of the red channel is below 0.3, then the region is classified as *normal*. If the red channel is above 0.3, then the region is classified as *lesion c.*; the rest of the tree follows the same logic. The decision tree is built automatically from the training dataset. There are many variants of decision trees and algorithms for the construction of decision trees. Given in intuitive terms, the most classic decision-tree building algorithm evaluates at each time which feature is most descriptive, that is, distinguishes better between classes. That feature is used as a decision node, and alternative (categorical) values of the feature (which can be intervals of numbers, individual values, or categories) correspond to different branches in the resulting subtree. Then, each possible path in the subtree is evaluated similarly.

Decision trees and decision-tree algorithms are wide subjects, with many variants and improvements, For example, Random Forests[15] having been proposed to improve accuracy and capacity to represent more difficult datasets.

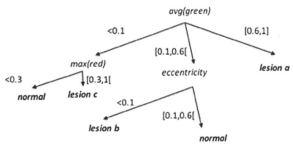

FIGURE 11.5   Example of the decision tree.

Neural Networks and backpropagation: An artificial neural network takes a feature vector as input and forwards the values to a set of neurons, which are computation units that transform the input signals using, for instance, a weighted sum-product of the values. A multilayer perceptron (MLP) is a feedforward artificial neural network with multiple fully-connected layers forming a directed graph.

Figure 11.6 is an example of an artificial neural network. Features f_1, f_n, and other features between those are forwarded to a set of neurons, each one doing a sum-product such as the one shown $(w_1 \times f_1 + \ldots + w_n \times f_n)$. The outputs of neurons (v in the figure) go through activation functions, also shown in the figure, and serve as inputs to the next layer of neurons. There may be many layers, but the last—output—layer is the one returning a class. The class may be returned as an activation of a specific output neuron, or as a specific code given by the combination of values of all output neurons. Based on the training dataset, the neural network must learn the coefficients (such as the weights w_i) that will result in correct class outputs for those training cases (model building). This is usually done based on the backpropagation algorithm.[20,37] Given an output for a specific feature vector and a correct classification for that vector, an error is the difference between the expected output and the given output. Backpropagation adjusts the network coefficients based on feeding the error back through the network and some adjustment function. After applying the backpropagation algorithm many times (epochs) for the training dataset, the neural network is expected to have learned appropriate coefficient values. The test dataset is used to assess the resulting accuracy.

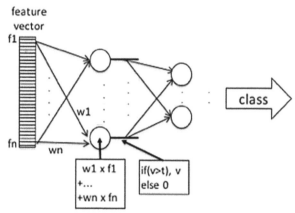

FIGURE 11.6   Artificial neural network.

Other classifiers: Other noteworthy classifier models include the Bayesian classifier,[7,11] a probabilistic approach based in Bayes theorem, support vector machines (SVM),[4,10] which determines data separation hyperplanes in the multidimensional space formed by the training dataset. A support vector is a multidimensional point (vector) closest to the separating hyperplane.

11.9 CONVOLUTION NEURAL NETWORKS

Multilayer perceptrons have nodes fully connected to inputs and between layers. This architecture does not scale well to images, since it means that all pixels of an $x \times y$ image are fed to all nodes in the first layer, resulting in a huge number of connections and weights to be adjusted. Also importantly, the locality can help reduce the number of connections and work, since nearby pixels can be analyzed locally (restricting connections to local pixels) prior to broader analysis. In a convolution neural network (CNN),[19,38] layers are stacked one after the other, but each neuron "sees" only its "receptive field," a small region from the previous layer or input pixels. The CNN has a set of convolution layers, followed by fully-connected layers. Convolution layers restrict their sum-product computations to the localized neuron receptive field. A typical CNN can receive the pixels of an image as input. Convolution layers will compute the weighted sum product of the inputs (receptive field) that correspond to a small region. Multiple filters can be used in these layers. ReLU layers apply activation functions on the output of the convolution layers, and pooling layers reduce the size of the output. There may be many convolutions, ReLU, and pooling layers, with varied architectures, until finally the output is fed to a fully-connected layer that determines the class or a class score. The convolution network is a type of neural network and such can be trained using the backpropagation algorithm. One important advantage of CNNs is that there is no need for prior feature extraction since the image itself is given as input and the CNN learns the weights of connections, which is equivalent to learning the feature extraction automatically.

11.10 CONCLUSIONS AND FUTURE CHALLENGES

Image processing techniques have important applications in medical imaging. We have described the steps involved in automated computerized image segmentation and classification of structures, objects, and lesions in the context of post-processing of medical images to detect and classify features of those images. We have also reviewed some of the alternative techniques to apply in each of the steps and concluded about the importance of each approach.

Nowadays, there is a significant amount of researchers in convolution neural networks. Region-based convolution neural networks[35] might also be of great use to improve object recognition capabilities in medical imaging. However, the main issues related to correctly identifying objects, structures, and lesions, in general, are still related to feature extraction mechanisms and feature engineering. While in very controlled setups it is possible to achieve top accuracy scores, in more general settings accuracy is still unsatisfactory. Another important research direction is to develop techniques that are specific to each context and that use contextual knowledge to improve accuracy.

KEYWORDS

- medical imaging
- image preprocessing
- classification
- machine learning
- data mining

REFERENCES

1. Achanta, R.; et al. Slic Superpixels. No. EPFL-REPORT-149300. 2010.
2. Altman, N. S. An Introduction to Kernel and Nearest-Neighbor Nonparametric Regression. *Am. Stat.* **1992**, *46*(3), 175–185.
3. Bay, H.; Ess, A.; Tuytelaars, T.; Van Gool, L. *Speeded Up Robust Features*; ETH Zurich, Katholieke Universiteit Leuven, 2006.
4. Chang, C.-C.; Lin, C.-J. LIBSVM: A Library for Support Vector Machines. *ACM Trans. Intell. Syst. Technol.* **2013**, *2*, 1–39.
5. Dalal, N.; Triggs, B. Histograms of Oriented Gradients for Human Detection. *IEEE Computer Society Conference on Computer Vision and Pattern Recognition (CVPR'05)*, IEEE, San Diego, CA, USA, USA, Vol. 1. 2005.
6. Deing, Y.; Manjunath, B. S. Unsupervised Segmentation of Color-Texture Regions in Images and Videos. *IEEE Trans. Pattern Anal. Machine Intell.* **2001**, *23*(8), 800–801.
7. DELL Software, Naive Bayes Classifier. [Online]. http://www.statsoft.com/Text-book/Naive- Bayes-Classifier (accessed Jan 20, 2016).
8. Emanuel, D. I'm Sorry to Say, But Your Understanding of Image Processing Fundamentals is Absolutely Wrong. *arXiv preprint arXiv,* **2008**, *0808.0056.*
9. Ester, M.; Kriegel, H.-P.; Sander, J.; Xu, X. (1996). Simoudis, Evangelos; Han, Jiawei; Fayyad, Usama M., eds. *A density-based algorithm for discovering clusters in large spatial databases with noise.* Proceedings of the Second International Confer-ence on Knowledge Discovery and Data Mining (KDD-96). AAAI Press. pp. 226–231. CiteSeerX 10.1.1.121.9220Freely accessible. ISBN 1-57735-004-9.
10. Fan, R.-E.; Chang, K.-W., Hsieh, C.-J.; Wang, X.-R.; Lin, C.-J. LIBLINEAR: A Library for Large 29 Linear Classification. *J. Mach. Learn.* **2008**, *9*, 1871–1874.
11. Frank, E.; Trigg, L.; Holmes, G.; Witten, I. H. Naive Bayes for Regression. *Mach. Learn.* **2000**, *41*(1), 5–15.
12. Han, J.; Pei, J.; Kamber, M. Data Mining: Concepts and Techniques. Elsevier, 2011.
13. Hawkins, D. M. The Problem of Overfitting. *J. Chem. Inf. Comput. Sci.* **2004**, *44*(1), 1–12.

14. He, D. C.;Wang, L. Texture Unit, Texture Spectrum, and Texture Analysis. *IEEE Trans. Geosc. Remote Sens.* **1990**, *28*, 509–512.
15. Ho, T. K. *Random Decision Forests (PDF).* Proceedings of the 3rd International Conference on Document Analysis and Recognition, Montreal, QC, August 14–16, 1995; pp. 278–282.
16. Hughes, G. F. On the Mean Accuracy of Statistical Pattern Recognizers. *IEEE Trans. Inf. Theory* **1968**, *14*(1), 55–63. DOI: 10.1109/TIT.1968.1054102.
17. Jolliffe I. T. *Principal Component Analysis, Series: Springer Series in Statistics*, 2nd ed.; Springer: NY, 2002, XXIX, 487 p. 28 illus; ISBN 978-0-387-95442-4.
18. Kass, M.; Witkin, A.; Terzopoulos, D. Snakes: Active Contour Models (PDF). *Int. J. Comput. Vision.* **1988**, *1*(4), 321.
19. Krizhevsky, A., Sutskever, I.; Hinton, G. E. Imagenet Classification with Deep Convolutional Neural Networks. Advances in neural information processing systems. 2012.
20. Li, Y.; Fu, Y.; Li, H.; Zhang, S. W. The Improved Training Algorithm of Back Propagation Neural Network with Self-adaptive Learning Rate. *2009 International Conference on Computational Intelligence and Natural Computing* **2009**, *1*, 73–76.
21. Liao, P.-S.; Chen, T.-S.; Chung, P.-C. A Fast Algorithm for Multilevel Thresholding. *J. Inf. Sci. Eng.* **2001**, *17*(5), 713–727.
22. Lowe, D. G. *Object Recognition from Local Scale-Invariant Features (PDF).* Proceedings of the International Conference on Computer Vision. 2. pp. 1150–1157. 1999 DOI: 10.1109/ICCV.1999.790410.
23. Lowe, D. Method and Apparatus for Identifying Scale Invariant Features in an Image and use of Same for Locating an Object in an Image, David Lowe's patent for the SIFT algorithm, U.S. Patent 6,711,293, March 23, 2004.
24. MacQueen, J. B. *Some Methods for Classification and Analysis of Multivariate Observations.* Proceedings of 5th Berkeley Symposium on Mathematical Statistics and Probability. April 04–07, 2009, 1. MR 0214227. Zbl 0214.46201, University of California Press: Berkeley, Calif., 1967; 281–297.
25. Marimont, R. B.; Shapiro, M. B. Nearest Neighbour Searches and the Curse of Dimensionality. *IMA J. Appl Math.* **1979**, *24*(1), 59–70.
26. Mark, H.; et al. The WEKA Data Mining Software: An Update. *ACM SIGKDD Explorations Newsletter* **2009**, *11*(1), 10–18.
27. McLaren, K. XIII—The Development of the CIE 1976 (L* a* b*) Uniform Colour Space and Colour-Difference Formula. *J. Soc. Dyers Colour.* **1976**, *92*(9), 338–341.
28. Medical Imaging in Wikipedia: https://en.wikipedia.org/wiki/Medical_imaging, (accessed 2016-11).
29. Najman, L.; Couprie, M.; Bertrand, G. Watersheds, Mosaics, and the Emergence Paradigm. *Discrete Appl. Math.* **2005**, *147*(2–3), 301–324.
30. Nock, R.; Nielsen, F. Statistical Region Merging (PDF). *IEEE Trans. Pattern Anal. Machine Intell.* **2004**, *26*(11), 1–7.
31. Ojala, T.; Pietikäinen, M.; Harwood, D. Performance Evaluation of Texture Measures with Classification Based on Kullback Discrimination of Distributions. *Proc. 12th IAPR Int. Conf. Pattern Recognit. (ICPR 1994).* **1994**, *1*, 582–585.

32. Ojala, T.; Pietikäinen, M.; Harwood, D. A Comparative Study of Texture Measures with Classification Based on Feature Distributions. *Pattern Recognit.* **1996,** *29,* 51–59.

33. Otsu, N. A Threshold Selection Method from Gray-Level Histograms. IEEE Trans. Sys. Man. Cyber. **1979,** *9*(1), 62–66. DOI: 10.1109/TSMC.1979.4310076.

34. Quinlan, J. R. Simplifying Decision Trees. *Int. J. Man-Mach. Stud.* **1987,** *27*(3), 221.

35. Ren, S.; et al. Faster R-CNN: Towards Real-Time Object Detection with Region Proposal Networks. Advances in Neural Information Processing Systems. 2015.

36. Roerdink, J. B. T. M.; Meijster, A. The Watershed Transform: Definitions, Algorithms, and Parallelization Strategies. *Fundamenta Informaticae* **2000,** *41,* 187–228.

37. Rumelhart, D. E.; Hinton, G. E.; Williams, R. J. Learning Representations by Back-Propagating Errors. *Nature.* **1986,** *323* (6088), 533–536.

38. Shih-Chung B. Lo; et al. Artificial Convolution Neural Network for Medical Image Pattern Recognition. *Neural Networks* **1995,** *8*(7–8), 1201–1214.

39. Vincent, L.; Soille, P. Watersheds in Digital Spaces: An Efficient Algorithm Based on Immersion Simulations. *IEEE Trans. Pattern Anal. Machine Intell.* **1991,** *13*(6), 583–598.

40. Wang, L.; He, D. C. Texture Classification Using Texture Spectrum. *Pattern Recognit.* **1990,** *23*(8), 905–910.

41. Witten, I. H.; Frank, E. Data Mining: Practical Machine Learning Tools and Techniques; Morgan Kaufmann: Burlington, 2005.

42. Zhang, H.; Fritts, J. E.; Goldman, S. A. Image Segmentation Evaluation: A Survey of Unsupervised Methods. *Computer Vision Image Understanding* **2008,** *110*(2), 260–280.

43. Zhu, N.; Wang, G.; Yang, G.; Weiming, D. A Fast 2d Otsu Thresholding Algorithm Based on Improved Histogram. Pattern Recognition, 2009. CCPR 2009. Chinese Conference on: 1–5.

CHAPTER 12

KINETICS OF ELLAGIC ACID ACCUMULATION BY SOLID-STATE FERMENTATION

ARMANDO ROBLEDO[1], ANTONIO F. AGUILERA-CARBO[2], ARELY PRADO-BARRAGAN[3], LEONARDO SEPULVEDA-TORRE[1], RAUL RODRÍGUEZ-HERRERA[1], JUAN C. CONTRERAS-ESQUIVEL[1] and CRISTOBAL N. AGUILAR[1,*]

[1]Food Research Department, School of Chemistry, Universidad Autónoma de Coahuila, Saltillo 25280, Coahuila, México

[2]Department of Food Science and Technology, Universidad Autónoma Agraria Antonio Narro, Buenavista, Saltillo, Coahuila, México

[3]Department of Biotechnology, Universidad Autonoma Metropolitana Unidad Iztapalapa, Mexico City, Mexico

*Corresponding author. E-mail: cristobal.aguilar@uadec.edu.mx

CONTENTS

ABSTRACT

The study investigated the process efficiency through the estimation of the kinetic parameters of production of ellagic acid (EA) by solid-state fermentation (SSF). EA is a potent antioxidant with anti-inflammatory and antiproliferative capacity. *Aspergillus niger* GH1 strain was grown on pomegranate husk residues as a substrate and support matrix. Logistic and Luedeking–Piret equations were used in order to estimate values of the following coefficients: maximal specific growth rate (μ_M), maximal biomass level (X_M), enzyme/biomass yield ($Y_{P/X}$) and secondary rate of production, or breakdown (k). It was showed that biomass aloud a high yield of product formation (EA) thus degrading ellagitannins (ETs). The fungus had a high degradation capacity of phenols (2.27 mg X/mg S h^{-1}) from pomegranate husk releasing EA during the bioprocess.

12.1   INTRODUCTION

Pomegranate (*Punica granatum* L.) husk, seed, and juice, have antioxidant capacity due to their tannin content. Ellagitannins (ETs), one of the principal groups of hydrolysable tannins, are esters of hexahydroxydiphenic acid (HHDP) and a polyol, usually glucose or quinic acid and are considered secondary plant metabolites found in cytoplasm and cell vacuoles.[13] When exposed to acids or strong bases, esters bonds are hydrolyzed and the HHDP is released, and spontaneously rearranged into the stable water-insoluble dilactone, namely, ellagic acid (EA).[11] ETs are principally obtained from bark and trunks of big trees[12] and also have been proved that fruit from bushy trees or berries trees, such as pomegranate,[3,14,18] cranberry,[20] straw-berry, raspberry, and blackberry[14] are also important sources of ETs and EA.

EA is a highly thermodynamically stable molecule, with four rings representing the lipophilic domain and four phenolic and two lactone groups (which can act as hydrogen bond donor and acceptor, respectively) representing the hydrophilic part. This structure provides EA a high anti-oxidant, anti-inflammatory, and antiproliferative capacity as well as the effect on subcellular signaling pathways, induction of cell cycle arrest and apoptosis.[14] EA also decreases incidence of congenital defects, promotes healing of wounds, reduces heart attacks, even can revert fibrosis of liver chemically induced, and stops proliferation of virus, such as VIH,[17] among others properties.[16]

Our research group has made an important contribution about the biodegradation of ETs using pomegranate husk as a support in a solid-state fermentation (SSF) bioprocess,[1,4,18] which has been optimized in terms of culture conditions[19] even with some progress in the mode of operation of the process.[7] However, the control and description of the bioprocess is essential to ensure the success of the technological development and the application of mathematical models for calculation of the kinetic parameters of the microbial process is used to predict future performance and efficiency. Hence, in this work, an attempt is made to define the kinetic parameters involved in accumulation of EA due biodegradation of the ETs present in pomegranate husk.

12.2 MATERIALS AND METHODS

12.2.1 POMEGRANATE HUSK

A lot of 50 kg of pomegranate fruits (*P. granatum* L., wonderful variety) was acquired from a local market located in Saltillo City, Coahuila, Mexico. Fruits were washed, peeled, and used to produce juice and the pomegranate husk was carefully collected and dehydrated at 60°C during 48 h into a conventional oven and, finally, pulverized to be used as a support for the growth of the fungus during the bioprocessing to produce EA.

12.2.2 MICROORGANISM

The *Aspergillus niger* GH1 strain (Food Research Department Collection, Universidad Autónoma de Coahuila, Mexico) was used in this study. Fungal strain was crio-conserved at −50°C in a medium containing glycerol–skimmed milk. Periodic reactivation was made on potato dextrose agar (PDA) slants and incubated for 5 days at 30°C. The fungus was maintained in PDA at 4°C. This strain has been previously reported as high-level tannin tolerant and ellagitannase producer in solid-state culture.[4,5,8,18]

12.2.3 INOCULUM PREPARATION

For inoculum preparation, the spores of *A. niger* GH1 were inoculated in 250 ml Erlenmeyer flasks containing 30 ml of PDA (PDA-Bioxon) medium, and incubated at 30°C for 5 days. The new spores were harvested with a sterilized solution of 0.01 % Tween-80, and then counted in a hemo-cytometer (Neubauer).

12.2.4   SOLID-STATE FERMENTATION (SSF)

Fungal growth was evaluated on Petri dishes and medium was prepared as follow: pomegranate residues were moisturized (70 %) with Czapek-Dox medium [(g/L): NaNO$_3$ (7.65); KH$_2$PO$_4$ (3.04); MgSO$_4$ (1.52); KCl (1.52)], using pomegranate residue as sole energy and carbon source. Spores of A. niger GH1 (2×10^7 spores) were inoculated at the center of the plates, which were incubated at 30°C. Samples were monitored kinetically during 192 h and consumption of total sugars[9] and ETs content[12] were determined, and fungal biomass was spectrophotometrically evaluated by the glucosamine content method[6] and reported as milligram of biomass per gram of dried solid support. Tannin acyl hydrolase was assayed by the high-performance liquid chromatography (HPLC) method reported by Aguilar et al.[2] Enzyme solution (0.05 ml) was incubated with 0.80 ml of 1.0 % (w/v) tannic acid in 0.2 M acetate buffer (pH 5.0) at 30°C for 30 min and then reaction was stopped by addition of 0.20 ml trichloroacetic acid (TCA). Reaction mixture was filtered (nylon membrane, 0.45 μm) and injected into HPLC equipment (Varian, ProStar system) with PDA detector at 254 nm. Separation was carried out with an Optisil ODS column (5 μm; 250×4.6 mm) at a temperature of 30°C. A tannase unit was defined as amount of enzyme able to release 1 μmol of gallic acid per minute under assay conditions. EA accumulation was also determined by HPLC.[18] Samples were analyzed in triplicates.

12.2.5   KINETIC PARAMETERS ASSOCIATED TO SOLID-STATE FERMENTATION (SSF) PROCESS

Within kinetic parameters are the specific growth rate (μ) obtained from growth plot linearization and slope from the straight line resulting by least square regression, and productivity (Γ), estimated in terms of grams of support used, and defined as follows:

$$\Gamma_{obs} = \text{maximum of} \left[\frac{p}{t} \right] \qquad (12.1)$$

That is, for a given fermentation curve, Γ_{Obs} will be the maximum of ratio between the product level (enzyme titer) per liquid broth volume, P, added to system and divided by fermentation time, t, evaluated at peak of enzyme or secondary metabolite production.

Viniegra et al.[22] mentioned about the relationship between biomass and productivity but related to a protein instead of a secondary metabolite as EA production. In this way, a process directed to a biomass production has a target to maximize biomass yield (Y_{XS}). On the other hand, if the interest is by-product, an increase of product yield ($Y_{P/X}$) should be performed.

The biomass yield refers to biomass quantity produced by gram of substrate used, expressed in mg X/mg S and calculated as follows:

$$Y_{X/S} = \frac{X_2 - X_1}{S_1 - S_2} \qquad (12.2)$$

where X_1 is the biomass initial condition and X_2 is the biomass concentration at the product maximum value; S_1 is the substrate initial condition and S_2 is the substrate concentration at the product maximum value.

The production yield is quantity of metabolite formed, expressed in mg AE/mg X, and calculated with the formula

$$Y_{P/X} = \frac{P_2 - P_1}{X_1 - X_2} \qquad (12.3)$$

where P_1 is the product initial concentration and P_2 is the maximum product concentration; X_1 is the biomass initial condition and X_2 is the biomass concentration at the product maximum value.

Biomass production was evaluated by the Verhulst–Pearl logistic equation,[2] originally developed for population growth.

$$\frac{dX}{dt} = \mu_M \left[1 - \frac{X}{X_{max}} \right] X \qquad (12.4)$$

where X is the biomass density (g per kg), μ_M is the maximum specific growth rate (h^{-1}), and X_M is the equilibrium level of X for which, $dX/dt=0$ for $X>0$. Solution of the above equation can be written as follows:

$$-\frac{dS}{dt} = \frac{1}{Y_{X/S}}\frac{dX}{dt} + mX \qquad (12.5)$$

where X_0 is the initial condition for X. Eq. (12.5) is useful to fit experimental data by Equation (12.4), finding the least value of the sum of squared errors as a function of parameters, X_0, X_M, and μ_M.

Substrate consumption was modeled using a two-term expression proposed by Pirt (1975) as follows:

$$-\frac{dS}{dt} = \frac{1}{Y_{X/S}}\frac{dX}{dt} + mX \qquad (12.6)$$

where S is the substrate concentration (g per kg), $Y_{X/S}$ is the biomass yield coefficient (mg X/mg S), and m is the maintenance coefficient (g S/g X h). Solution of Equation (12.6) can be obtained as a function of X as follows:

$$S(t) = S_0 - \left(\frac{X - X_0}{Y_{X/S}}\right) - \left(\frac{X_{max}*m}{\mu}\right)\ln\left[\frac{X_{max} - X_0}{X - X_0}\right] \qquad (12.7)$$

where S_0 is the initial condition for substrate level, S. Equation (12.7) helps to test the importance of maintenance coefficient, m, because a state plot of $S(t)$ versus $X(t)$ will yield a straight line with slope, $1/Y_{X/S}$, whenever m is negligible. Otherwise, a logarithmic correction will appear with coefficient, mX_M/μ_M.

Kinetics of product formation can be modeled using the Luedeking and Piret[15] equation as follows:

$$\frac{dP}{dt} = Y_{P/X}\frac{dX}{dt} + kX \qquad (12.8)$$

where P is the product concentration, $Y_{P/X}$ is the product yield in terms of biomass (units of product per unit of biomass) and k is the secondary coefficient of product formation or destruction. Equation (12.8) is similar to Equation (12.6), but here coefficient k can be negative, zero, or positive, since product formation or destruction is not necessarily related to growth. Again, it is possible to solve Equation (12.8) as a function of biomass.

$$P(t) = P_0 + Y_{P/X}(X - X_0) + \frac{kX_M}{\mu_M}\ln\left[\frac{X_M - X_0}{X - X_0}\right] \qquad (12.9)$$

In terms of specific growth rate (μ_M), the specific production rate of enzyme, q_P, can be defined as follows:

$$q_P = \mu_M \cdot Y_{P/X} \qquad (12.10)$$

and the specific substrate uptake rate, q_S, can be defined as follows:

$$q_S = \mu_M / Y_{X/S} \qquad (12.11)$$

$Y_{P/X}$ and $Y_{X/S}$ were estimated from linear correlation between EA and biomass concentration, and biomass and pomegranate husk powder, respectively.

12.2.6 EXPERIMENTAL DESIGN AND DATA ANALYSIS

SSF experiments were conducted by triplicate and average values are reported. Data were analyzed using a unidirectional analyses of variance (ANOVA) procedure in Minitab® 15.1.20.0. When needed, treatment means were compared using the Tukey's range procedure ($p \leq 0.05$).

12.3 RESULTS AND DISCUSSION

12.3.1 SOLID-STATE FERMENTATION (SSF) PROCESS ON POMEGRANATE HUSK

SSF permitted release and recovery of potent phenolic antioxidants from agro-industrial waste. EA production through pomegranate husk fermentation by *A. niger* GH1 was investigated to estimate the kinetic parameters of ET's degradation and EA accumulation. The maximum biomass accumulation during growth kinetic (Fig. 12.1) was showed at 168 h (390 mg/gS) without a significant statistical difference with the value obtained at 96 h (353 mg/gS). Notably, natural SSF substrates primarily have more than one carbon source that can be employed for microorganism growth. Obtained biomass values from pomegranate husk fermentation were adjusted through the Verhulst–Pearl logistic equation (Eq. 12.4) to obtain X_0, X_{max}, and μ_M as biomass kinetic parameters. Since consumption rate for different substrates may be different, a deviation from classical growth curves (with one exponential growth phase) may appear. In this case, the specific growth rate achieved a value of 0.3527 h^{-1} between 24 and 48 h of fermentation, decreasing to 0.0045 h^{-1} from 48 to 168 h, that could be due to EA presence in the media, which may acts as growth inhibitor. These data match with EA production which reaches its maximal value at 96 h.

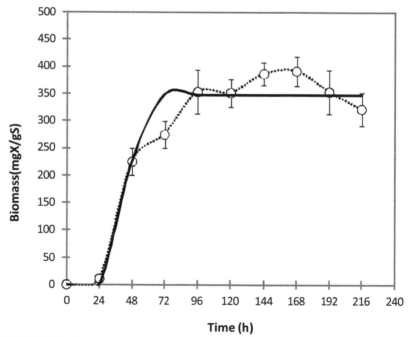

FIGURE 12.1   Cell growth curve of the batch fermentation of *Aspergillus niger* GH1 on pomegranate husk powder. (—) theoretical; (⋯) experimental.

Total hydrolysable phenols (THP) were considerate as substrate for EA accumulation, and their consumption is showed in Figure 12.2. THP content had an increase of 20% at the first day of fermentative process, probably because they get dissolved into the media during incubation time, after which value decline to keep between 60–80 mg/gds. After the second day, consumption of THP reaches 40% and keeps around this value at the end of fermentation process. During this time, a generation and consumption of polyphenols monomers could occur.

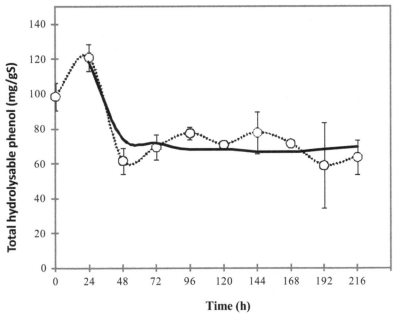

FIGURE 12.2 Consumption of total hydrolysable phenols (THP) during *Aspergillus niger* GH1 fermentation on pomegranate husk powder. (—) theoretical; (···) experimental.

Maximum concentration of EA accumulation (Fig. 12.3) was reached at 96 h of fermentation (11.27 mg/gds). Vattem and Shetty[20] reports 0.350 mg/gds using *Lentinus edodes* on cranberry pomace at 120 h of culture; Ventura et al.[21] reached values of 4.74 mg/gds of creosote bush and 7.56 mg/g of tar bush using *A. niger PSH* after four days of culture. The decreasing value of EA concentration could be due to the complex formation ability with proteins of this reagent.

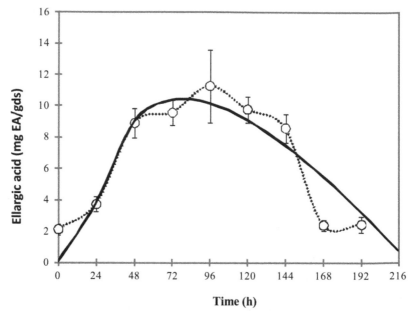

FIGURE 12.3   Ellagic acid (EA) accumulation during *Aspergillus niger* GH1 fermentation on pomegranate husk powder. (—) theoretical; (···) experimental.

12.3.2   KINETIC PARAMETERS DURING SOLID-STATE FERMENTATION (SSF)

Microorganism yields give an idea of the production process efficiency. In this way, a process focused on biomass production should maximize $Y_{X/S}$. Furthermore, if the interest is the product, increasing of $Y_{P/X}$, minimizing as much as possible the $Y_{X/S}$ value, is needed.

Kinetic parameters related with the fermentative process (Table 12.1) show that the amount of EA obtained by milligram of biomass is high (0.0258 mg EA/mg biomass). Viniegra-Gonzalez et al.[22] established a relation among better productivity due to higher biomass production. According to the Luedeking and Piret[15] model, EA formation rate depends on both instantaneous biomass concentration and growth rate.[10] In this case, an estimation of ellagitannase yield should be made in order to correlate this assumption.

TABLE 12.1   Kinetic Parameters of Pomegranate Husk Powder Fermentation Obtained in This Study.

Parameter	Units	Value
Specific growth rate, μ_{max}	1/h	0.353
Biomass yield, $Y_{X/S}$	mg X/mg S	17.695
Product yield, $Y_{P/X}$	mg AE/mg X	0.028
Specific production rate, q_P	mg AE/mg X h^{-1}	0.221
Specific substrate uptake rate, q_S	mg S/mg X h^{-1}	2.278
Maintenance coefficient, m	G S/g X h^{-1}	0.7239
Product coefficient, k		-0.037

The microorganism showed high substrate absorption (2.2781 mg X/ mg S h^{-1}), for this kind of polyphenols. Small values of maintenance coefficient (m) indicated a fungal growth in relation of substrate consumption. Maintenance coefficient value (0.7239 g S/g X h^{-1}) from fermentation shows that the process characteristic is product formation, result supported by high productivity, where hydrolysable phenols conversion of 87% into EA can be seen. Finally, EA accumulation is indicated by a k value of -0.0369, where if $k < 0$, the system will have a convex fermentation curve indicating a secondary specific rate of enzyme decomposition that may balance production rate associated with vegetative growth (q_p). This factor is responsible for the presence of peak values during fermentation. Moreover, if there is a secondary rate of production ($k > 0$), the curve will be convex with no peak values. From the production point of view, a nonnegative value of k helps to identify fermentation conditions in which the excreted enzyme activity will be stable in fermentation broth and may be a significant factor for better enzyme productivity.[2]

12.4   CONCLUSIONS

Bioconversion of ETs to EA represents an interesting method of producing a commercially important metabolite (EA) from an agro-waste product. A maximum biomass concentration of 390 mg/g S and EA concentration of 11.27 mg/gds could be obtained in the bioreactor giving the highest EA yield achieved so far of 0.0258 mg AE/mg X, for this strain. ETs conversion of 87% into EA was achieved. Kinetics data obtained would be particularly useful for monitoring and control of EA production in a batch mode for the operation of the bioprocess and serve as a guide for designing various reactor-operating strategies for further improving EA concentration.

12.5 ACKNOWLEDGMENT

Authors thank CONACYT for the financial support through research project: SEP-CONACYT CB-2011-01-167764.

KEYWORDS

- kinetic parameters
- ellagic acid
- ellagitannins
- solid-state fermentation
- biodegradation

REFERENCES

1. Aguilar, C. N.; Aguilera-Carbo, A.; Robledo, A., Ventura, J., Belmares, R., Martinez, D., Rodríguez-Herrera, R., Contreras, J. Production of Antioxidant Nutraceuticals by Solid-State Cultures of Pomegranate (*Punica granatum*) Peel and Creosote Bush (*Larrea tridentata*) Leaves. *Food Technol. Biotechnol.* **2008**, *46*, 218–222.
2. Aguilar, C. N.; Augur, C.; Favela-Torres, E.; Viniegra-González, G. Production of Tannase by *Aspergillus Niger* Aa-20 in Submerged and Solid State Fermentation: Influence of Glucose and Tannic Acid. *J. Ind. Microbiol. Biotechnol.* **2001**, *26*, 296–302.
3. Aguilera-Carbo, A.; Augur, C.; Prado-Barragan, L.; Aguilar, C; Favela-Torres, E. Extraction and Analysis of Ellagic Acid from Novel Complex Sources. *Chem. Pap.* **2008**, *62*, 440–444.
4. Aguilera-Carbo, A.; Hernández, J.; Augur, C.; Prado-Barragan, L.; Favela-Torres, E.; Aguilar, C. N. Ellagic Acid Production from Biodegradation of Creosote Bush Ellagitannins by *Aspergillus Niger* in Solid State Culture. *Food Bioprocess Technol.* **2009**, *2*, 208–212.

5. Ascacio-Valdés, J.; Aguilera-Carbó, A.; Martínez-Hernández, J.; Rodríguez-Herrera, R.; Aguilar, C. *Euphorbia Antisyphilitica* Residues as a New Source of Ellagic Acid. *Chem. Pap.* **2010,** *64,* 528–532.
6. Boone-Villa, V. D.; Contreras-Esquivel, J. C.; Rodriguez-Herrera, R.; Aguilar, C. N. Comparison of Cellular Components Analysis Techniques to Estimate Fungal Growth in Cultures on Inert Supports; In *Proceedings of the 1st Food Science and Food Biotechnology in Developing Countries,* Durango, Dgo, México. FE15, 2004.
7. Buenrostro-Figueroa, J.; Huerta-Ochoa, S.; Prado-Barragán, A.; Ascacio-Valdés, J.; Sepúlveda, L.; Rodríguez, R.; Aguilar, C. N. Continuous Production of Ellagic Acid in a Packed-Bed Reactor. *Proc. Biochem.* **2014,** *49*(10), 1595–1600.
8. Cruz-Hernandez, M. A.; Contreras-Esquivel, J. C.; Lara, F.; Rodríguez-Herrera, R.; Aguilar, C. N. Isolation and Evaluation of Tannin Degrading Strains from the Mexican Desert. *Z. Naturforsch. C* **2005,** *60,* 844–848.
9. Dubois, M.; Guiles, K. A.; Hamiton, J. K.; Rebers, P. A.; Smith, F. Colorimetric Method for Determination of Sugar and Related Substances. *Anal. Chem.* **1956,** *21,* 145–149.
10. 10. Feng, J.; Zhan, X. B.; Wang, D.; Zhang, L. M.; Lin, C. C. An Unstructured Kinetic Model to Study NaCl Effect on Volatile Ester Fermentation by *Candida etchellsii* for Soy Sauce Production. *Biotechnol. Bioproc. Eng.* **2012,** *17,* 242–249.
11. Gross, G. G. Biosynthesis of Ellagitannins: Old Ideas and New Solutions. In *Chemistry and biology of ellagitannins: An Underestimated Class of Bioactive Plant Polyphenols*; Quideau, S. Ed.; World Scientific Publishing: Singapore, 2009; pp 94–118.
12. Huang W; Ni J; Borthwick, A.G. L Biosynthesis of Valonia Tannin Hydrolase and Hydrolysis of Valonia Tannin to Ellagic Acid by *Aspergillus niger* SHL6. *Proc. Biochem.* **2005,** *40,* 1245–1249.
13. Khadem, S.; Marles, R. J. Monocyclic Phenolic Acids; Hydroxy- and Polyhydroxybenzoic Acids: Occurrence and Recent Bioactivity Studies. *Molecules* **2010,** *15,* 7985–8005.
14. Landete, J. M. Ellagitannins, Ellagic Acid and Their Derived Metabolites: A Review About Source, Metabolism, Functions and Health. *Food Res. Inter.* **2011,** *44,* 1150–1160.
15. Luedeking, R.; Piret, E. L. A Kinetics Study of the Lactic Acid Fermentation. Batch Process at Controlled pH. *J. Biochem. Microbiol. Technol. Eng.* **1959,** *1,* 393–412.
16. Manach, C.; Scalbert, A.; Morand, C.; Rémésy, C.; Jiménez, L. Polyphenols: Food Sources and Bioavailability. *Am. J. Clin. Nutr.* **2004,** *79,* 727–747.
17. Neurath, R.; Nathan, S.; Yun-Yao, L.; Debnath, A. K. *Punica granatum* (Pomegranate) Juice Provides an HIV-1 Entry Inhibitor and Candidate Topical Microbicide. *BMC Infect. Dis.* **2004,** *4,* 41.
18. Robledo, A.; Aguilera-Carbó, A.; Rodriguez, R.; Martinez, J.; Garza, Y.; Aguilar, C. Ellagic Acid Production by *Aspergillus niger* in Solid State Fermentation of Pomegranate Residues. *J. Ind. Microbiol. Biotechnol.* **2008,** *35,* 507–513.
19. Sepúlveda, L.; Aguilera-Carbó, A.; Ascacio-Valdés, J. A.; Rodríguez-Herrera, R.; Martínez-Hernández, J. L.; Aguilar, C. N. Optimization of Ellagic Acid Accumulation by *Aspergillus niger* GH1 in Solid State Culture Using Pomegranate Shell Powder as a Support. *Proc. Biochem.* **2012,** *47*(12), 2199–2203.

20. Vattem, D. A.; Shetty, K. Ellagic Acid Production and Phenolic Antioxidant Activity in Cranberry Pomace (*Vaccinium macrocarpon*) Mediated by *Lentinus edodes* Using a Solid-State System. *Proc. Biochem.* **2003,** *39,* 367–379.
21. Ventura, J.; Belmares, R.; Aguilera-Carbo, A.; Gutiérrez-Sanchez, G.; Rodríguez-Herrera, R.; Aguilar, C. N. Fungal Biodegradation of Tannins from Creosote Bush (*Larrea tridentata*) and Tar Bush (*Fluorensia cernua*) for Gallic and Ellagic Acid Production. *Food Technol. Biotechnol.* **2008,** *46,* 213–217.
22. Viniegra-González, G.; Favela-Torres, E.; Aguilar, C. N.; Rómero-Gomez, S.; Díaz-Godínez, G.; Augur, C. Advantages of Fungal Enzyme Production in Solid State Over Liquid Fermentation Systems. *Biochem. Eng. J.* **2003,** *13,* 157–167.

CHAPTER 13

PLANT GROWTH REGULATORS

RAJEEV SINGH[1], NEELAM GAUTAM[2] and ANAMIKA SINGH[3,*]

1Department of Environmental Studies, Satyawati College, University of Delhi, Delhi, India

2Botanical Survey of India, Allahabad, India

3Department of Botany, Maitreyi College, University of Delhi, Delhi, India

*Corresponding author. E-mail: arjumika@gmail.com

CONTENTS

ABSTRACT

Plant hormones are naturally occurring chemicals formed inside plants. They play vital role in various biological activities in plant. These plant regulators are active at very low concentration. They are also used in as pesticides and promote growth of plants. They are called growth regulators as they help in increase of cell size, volume, and weight of any part of plant's body by cell division and cell enlargement, and development of irreversible change in state. In this chapter, we highlight nature, activity, structure, and the important biological roles of plant hormones. These regulators are now-a-days widely used for commercial uses in nurseries, gardens, and crop fields for better yield.

13.1   INTRODUCTION

The term "phytohormone" (plant hormone) was coined by Thiemann in 1948. Plant hormones are actually growth factors and small signaling molecules which help plant regulate growth and other functions. They are actually chemical compounds, and found in very low concentrations. Similar to animals, they have their specific targets and a particular response.

Flowering, shedding of leaves, ripening of fruits, and stem leaves growth are due to hormonal actions. In animals there are glandular systems, while in plants every cell is capable of producing hormones. Plant hormones also affect seed growth, shape of plant, flowering time, fruit formation, senescence of leaves, bipolar tissue growth, longevity, and death of plant. If plants do not produce these hormones, they will develop as a mass of tissues without differentiation. Plant hormones are vital to plant growth, and they are found in algae, fungi, bacterial cells, and in microorganisms. There are different hormones found in plants that are discussed in detail in subsequent text.

13.2   AUXINS

Auxins are plant growth regulators which are essential for plant growth and its behavior. Dutch scientist Frits Warmolt Went first described the role of auxins in plants. Kenneth V. Thiemann isolated auxins first, and gave its chemical structure as indole-3-acetic acid (IAA). The details of auxins were published in *Phytohormones* (book) in 1937, coauthored by Went and Thiemann.

13.2.1   DISCOVERY OF AUXINS

Charles Darwin in 1881 and his son Francis performed experiments on coleoptiles tip. In the experiment, they exposed the coleoptiles tip to light from a unidirectional source, and observed that the tip bends towards the light. Darwin identified that the light is detected by the coleoptiles tip, but the bending of tip occurs in the hypocotyls. However the seedlings showed no signs of development towards light. In the second step, when he covered the coleoptiles tip with an opaque cap, no bending was observed, and similar results were observed for the cut tip. So he concluded that the tip of the coleoptiles was actually responsible for sensing light, and it produces a particular messenger that moves in the downward direction and causes bending of tip.

Danish scientist Peter Boysen-Jensen, in 1913, proved that the signal produced during this action is mobile in nature.

1. He separated the tip from coleoptiles and placed it on a gelatin cube. Further he observed that the response to light was normal as gelatin gives a passage for the chemicals synthesized at the tip to pass to the other parts.
2. In his second experiment, he separated the tip by an impermeable substance, and found that they did not bend toward light side.

These two simple methods demonstrated that the chemicals synthesized at the tip are moving toward lower side. In 1926, the Dutch botanist Frits Warmolt Went showed that a chemical messenger produced at the tip gets diffused from coleoptiles. His experiment proved how coleoptiles move toward light.

13.2.1.1   AUXIN SYNTHESIS AND TRANSPORT

Indole acetic acid (IAA) is found in the cell naturally. It was the first phytohormone to be discovered (Fig. 13.1). It is synthesized in the meristematic cells. Shoot apices synthesize more auxin than the root apices. Thus, auxins are synthesized in cells and transported to the different sites. Auxins are generally not synthesized in every cell and for that they are usually transported toward the required site, so it is transported from the site of synthesis to the site of action, which is not far away. The transportation of auxin is polar, that is, from apex to the base, which is called basipetal movement. These auxins may be transported to short distances via polar transport. For long distances, relocation occurs via sieve tubes, and it is a facilitated mechanism. Polar transport of auxin is directional and regulated by an efflux carrying protein which is unevenly distributed in the plasma membrane and these carrier proteins send auxins in the proper direction.

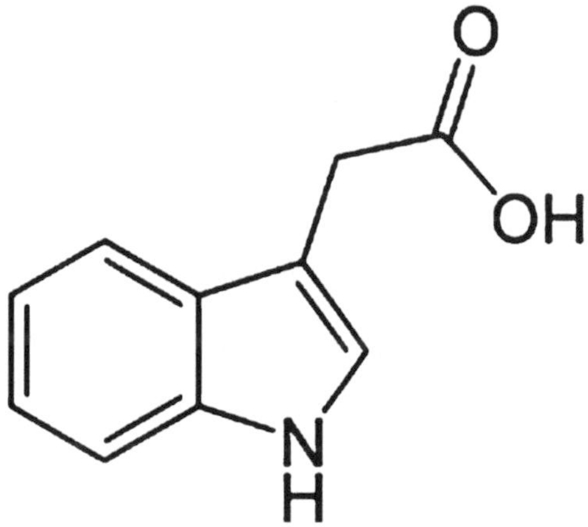

FIGURE 13.1   Indole acetic acid: natural auxin.

13.2.2   EFFECTS OF AUXINS

13.2.2.1   CELLULAR GROWTH

Auxins are mainly responsible for cell division and expansion. Differentiation of cells also depends upon the concentration of auxins. It helps in shoot elongation. Factors such as soil, environment, humidly, and others along with concentration of auxins affect the overall growth and development of plant. Auxin promotes growth of shoots, that is, axial growth. It helps in cell division along with cell expansion.

13.2.2.2   ORGAN PATTERNS

Growth and division of cells lead to development of tissue and finally organ development. Plant size increases due to the growth of cells, uneven growth results in bending, turning, and directional development of organ. These few features are due to auxins, such as *phototropism*: bending of the stem toward light source, *gravitropism*: growth of roots toward gravity, and few other types of tropism due to one side growth of cell in organ. Therefore, auxin concentration within a cell results in plant growth and finally organization of a plant.

13.2.2.3   APICAL DOMINANCE

Auxin is a very important hormone for normal plant growth and it helps in organ shaping. For the normal growth and development of plant, auxin is very much required. Absence of auxin leads to the growth of an undifferentiated mass of cells. Auxin requirement starts from the embryo phase itself to help differentiate the two poles, later it helps to develop normal root, cotyledon, leaves, and so forth. Most important function of auxin is based upon its distribution. This function is known as apical dominance. Auxin produced by the apical buds (meristematic cell of growing tip) diffuses downwards and inhibits the growth of lateral buds. Removal of apical tip allows tremendous growth of lateral buds which were previously in dormant condition. This is a complex process as auxin is synthesized in the tips and transported downward. During its transportation, it reacts with many intermediate hormones such as cytokinins or strigolactones. For the development of more lateral branches, it is important to cut the apex. This process is known as pruning. It is a very important technique in horticulture. Higher concentration of auxin directly stimulates ethylene synthesis in lateral buds, which causes inhibition of their growth and potentiation of apical dominance. When the apex of the plant is removed, the inhibitory effect is removed and the growth of lateral buds is enhanced.

13.2.2.4   CELL ELONGATION

Auxin stimulates cell elongation due to a wall loosening factor known as elastins. This effect increases more in the presence of gibberellin. Auxin also stimulates cell division in the presence of cytokinins. In a growing callus if different concentrations of auxins and cytokinins are applied, different results are seen. If auxin concentration is more than cytokinin, root development takes place. Xylem tissues develop when the concentration of auxin and cytokinin is equal.

13.2.2.5   WOUND RESPONSE

Auxin induces the formation and organization of xylem and phloem tissues. In the wounded condition, differentiation and regeneration of vascular tissues occur.

13.2.2.6   ROOT DEVELOPMENT

Auxins promote root initiation and development. They induce growth of existing and adventitious root formation, that is, branching of the roots occurs due to auxins. If more auxin is transported down the stem to the roots, development of the roots is stimulated. If the tip of the stem is removed, the growth of stem is more as compared to root growth. Higher concentration of auxin inhibits root elongation but enhances root formation. Root tip removal causes inhibition of secondary roots.

13.2.2.7   FRUIT DEVELOPMENT

Auxin plays a very important role in fruit growth and in delay of fruit senescence. Auxin promotes fruit development in many adverse conditions like if we removed seeds from fruits, external application of auxins leads to development of fruits. Parthenocarpy is due to external auxin application. Fruits form abnormal morphologies when auxin transport is disturbed.

13.2.2.8   FLOWERING

Auxin also plays a minor role in the initiation of flowering and development of reproductive organs. In very low concentrations, it can delay senescence of flowers.

13.2.2.9   ETHYLENE BIOSYNTHESIS

In very low concentrations, auxin can inhibit ethylene formation and transport of precursors in plants, while higher concentrations can induce the synthesis of ethylene. Therefore, high concentration can induce femaleness of flowers in some species. Auxin inhibits abscission prior to formation of abscission layer, and thus inhibits senescence of leaves.

13.2.2.10   SYNTHETIC AUXINS

Many of these have been found to have economical potential for man-controlled growth and development of plants in agronomy. Auxin has been identified mainly as IAA, but for biological research, plant biochemists started looking for similar compounds in nature and in laboratories. They found many known compounds with noticeable auxin activity, which can be synthesized. Synthetic auxins have been discovered and they were observed to have similar functions like auxins as growth promoting hormones. Indole propionic acid, indole butyric acid, naphthalene acetic acid, phenyl acetic acid, 2,4 dichlorophenoxy acetic acid (2,4-D) are just few of the known synthetic auxins (Fig. 13.2). Auxins show toxic effects in a higher concentration in plants. Toxicity is more in dicots as compare to monocots. Due to these features, they may act as herbicides includes 2,4-D and 2,4,5-trichlorophenoxyacetic acid (2,4,5,-T). 2,4-D was the first widely used herbicide. 1-naphthalene acetic acid (NAA) and indole-3-butyric acid (IBA) are commonly used to stimulate root growth. At higher concentrations, auxin stimulates ethylene production. Excess of ethylene production may lead to inhibition of elongations, falling of leaves, and even death of plant.

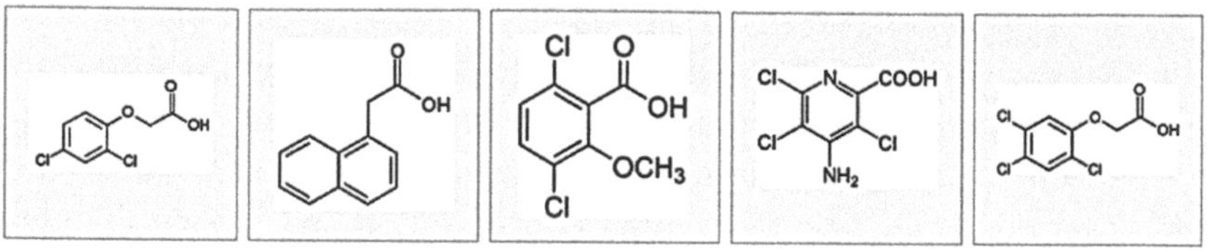

| 2,4-Dichlorophenoxyacetic acid (2,4-D); active herbicide and main auxin in laboratory use | α-Naphthalene acetic acid (α-NAA); often part of commercial rooting powders | 2-Methoxy-3,6-dichlorobenzoic acid (dicamba); active herbicide | 4-Amino-3,5,6-trichloropicolinic acid (tordon or picloram); active herbicide | 2,4,5-Trichlorophenoxyacetic acid (2,4,5-T) |

FIGURE 13.2   Showing different synthetic auxin.
Courtsey: https://en.wikipedia.org/wiki/Auxin#cite_note-shaping-4.

13.2.3   IMPORTANT POINTS

- Auxins are a class of plant growth substances.
- They were first discovered by a Dutch scientist named Fritz Went (1903–1990).
- They are transported mainly by active transport and for long distance by facilitated diffusion.
- IAA is a naturally found auxin.
- Synthetic auxins include 1-naphthaleneacetic acid (NAA), 2,4-dichlorophenoxyacetic acid (2,4-D) and so on.

13.3   GIBBERELLINS

Gibberellins are plant hormones that regulate stem elongation, enzyme induction, fruit senescence. Thus, they are mainly responsible for developmental process of plant. Japanese scientist Eiichi Kurosawa, in 1926, first recognized it when he was studying foolish seedling disease in rice. Later Yabuta and Sumuki in 1935 isolated a crystalline substance named, gibberellin from fungus *Gibberella fujikuroi*. E. Kurosawa in 1926 observed abnormally tall yellow plants of paddy which were devoid of seeds. Gibberellin is mainly distributed in meristematic regions of the plants mainly root apex, shoot apex, buds, embryos, seeds, and young developing organs. Gibberellin promotes elongation in stems due in part to activation of the intercalary meristem. Another important role of gibberellins is the induction of hydrolytic enzymes such as α-amylase and protease in the seeds of grasses and cereals, which facilitate endosperm mobilization.

13.3.1 STRUCTURE

The basic structure of gibberellic acid (GA) consists of gibbane skeleton. GAs are known to occur in different forms such as GA3, GA4, GA1, GA2, and so forth; among them GA3 is most common and widely found (Fig.13.3). There are a few more structures in nature which do not have Gibbane-like structure but show similar activity as gibberellin. These compounds are phaseolic acid, helminthosporal, ecdysone, and steviol. Helminthosporal is extracted from *Helminthosporium sativum* and it promotes stem growth of dwarf variety of rice plant only. Phaseolic acid is extracted from seeds of *Phaseolus* and it promotes stem growth in dwarf maize and pea. Ecdysone is a hormone found in insects which controls molting, and it promotes growth of dwarf maize seedlings. Gibberellin is synthesized at tips of the shoot, root, leaf, buds, and developing seeds.

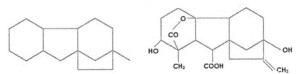

FIGURE 13.3   Showing gibbane ring and gibberellic acid (GA3).

13.3.2 EFFECT OF GIBBERELLINS

13.3.2.1 DWARFISM

Gibberellin application can revert back the dwarfism in plants. In dwarf plants, internodes get elongated and they become normal tall plants.

13.3.2.2 BOLTING

In certain plants dwarf plants grow only a rosette of leaves during first year of growth and dwarfing, during second year internodes elongation occurs and this process is called Bolting. Gibberellins induce stem elongation in rosette plants. Cabbage is a rosette plant having profuse leaf growth and retarded internodes length. Just prior to flowering, internodes elongate enormously. Bolting either needs long days or cold nights. When a cabbage head is kept under warm nights, it retains its rosette habit. Bolting can be induced artificially by the application of gibberellins under normal conditions. Low doses of gibberellins are introduced in plants which favor bolting and if high doses of gibberellins are introduced in plants it will favor flowering.

13.3.2.3 SEED GERMINATION

It is applicable for those seeds which are light sensitive such as tobacco and lettuce. These seeds can germinate in the presence of light only, but they can also germinate on treatment with GA3. At the time of seed germination plant embryo produces gibberellins, and it affects the aleurone cells. GA acts on hydrolytic enzymes and these hydrolytic enzymes are synthesized in aleurone cells (amylase, protease, ribonuclease, and so forth). Activity of hydrolytic enzyme increases and the stored food material is hydrolyzed into soluble amino acid nucleosides by hydrolytic enzymes and seedlings emerge.

13.3.2.4 BREAKING BUD AND SEED DORMANCY

Gibberellins can break bud dormancy, for example, in birch buds which are produced during winter, dormancy is maintained until spring, but this dormancy can be broken by using gibberellins. Gibberellins break dormancy of buds and tubers. Although in root tubers, it inhibits the development of the root tuber.

13.3.2.5 PARTHENOCARPY

It is a process where fruit is formed without fertilization of ovules naturally or artificially, fruit is therefore seedless. According to Davison[2] and Bradley and Crane[1], gibberellin is capable of producing parthenocarpic fruits in cases like apple and stone fruits. Gibberellins cause parthenocarpy in apple and pear.

13.3.2.6 INDUCTION OF FLOWERING

In certain long-day herbaceous plants, flowering can be induced by exogenous application of gibberellin under short-day conditions. But in only a few short-day plants such as *Bryophyllum* spp, *Raphanous sativus*, and so forth, flowering can be induced by gibberellins and it also inhibits flowering in some woody plants like *apple, salix, bouginvillea.*

13.3.2.7 ROLE IN ABSCISSION

GA3 treatments accelerated the rate of abscission in explants of bean and coleus.

13.3.2.8 SEX EXPRESSION

Gibberellins are also capable of altering the sex of the flowers. In *Cucumis*, it could induce maleness by foliar application of GA3 to the female flowers. Moreover, antheridial induction has been developed in many fern gametophytes by GA3 treatment.

13.3.2.9 JUVENILITY

Many plants have two stages in their life cycle: a juvenile stage and an adult stage. For example, in a species of eucalyptus (*Eucalyptus globulus*), in juvenile stage the leaves are shorter and oppositely placed, softer, and with an emarginate apex whereas the leaves of the adult stages are spirally arranged, larger, harder, and acicular with pointed apex. Here, application of gibberellins may help determine whether a particular part of a plant is juvenile or adult. Treating them with gibberellin causes them to grow into juvenile branches.

13.3.3 IMPORTANT POINTS

- It is used in horticultural techniques or it induces plant regeneration and elongation of internodes.
- Promotes growth of a variety of fruit crops and increases sugar yield in sugarcane.
- The alternate fruit bearing of some cultivars can be overcome by applying GA4 in the "off" year to promote the formation of flower buds, and subsequent fruit set.
- Commercially they are used for breaking dormancy of buds.
- Gibberellins can fasten flowering and fruiting in plants.
- They can also stimulate production of seedless fruits in absence of pollinators.
- They can be used to control weed (unwanted plants growing in fields) growth.

13.4 CYTOKININS

Auxins and gibberellins are the two hormones that, besides inducing cell elongation, also promote cell division (cytokinesis) under certain conditions. In 1941, Van Overbeek et al. found that coconut milk acts as an active stimulant of cell division. Later, in 1955, Carlos Miller et al. isolated a compound from yeast DNA which acts as "cell division stimulating factor." It was named as kinetin because of its amazing power to stimulate cell division (cytokinesis) in the presence of an auxin. Later many artificial compounds were synthesized. In 1956, Miller and his associates grouped all compounds, which had cell division activity and named them as kinetin under a generic name kinin. First natural cytokine discovered was from maize plant called zeatin. D. S. Leetham[4] of New Zealand proposed the term cytokinins for such substances. This term is the most acceptable one. Fairley and Kilgour[3] used the term "phytokinins" for such substances in order to distinguish them from the peptide hormones of animal gastrointestinal tract. Cytokines are widely distributed in plants in both free and bound state. In brown and red algae, diatoms, many angiosperms, and few gymnosperms, cytokines are found in free state while in bound state they are synthesized in the root tips and transported upward through xylem. Large amount of cytokines is found in germinating seeds, young developing fruits, bleeding sap, embryo, and so forth.

All cytokines have basic structure of isopentenyl adenine. Naturally occurring cytokines are zeatin, isopentyladenine, ciszeatin, dihydrozeatin, zip, and so forth. Synthetic cytokines are adenine, kinetin, 6-benzylamino-purine (benzyl adenine), benzimidazole, and 6-benzyladenine (Fig. 13.4). Adenine also has some cytokinin activity. Cytokinins are structurally related to the purine derivative, adenine, and they have side chains rich in carbon and hydrogen and attached to nitrogen protruding from the top of the adenine ring. Chemically, kinetin ($C_{10}H_9ON_5$) is 6-furfurylamino-purine. It is formed from deoxyadenosine which is a degradation product of DNA.

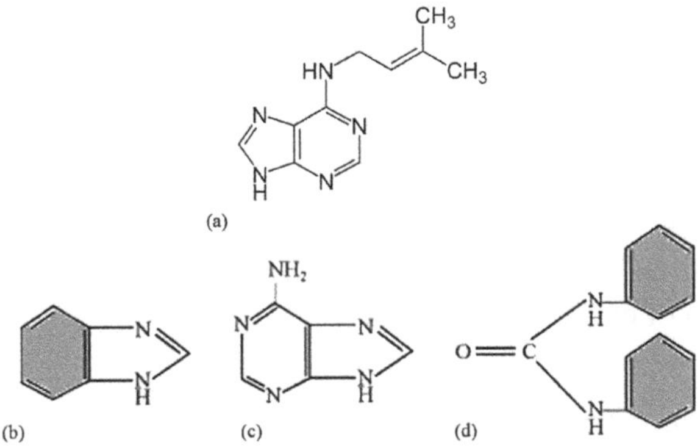

FIGURE 13.4 Structures of different cytokinins: (a) isopentanyl adenine (b) benzimidazole (c) adenine (d) diphenylurea.

13.4.1 EFFECT OF CYTOKININ

13.4.1.1 CELL DIVISION

Auxin and cytokinin ratio decides the growth of cells. If a mixture of cytokinin and auxin is added to unspecialized cells, they will start differentiating into different plant organs. If cytokinin auxin ratio is high then shoots, buds and leaves differentiation starts while at low ratio root develops. If one treatment is followed by the other, it provides a means of forming small plantlets. Cell division is completed in three steps: (1) DNA synthesis, (2) mitosis, (3) cytokinesis. Studies suggested that IAA influences the first two steps, that is, DNA synthesis and mitosis; while cytokinin induces cell division. It has been suggested that the adenine moiety of the kinetin molecule is essential for cell division.

13.4.1.2   CELL ELONGATION

Cytokines promote cell elongation in cortical cells of tobacco roots. Cell elongation is mainly induced by kinetin and it is regarded exclusively as a cell division factor.

13.4.1.3   COTYLEDONS AND LEAVES EXPANSION

These induce expansion of excised cotyledons in dicot plants, such as cucumber, lettuce, mustard, radish, and so forth. Cytokinins promote cell division and expansion in cotyledons because they influence wall plasticity. Cytokinins also increase the amount of sugars (especially glucose and fructose) in cells which creates an osmotic influx of water and it results into expansion of cytokinin treated cells in cotyledons.

13.4.1.4   PIGMENT SYNTHESIS

Cytokines increase the production of anthocyanin in petals of *Impatiens balsamina* (garden balsam, garden jewelweed, rose balsam, spotted knapweed, touch-me-not) by many folds.

13.4.1.5   CHLOROPLAST DEVELOPMENT

Exogenous cytokine application on plants promotes chloroplast development in callous tissue of excised cotyledons.

13.4.1.6   MORPHOGENESIS OR ORGANOGENESIS

Morphogenesis is the process of organ formation and auxins, cytokines ratio plays an important role in it. When auxin concentration is more as compared to cytokine's concentration, root formation is favored in solution of callus but if cytokine's concentration is more, shoot formation is promoted. Cytokinins also stimulate production of buds in leaf segments of various plants such as *Saintpaulia ionantha*, *Bryophyllum* sp., and *Begonia* sp. In addition to the root and shoot differentiation, the cytokinins also helps in morphogenetic responses such as proplastids maturation, differentiation of tracheids, induction of parthenocarpy, and flowering.

13.4.1.7   APICAL DOMINANCE

It is phenomena in which apical bud keeps on growing and suppresses growth of lateral buds. Cytokines are antagonists to auxins, as cytokines promote growth of lateral branches and nullify apical dominance. If the apical bud is present, the lateral buds do not develop, but the removal of the apical bud leads to the stimulation of growth of the lateral buds. If, the intact shoot is soaked in kinetin (cytokinin) solution, the inhibition of lateral buds is checked or the lateral buds tend to develop, although less vigorously, as in case where apex of the shoot has been cut off. Thus, apical dominance is mainly maintained by a balance between auxins and endogenous cytokinins (Kinetin-like substance). That is why it is treated as strong promoter of lateral bud growth.

13.4.1.8   DELAY OF SENESCENCE

Cytokinins treatment extends life span of detached leaves of *Xanthium* by delaying chlorophyll and proteins degradation.

13.4.1.9   DORMANCY BREAKAGE OF SEEDS

In light sensitive seeds, such as lettuce, cytokinin promotes germination of seeds after breaking dormancy of seeds. Cytokinin treatment enables them to germinate even in dark. Cytokinins are also effective in breaking seed dormancy in lettuce, tobacco, white clover, and carpet grass. Thimann[5] suggested that the site of cytokinin action in such cases is the cotyledon. Furthermore, the inhibitory effect of infrared light on germination of lettuce seeds is also alleviated by kinetin treatment.

13.4.1.10   ROLE IN ABSCISSION

Cytokinins can accelerate as well as retard the process of abscission in leaf petioles depending on the site of their application.

Box 1: RICHMOND—LANG EFFECT

In 1957, A. E. Richmond and A. Lang demonstrated that cytokinins treatment extended life span of detached leaves of *Xanthium* as it delays the degradation of chlorophyll and proteins. This phenomenon is called as "Richmond–Lang effect." On cytokines treatment, nutrients from adjoining leaves are withdrawn by cytokine-treated leaves. Cytokine may either act by depressing protein degradation or by increasing protein synthesis.

13.4.2   IMPORTANT POINTS

- It is used in horticultural technique as it promotes cell division and shoot indication.
- Cytokinin auxin ratio determines development of root or shoot in callus concentration.
- High auxins concentration forms roots and high cytokines concentrations forms stems.
- Cytokinin delays senescence in detached leaves by slowing down the loss of chlorophyll.
- Cytokinin breaks seed dormancy and promotes seed germination.
- Colored pigment synthesis like anthocyanin and flavanoid is enhanced by cytokinins.
- Cytokinin is capable of stimulating nutrients mobilization in plants body.
- Openings of stomata and increased resistant to disease is also controlled by cytokines.

- It is a very useful hormone to overcome phenomena of apical dominance, that is, it promotes development of lateral branches rather than apical bud which is useful for commercial crops like tea plantations.
- Commercially applicable for maintaining fruit shape.
- In potato, cytokines induce tuber formation and inhibits stolon elongation.

KEYWORDS

- **phytohormones**
- **agrochemicals**
- **plant growth regulators**
- **herbicides**

REFERENCES

1. Bradley, M. V.; Crane, J. Gibberellin-Induced Inhibition of Bud Development in Some Species of *Prunus. Science* **1960,** *131,* 825–826.
2. Davison, R. M. Fruit-setting of Apple using Gibberelic Acid. *Nature* **1960,** *188,* 681–682.
3. Fairley, J. L.; Kilgour, G. L. *Essentials of Biological Chemistry.* Affiliated East-West Press Pvt. Ltd.: London, 1966.
4. Letham, D. S. Zeatin. A Factor Inducing Cell Division Isolated from *Zea mays. Life Sci.* **1963,** *2,* 569.
5. Thimann, K. Plant Growth Substances: Past, Present and Future. *Ann. Rev. Plant Physiol.* **1963,** *14,* 1–18.

SUGGESTED READINGS

1. Salisbury, F. B.; Ross, C. W. *Plant Physiology, Hormones and Plant Regulators: Auxins and Gibberellins,* 4th ed.; Wadsworth Publishing: Belmont, 357–381.
2. Lambers, H. *Plant Physiological Ecology;* Springer-Verlag: New York, 1998. ISBN: 0-387-98326-0.

3. Larcher, W. *Physiological Plant Ecology,* 4th ed.; Springer: Berlin, 2001. ISBN 3-540-43516-6.
4. Stern, K. R.; Jansky, S. *Introductory Plant Biology;* WCB/McGraw-Hill: USA, 1991; p 309. ISBN: 978-0-697-09948-8.

CHAPTER 14

INFORMATICS APPROACH AND ITS IMPACT FOR BIOSCIENCE: MAKING SENSE OF PHYSICAL CHEMISTRY INNOVATION

HERU SUSANTO*

Department of Computer Science & Information Management, Tunghai University, Taichung, Taiwan

Computational Science, The Indonesian Institute of Sciences, Serpong, Indonesia

Corresponding author. E-mail: heru.susanto@lipi.go.id, susanto.net.id@gmail.com

CONTENTS

ABSTRACT

In today's society, bioinformatics research is putting a great emphasis on answering "when," "what if," and "why" questions with the help of information system and technology, and some researchers have argued that it could be the key factor in facilitating and attaining efficient decision-making in medical research. Hence, the main purpose of this chapter is to explore the application of information system in biological world and to study the extent to which technology could bring opportunities as well as challenges in science. This chapter will examine the importance and evolution of bioinformatics over the past decades.

With the current deluge of data, computational methods have become indispensable to biological investigations. Originally developed for the analysis of biological sequences, bioinformatics now encompasses a wide range of subject areas including structural biology, genomics, and gene expression studies. Additionally, nowadays, biological data is proliferating rapidly. With the advent of the World Wide Web and fast internet connections, the data contained in these databases and a considerable amount of special-purpose programs can be accessed quickly and efficiently from any location in the world. As a consequence, computer-based tools now play an increasingly significant role in the advancement and development of biological research. Hence, this chapter will investigate the relationship between information system and science as well as the consequences and implication of technology in supporting medical research.

14.1   INTRODUCTION

Information system is a part of information technology. It has been well defined in terms of two perspectives: one relating to its purpose; the other relating to its structure. From a functional perspective, an information system is a technologically implemented medium for the purpose of recording, storing, and disseminating linguistic expressions as well as for the supporting of inference making, while from a structural perspective, an information system consists of a collection of people, processes, data, models, technology, and partly formalized language, forming a cohesive structure which serves some organizational purpose or function. However, it can also be defined as a set of interconnected components that assemble (or retrieve), process, store, and allocate information in order to support decision-making and control in an organization. In addition to support decision-making, coordination, and control, information systems may also aid in helping workers in analyzing problems, visualizing complex subjects, and creating new products.

14.2 THE GENERAL IMPORTANCE OF INFORMATION SYSTEM IN SCIENCE

Owing to the availability of large data sets of digital medical information, the use of informatics to improve healthcare and medical research has made possible where they provide a new trail for investigation and medical discovery. This is because informatics focuses on developing new and effective methods of using technology to process information. In today's society, informatics is being applied at every stage of health care from basic research to care delivery and includes many specializations such as bioinformatics, medical informatics, and biomedical informatics.

The field of bioinformatics has exploded within the past decade to keep pace with advancements and developments in molecular biology and genomics research where researchers could use bioinformatics to obtain an effective understanding of complex biological processes which include examining DNA sequences or restructuring protein structures.

Furthermore, informatics has also had huge impact on the field of systems biology as systems biology could use computer modeling and mathematical simulations to predict how complex biological systems will behave. National Institute of Health has claimed that researchers have created models to simulate tumor growths. By applying the computer models in the study, researchers can obtain a better and more comprehensive understanding of how diseases affect an entire biological system in addition to the effects on individual component.

The use of informatics to improve healthcare and medical research has made possible because of the availability of large data sets of digital medical information. This is due to the development of a new trail for investigation and medical research. Informatics highlights on improving a new and effective method of using technology to process information. In today's society, informatics is being applied at all health care phases from elementary study to care delivery, including a considerable amount of specialization such as bioinformatics, medical informatics, and biomedical informatics.

Within this past decade, the study of bioinformatics has exploded. This is to keep pace with progression and development in molecular biology and genomics research. Thus, researchers could use bioinformatics to obtain an effective understanding and knowledge of complex biological processes which include examining DNA sequences or modifying the protein structures.

14.3   THE RELATIONSHIP BETWEEN INFORMATION SYSTEM AND BIOINFORMATICS

According to Cannataro et al.,[3] bioinformatics is the application of computational tools and techniques to the management and analysis of biological data. Over the past few decades, rapid developments in genomic and other molecular research technologies as well as developments in information technologies have combined to produce a tremendous amount of information related to molecular biology. The primary goal of bioinformatics is to increase the understanding of biological processes.

Bioinformatics develops algorithms and biological software of computer to analyze and record the data related to biology including the data of genes, proteins, drug ingredients, and metabolic pathways. A study has concluded that the creation and analysis of a group of sequences, large data sequences, and adding new modules for visual representation of input data show output results on the Microsoft windows platform. Bioinformatics is the field of science in which biology, computer science, and information technology merge to form a single discipline.[13] Biological data is in need of a certain storage house in which the data can be stored, organized, and manipulated. Thus, biological software and databases provide the scientists and researchers this opportunity, enabling them to extract data from these databases efficiently and effectively.

Bioinformatics can be considered to be a combination of several scientific disciplines that include biology, biochemistry, mathematics, and computer science. This is due to the availability of enormous amounts of public and private biological data as well as the compelling need to transform biological data into useful information and knowledge. Additionally, understanding the correlations, structures, and patterns in biological data is the most important task in bioinformatics. Thus, the knowledge and understanding obtained from these disciplines could be sensibly used for applications that cover drug discovery, genome analysis, and biological control. Furthermore, it involves the use of computer technology and statistical methods to manage and analyze a huge volume of biological data regarding DNA, RNA, protein sequences, protein structure, gene expression profiles, and protein interactions.

14.4   AIMS OF BIOINFORMATICS

There are three aims in using bioinformatics. First, bioinformatics is used as a data organizer in a way that it allows researchers to access existing information as well as making new entries of fresh data. However, information stored in bioinformatics databases will not be useful unless it is analyzed to extend the purpose of bioinformatics. Second, bioinformatics is also used as developing tools and resources to analyze the information. For example, the sequence of a particular protein needs more than a simple text-based search and program which needs to be supported by a biologically significant match. Additionally, this development process needs an expertise not only in computers, but also in the understanding of medical research. The third aim of bioinformatics is to use the developing tools in analyzing the data and interpreting the result in a biologically meaningful manner. Traditionally, biological studies are conducted on individual system and comparison process. With the help of bioinformatics system, the analysis process can be conducted globally with the available large range data and the aim of open common principle across many systems.

14.5   THE PROGRESS OF BIOINFORMATICS

Grid infrastructures played an important role in the recent decade in supporting scientific computer-based analysis. However, the increasing complexity of bioinformatics resulted in finding new solutions to speed up computational time. Grid infrastructure is not completely satisfactory in terms of providing services and managing data that is reliable for presenting bioinformatics.

Another key issue is represented by the fact that the grid offers poor chances to customize the computational environment. In fact, it is quite common in computational biology to make use of relational databases and/ or web-oriented tools to perform analyses, store output files, and visualize results, which are difficult to exploit without having administration rights on the used resources. Another related problem derives from the huge amount of bioinformatics packages available in different programming environments (such as R, Perl, Python, and Ruby) that typically require many dependencies and fine-tuned customizations for the various users.

These are the reasons why cloud computing is the best solution. Computation is moving from in-house computing infrastructure to cloud computing delivered over the internet. Cloud computing provides cheap, reliable large scale data where a small-sized organization can get the same information as a well-funded organization. Bioinformatics grew with the rising use of the internet which allowed creation, shared large biological data, and offered rapid publication of research results. The internet also provides the researchers with a supercomputing system that is complex, such as grid infrastructure.

14.6   THE APPLICATION OF BIOINFORMATICS

Some of the grand areas of research in bioinformatics include:

14.6.1   SEQUENCE ANALYSIS

It is the most primitive operation in computational biology where the operation includes finding which part of the biological sequences are alike and which part differs during medical analysis and genome mapping processes. Hence, the sequence analysis implies subjecting a DNA or peptide sequence to sequence alignment, sequence databases, repeated sequence searches, or other bioinformatics methods on a computer.

14.6.2   ANALYSIS OF MUTATIONS IN CANCER

The arrangement of genomes of the affected cells is complex where a huge sequencing strength is needed to identify previously unknown point mutations in a variety of genes in cancer. By producing specialized automated systems, the sheer volume of sequence data produced could be managed and new algorithms and software can be created for comparing the sequencing results to the growing collection of human genome sequences and germ line polymorphisms. Another type of data that requires novel informatics development is the analysis of lesions found to be recurrent among many tumors.

14.6.3 MODELING BIOLOGICAL SYSTEMS

Modeling biological systems is significant in biology and mathematical biology, where computational systems biology aims to develop and use efficient algorithms, data structures, visualization, and communication tools for the integration of large quantities of biological data with the goal of computer modeling. It involves the use of computer simulations of biological systems, including cellular subsystems such as the networks of metabolites and enzymes, signal transduction pathways, and gene regulatory networks to both analyze and visualize the complex connections of these cellular processes.

14.6.4 HIGH-THROUGHPUT IMAGE ANALYSIS

Computational technologies are used to accelerate and facilitate the processing, quantification, and analysis of a considerable amount of high-information-content biomedical images. Additionally, modern image analysis systems enhance an observer's ability to make measurements from a large or complex set of images. A fully developed analysis system may completely replace the observer. Biomedical imaging is becoming more important for both diagnostics and research. Some of the examples of research in this area are clinical image analysis and visualization, inferring clone, overlaps in DNA mapping, and bioimage informatics.

14.6.5 DRUGS DISCOVERY

Traditionally, pharmaceutical companies were only attracted in introducing new drugs when any well-known pharmaceutical company had been successful in developing them. However, in today's society, pharmaceutical companies have invested heavily on approaches that can speed up the development process. The pressure of producing drugs in a short period of time with concern for a high standard of safety has resulted in extremely enhanced interest of the researchers in bioinformatics. Bioinformatics acts as an identification of biological candidate and could be the storage of information. Drugs can only be produced if the drug target is studied and identified. For example, human genome sequence information can be found in the system that can help in the drug-making process.

14.6.6   PREVENTION AND TREATMENT OF DISEASES

Bioinformatics is a scientific discipline that deals with earning, analyzing, distributing, processing, and storing of biological information. It uses scientific knowledge such as algorithm and computer science in order to understand the biological significance of a wide variety of data. With this, it enables researchers to find new strategies to look for clues in the prevention and treatment of diseases. Bioinformatics has turned into a key ingredient with the alliance of genomics, proteomics, and drugs in today's world.

In fact, bioinformatics owes its creation to the need to handle large amounts of data produced by these "-omic" technologies (genomics, proteomics, and more recently metabolomics). This method of information is generated by high-performance methods such as gene sequencing, DNA microarrays, and mass spectroscopy. For this reason, bioinformatics can be called a transverse activity because it is applicable to all the subsectors of biotechnology and life sciences. However, its main application is biomedicine. Bioinformatics manages and decodes "-omic" data and facilitates the translational medicine concept by distributing information throughout the entire health care value chain. This covers the discovery and analysis of genes, the protein structures coded by these genes, and the design of molecules and drugs to counter these proteins, up to their clinical application, which is where bioinformatics plays a leading role in the development of specific medicine.

14.6.7   STUDYING GENETIC DISEASE

There is a growing market in the use of microarrays for studying diseases associated with genetic characteristics. The widespread acceptance of this technique is driving demand for a more user-friendly version of the software, and bioinformatics companies are supporting this in their latest product developments. The big pharmaceutical companies are using systems biology in their drug discovery processes. For example, Novartis has created Novartis Biologics: a new division that incorporates bioinformatics at all levels of the drug creation value chain. Programmers have recently developed an extended markup language exclusively for systems biology called systems biology markup language (SBML).

This language makes it possible to integrate the software applications of different providers. As a result, bioinformatics is also moving toward standardization of the language used for developing software. This will accelerate the production of new applications and utilities by small (nonindustrial) developers, using an open-source environment. In fact, experts expect that within a few years, all legacy applications in bioinformatics will be available via the internet and will run in ordinary browsers. Consequently, it will be important for bioinformatics companies to adapt their existing products for online use or to develop new applications that are suitable for this purpose.

14.7 THE BENEFITS OF USING INFORMATION SYSTEMS IN BIOINFORMATICS

Bringing together large sets of medical data and tools to analyze the data offers the potential to enlarge the research capabilities of researchers where they could use this vast source of biological and clinical data to discover and develop new treatments and better understand illnesses. Pharmaceutical companies could use the biomedical data to create drugs targeted at specific populations. Furthermore, health care providers can use the data to better inform their treatments and diagnoses.[4]

Etheredge as cited in Castro[4] claimed that applying informatics to health care creates the possibility of enabling "rapid learning" health applications to aid in biomedical research, effective research, and drug safety studies. For example, using this technology, the side effects from the drugs newly introduced to the market can be monitored in real time, and problems, such as those found with the recently withdrawn prescription drug Vioxx, can be identified more quickly. Moreover, the risks and benefits of drugs can be studied for specific populations yielding more effective and safer treatment regimens for patients.

Etheredge had concluded that using rapid learning techniques can not only improve patient safety, but can also lead to substantial improvements in the quality and cost of care by turning all of the raw digital data into knowledge where these rapid learning health networks can enable doctors and researchers to better practice evidence-based medicine. Evidence-based medicine is the use of treatments judged to be the best practice for a certain population on the basis of scientific evidence of expected benefits and risks.

14.8   THE LIMITATIONS OF INFORMATION SYSTEM IN BIOINFORMATICS

Achieving the vision of an intelligent and fully connected health research infrastructure has not been realized yet. While various pilot projects have shown success and have demonstrated the potential benefits that can emerge from a ubiquitous deployment of informatics in health research, many technical obstacles still need to be overcome. Doolan as cited in Castro[4]believes that these obstacles include making data accessible, connecting existing data sources, and building better tools to analyze medical data and draw meaningful conclusions. Much medical research data is not accessible electronically.

Achieving the widespread use of electronic health records is a necessary requirement for creating the underlying data sets needed for bioinformatics research. Access to the electronic health records of large populations will help researchers apply informatics to various problems including clinical trial research, comparative effectiveness studies, and drug safety monitoring. However, collecting medical data in electronic format is only the first step. Interoperability poses a substantial challenge for biomedical research. This is because the vast amount of electronic medical data cannot fully be utilized by researchers because the data resides in different databases. Even when the organizations that collect and distribute biomedical data are willing to share data, incompatible data formats or data interfaces can create challenges for analyzing data across multiple data sets.

Thus, Stein as cited in Castro[4] claims that researchers wishing to use multiple data sets must devote significant resources simply to manage the differences between the data and, as a result, have fewer resources available for working with the data.

Highly trained workers that are familiar with life sciences are needed to be able to maintain the system in bioinformatics. In addition, researchers will also need to be trained that may cost the organization.

14.9   THE EVOLUTION OF BIOINFORMATICS

Bioinformatics deals with computer management and analysis of biological information: genes, genomes, proteins, cells, ecological systems, medical information, robots, and artificial intelligence as there are many applications of bioinformatics from the combination of computer and biology. The evolution of technology helps in supporting bioinformatics in discovering diseases and application in forensics using software packages and bioinformatics tools, for example, the evolution of technology by bioinformatics such as Illumina next-generation sequencing (NGS) to provide accurate sequencing. NGS technology can provide valuable and useful information for a better understanding in health and diseases.

The use of bioinformatics can also be useful in determining the order of the four chemical building blocks called bases that make up the DNA molecule. This is because the sequence provides scientists regarding what kind of genetic information is carried in a particular DNA segment. Moreover, the sequence data can highlight the changes in a gene that may cause disease.

14.9.1   FORENSIC DNA AND BIOINFORMATICS

Bioinformatics and forensic DNA are fundamentally similar fields and draw their techniques from statistics and computer science which facilitate in solving the problems in law and biology. Identifying the victim and suspecting with personal relatedness to other individuals are the two major focuses of forensic DNA analysis. It is a common event in forensic analysis especially by crime and investigation unit or CSI to look at close connections; for example, paternity disputes, suspected incest case, corpse identification, alimentary frauds (such as, genetically modified organism (OGM), poisonous food, and so forth), semen detection on underwear for suspected infidelity, insurance company fraud investigations when the actual driver in a vehicle accident is in question, criminal matters, and autopsies for human identification following accident investigations. All of these problems may be solved by using bioinformatics methods.[7]

Genetic tests have been widely used for major catastrophic events as well such as terrorist attacks, airplane crashes, and tsunami disasters. It can be used for mass fatality identification and forensics evidences. Personal identification relies on identifiable characteristics as the human body has a personal identity that is unique biologically (such as blood, saliva, DNA), physiologically (such as fingerprints, irises and retinas, hand palms and geometry, and facial geometry), and also behaviorally (such as body posture, habits, signature, keystroke dynamics, and lip motion, and on combination of physiological and dynamic characteristics such as the voice).

Hence, genetic testing results are integrated with the information collected by multidisciplinary teams composed of medical examiners, forensic pathologists, anthropologists, forensic dentists, fingerprint specialists, radiologists, and experts in search and recovery of physical evidence. Officers could have access to the personal information where biological data can be obtained from hospital records and behavioral data may be collected from banks or office documents such as fingerprint or signature just by looking at the database.

Therefore, the application of genetic testing in large scale tissue sampling and long-term DNA preservation plays an important role in mass fatalities which have been recently labeled.[7] Thus, DNA has become the most important personal identification characteristic because all genetic differences, whether being expressed regions of DNA (genes) or some segments of DNA, are characteristic of a person. DNA possesses coding pattern of inheritance which can be monitored and used as markers.

14.9.2   BIOINFORMATICS AND CANCER

According to the Cancer Research UK,[2] cancer is one of the leading causes of death worldwide; there were 14.1 million cases of cancer were recorded and about 8.2 million deaths worldwide were estimated in 2012. A leading cause of cancer is any malignant growth or tumor caused by abnormal and uncontrolled division due to the changes of DNA in cell by mutation. Errors in the genes may also cause this abnormal behavior to be cancerous. These changes develop when exposed to a certain type of cancer causing substance.

The post genome era holds phenomenal promises for identifying the mechanistic bases of organismal development, metabolic processes, and diseases. Bioinformatics research will lead to a wide understanding of the regulation of gene expression, protein structure determination, comparative evolution, and drug discovery. Presently, 2D gel protein pattern can be easily analyzed using bioinformatics technology where these software applications possess user-friendly interfaces that are incorporated with tools for linearization and merging of scanned images.

New techniques and collaborations between computer scientists, biostatisticians, and biologists are required in today's research. There is a need to develop and integrate database repositories for the various sources of data being collected, to develop tools for transforming raw primary data into forms suitable for public dissemination or formal data analysis, to obtain and develop user interfaces to store, retrieve, and visualize data from databases as well as to develop efficient and valid methods of data analysis.[1]

Cancer DNA sequencing using NGS provides better information and is less time-consuming compared to normal gene sequencing using gel structure. With NGS, researchers can perform whole-genome studies, targeted gene profiling and tumor-normal comparisons. Therefore, it is easy to detect tumor and DNA fragments with detailed quantitative measurements from the database.

Furthermore, the prediction of genes is likely to be linked to a new developing disease or a modified version of an old disease that has evolved or mutated. The use of bioinformatics can easily recognize related genes as similar to any function or characteristic of an original gene such as the similarity in percentage of DNA sequence. The highest challenge is to identify enormous markers of DNA as the application of molecular links to diseases will continue to face technological as well as biological, and algorithmic challenges. The human body consists of very complicated and diverse features because it is continually evolving, and responding to changes.

As for using bioinformatics to replicate the structure of new DNA structure provides a challenge in technology. This is because of other interrelationships such as cells that may not be visible through the microscopic view. Thus, the already designed computer frameworks or databases may not cope with the expanding network-level measurements and information.

14.9.3 ETHICAL ISSUE

According to Johnson,[6] "computer ethics has followed computer technology in its evolution, and for the same reason computer ethics as a separate discipline will disappear in the near future. In fact, when computing becomes a mature technology, the problem of its (urgent) ethical and social impacts due to policy vacuums (according to Moor[10]) will diminish, and using computers as a means of achieving some goals will become part of ordinary human action."

What he said was, as time changed from period to period, technology changed. He believes that when the technology changes, the ethics of computer also change when there is an adaptation of easily accessible technology.

Another citation from Johnson, "Once the new instrumentation is incorporated into ethical thinking, it becomes the presumed background condition.... What was for a time, an issue of computer ethics becomes simply an ethical issue. Copying software simply becomes an issue of intellectual property. Selling software involves certain legal and moral liabilities. Computer professionals understand they have responsibilities. Online privacy violations are simply privacy violations. So as we come to presume computer technology as part of the world we live in, computer ethics as such is likely to disappear."

14.9.4   INFECTIOUS DISEASES ETHICS

The emphasis of human bioethics in the 1950s and 1960s coincided with a widespread belief in particular area and time (but with hindsight, unwarranted and dangerous) that the problems of infectious diseases had been solved by sanitation, immunization and antibiotic therapy. The much-quoted pronouncement that "it is time to close the book on infectious disease" is usually attributed to former US Surgeon General William Stewart. Although there appears to be no evidence that he ever actually said this, the sentiment was certainly widely shared at the time.[14] This widespread complacency remained largely unchallenged throughout most of the 20th century. It was dispelled by the unfolding of Human Immunodeficiency virus (HIV) pandemic and the plethora of other emerging and re-emerging infectious diseases that followed (or in some cases preceded) it, but it had already contributed to the gross neglect of infectious diseases by bioethicists.[5,15,17]

Aquired immunodeficiency syndrome (AIDS) was a rare exception, but many of the ethical issues it raised—confidentiality, discrimination, patients' rights, and sexual freedom—were not specifically related to its status as an infectious disease. Belatedly, this neglect is now being addressed; infectious diseases have at last come to the attention of bioethicists. In the 21st century, public health ethics have become a rapidly growing subdiscipline of bioethics, and much of the public health ethics literature has focused on infectious diseases in particular. In addition to

AIDS, attention has especially focused on severe acquired respiratory syndrome (SARS), pandemic influenza planning, and issues related to bioterrorism.[9,12,18]

There has also been debate about the ethical issues such as: intellectual property rights related to antimicrobial agents and their implications for the access to essential treatment of infectious diseases,[11] and the relationship between marketing of antimicrobials, and the emergence of antibiotic resistance.[16]

By the citation of the researchers, it can be argued that, technology can make bioinformatics more efficient, and much more reliable. But it might as well give people a negative impact such as the confidentiality as well as the consent of the participants.

14.10   EXAMPLES OF BIOINFORMATICS IN INFORMATION CONCEPT SYSTEM

Generally, information system concept in bioinformatics has the same aim, and hence has similar flow of procedure. It organizes data which all users had input, and access existing data, analyze each input, and interpret the results in a biological manner.

14.10.1   EBI

The European Bioinformatics Institute (EBI) is a research and services center in bioinformatics. This database provides researchers with molecular biology, genetics, medicine, biotechnology, and industries related to pharmaceuticals and chemicals.

There are various ways for data entry. Data input can be done via web, accessing their website; or via Sequin, a developed tool accessed via an FTP server; or via e-mail to users whose internet access is through e-mailing services.

Data input by users is then analyzed whether it is new or existing data. For instance, a sample of an unknown virus shows similar signs and symptoms as that of an existing virus. This data is then compared with the existing database producing the results which are further elaborated, and interpreted by the user.

14.10.2   PanCan RISK

PanCan risk is a European project which aims to identify cancer vulnerability, and clinical management via bioinformatics. With this, they are able to predict the treatments of cancer as the cancer genome sequencing is very challenging to be understood.

The company intends to give a deliberate, cross-disciplinary structure for superior comprehension, joining and utilization of tumor clinical information in the assessment of a large number of hereditary variations, and changes included in growth vulnerability for the immediate advantage of diseased patients.

Similar to that of EBI, PanCan risk uses existing data to compare to newly provided sample and looks for varieties of genotypes vulnerable to cancer.

14.10.3   GENOGRAPHIC

The project is anonymous, nonmedical, nonprofit, and all results will be placed in the public domain following scientific peer publication. It is sponsored by National Graphic Society and Waitt Family foundation which helps with the migratory history of the human species. This is, so the project will be able to compile the data in collaboration with the indigenous and traditional people globally. This will study historical DNA patterns from contributors worldwide to better recognize our anthropological genetic heritages. All results are published and accessible to the public.

14.10.4   GEMINI

Gemini is a flexible software for exploring all forms of human genetic variation. It is designed for reproducibility and flexibility of biologists, and researchers with a standard framework for medical genomics. Gemini incorporates genetic variation with an adjustable and variable set of genome annotations into a unified database to enable interpretation, and data exploration.

Among many bioinformatics service providers and softwares, these are the four which stand out, and still have improvement to be done. The development not only will take time but will be very costly as well. Most of the concerns raised along with the advancement of the system, are related to the purchase of the machines required to run such experiments for researchers and students majoring in bioinformatics.

14.11 OPINION

We believe that bioinformatics deals with computer management and analysis of biological information: genes, genomes, proteins, cells, ecological systems, medical information, robots, and artificial intelligence as there are many applications of bioinformatics from the combination of computer and biology. The evolution of technology helps in supporting bioinformatics in discovering diseases, and application in forensics using software packages and bioinformatics tools. We also believe that information system could be the key factor in facilitating and attaining an efficient decision-making in medical research as the knowledge and understanding obtained from bioinformatics could be sensibly used for applications that cover drug discovery, genome analysis, and biological control.

14.12 CONCLUSION

In conclusion, with the current deluge of data, computational methods have become indispensable to biological investigations. Thus, bioinformatics tools hold a huge potential for use in medical research and clinical practice as the analysis of genetic information offered by bioinformatics, and the study of systems behavior with detailed mathematical models may lead to huge benefits for drug development and personalized health care. Moreover, the research and education in life sciences is increasingly dependent on bioinformatics and advanced information system to support the evidence using a large set of data.

KEYWORDS

- computational technologies
- information systems
- bioinformatics
- DNA sequences
- protein structures
- sequences analysis

REFERENCES

1. Bensmail, H.; Haoudi, A. Postgenomics: Proteomics and Bioinformatics in Cancer Research. *BioMed Res. Int.* **2003**, *2003*(4), 217–230.
2. Cancer Research UK. Worldwide Cancer Statistics, 2014. http://www.cancerresearchuk.org/health-professional/worldwide-cancer-statistics.
3. Cannataro, M.; Santos, R.W.; Sundnes, J. Bioinformatics' Challenges to Computer Science: Bioinformatics Tools and Biomedical Modeling, Part I, LNCS 5544, 2009, pp. 807–809.
4. Castro. D. Building the Digital Platform for Medical Research. The Role of Information Technology in Medical Research, Washington. *Exploration of Genetic Variation and Genome Annotations. PLoS Comput. Biol.* **2009**, *9*(7): e1003153. DOI: 10.1371/journal.pcbi.1003153.
5. Francis, C. A.; Roberts, K. J.; Beman, J. M.; Santoro, A. E.; Oakley, B. B. Ubiquity and Diversity of Ammonia-Oxidizing Archaea in Water Columns and Sediments of the Ocean. *Proc. Natl. Acad. Sci. U. S. A.* **2005**, *102*(41), 14683–14688.
6. Johnson, W. C. Analyzing Protein Circular Dichroism Spectra for Accurate Secondary Structures. *Proteins: Struct., Funct., Bioinf.* **1999**, *35*(3), 307–312.
7. Lucia, B.; Pietro, L. Forensic DNA and Bioinformatics. *Briefings Bioinf.* **2007**, *8*(2), 117–128.
8. Luscombe, N. M.; Greenbaum, D.; Gerstein, M. *What is Bioinformatics? An Introduction and Overview*; Department of Molecular Biophysics and Biochemistry, Yale University: New Haven, USA, 2001.
9. Miller, J. R.; Delcher, A. L.; Koren, S.; Venter, E.; Walenz, B. P.; Brownley, A.; Sutton, G. Aggressive Assembly of Pyrosequencing Reads with Mates. *Bioinformatics* **2008**, *24*(24), 2818–2824.
10. Moor, J. H. What is Computer Ethics? *Metaphilosophy* **1985**, *16*(4), 266–275.
11. Ng, P.; Wei, C. L.; Sung, W. K.; Chiu, K. P.; Lipovich, L.; Ang, C. C.; Liu, E. T. Gene Identification Signature (GIS) Analysis for Transcriptome Characterization and Genome Annotation. *Nat. Methods* **2005**, *2*(2), 105.
12. Reid, L. Diminishing Returns? Risk and The Duty to Care in The SARS *Epidemic. Bioethics* **2005**, *19*(4), 348–361.
13. Santhaiah, C.; Reddy, R. M. Role of Computers in Bioinformatics by Using Different Biological Datasets. *J. Comput. Eng.* **2014**, *16*(2), 80–83 (2278–8727).
14. Sassetti, C. M.; Rubin, E. J. The Open Book of Infectious Diseases. *Nature medicine* **2007**, *13*(3), 279.
15. Selgelid, M. J. Ethics and Infectious Disease. *Bioethics* **2005**, *19*(3), 272–289.
16. Selgelid, M. J. Ethics and Drug Resistance. *Bioethics* **2007**, *21*(4), 218–229.
17. Smith, L.; Rindflesch, T.; Wilbur, W. J. MedPost: A Part-of-Speech Tagger for BioMedical Text. *Bioinformatics* **2004**, *20*(14), 2320–2321.
18. Thompson, D. G.; Solomon, K. R.; Wojtaszek, B. F.; Edginton, A. N.; Stephenson, G. R.; Relyea, R. A. The Impact of Insecticides and Herbicides on the Biodiversity and Productivity of Aquatic Communities: [with Response]. *Ecol. Appl.* **2006**, *16*(5), 2022–2034.

PART III
Multidisciplinary Perspectives

CHAPTER 15

EPR PARADOX, QUANTUM DECOHERENCE, QUBITS, GOALS, AND OPPORTUNITIES IN QUANTUM SIMULATION

FRANCISCO TORRENS[1,*] and GLORIA CASTELLANO[2]

[1]*Institut Universitari de Ciència Molecular, Universitat de València, Edifici d'Instituts de Paterna, P. O. Box 22085, E-46071 València, Spain*

[2]*Departamento de Ciencias Experimentales y Matemáticas, Facultad de Veterinaria y Ciencias Experimentales, Universidad Católica de Valencia San Vicente Mártir, Guillem de Castro-94, E-46001 València, Spain*

Corresponding author. E-mail: torrens@uv.es

CONTENTS

ABSTRACT

In 1935, three physicists (Albert Einstein, Boris Podolsky, and Nathan Rosen) proposed a paradox that questioned the interpretations of quantum mechanics (QM). The fact that, apparently, quantum information had to be transmitted more rapidly than the speed of light seemed to breach of wave functions (WFs) that collapsed. Quantum systems (QS) easily entangle each other so that their WFs combine. The fact that they do or not do in phase dictates the result. Thus, quantum information can easily escape, which leads to the loss of cohesion of a quantum state (QSt). Large objects get decoherence more rapidly than smaller ones. Quantum computers (QCs) can someday succeed in substituting Si-based technologies. They can be potent enough to decode any code. They are already only proto-types and handle binary data fragments in the form of quantum bits or atomic states. Based on QM, they could exploit phenomena, for example, entanglement, in order to carry out millions calculations at the time. At supercold temperatures, some metals, alloys, and ceramics completely lose their electric resistance. Currents are free of flowing during thousands of millions years without losing any energy. The reason is QM. On matching, and with a slight shake of the cations lattice, electrons can be kept together. Feynman's 1981 conjecture, in which QCs can be programmed to simulate any local QS, is correct. Quantum simulators are controllable QSs that could be used to simulate other QSs. Being able to tackle problems that are intractable on classical computers, quantum simulators would provide a means of exploring new physical phenomena. How may quantum simulators become a reality in the near future, as the required technologies are now within research? Quantum simulators, relying on the coherent control of neutral atoms, ions, photons, or electrons, would allow studying problems in a number of fields, for example, condensed matter physics, high-energy physics, cosmology, atomic physics, and quantum chemistry. The long-term promises of quantum simulators are far-reaching but the field needs clearly defined short-term goals.

15.1 INTRODUCTION

In quantum theory and information background, quantum mechanics (QM) offers new forms of processing and transmission of information. In order to implement them, one must combat decoherence, the noise that lowers the quantum properties (QPs) of every system. Quantum laws involve that secure cryptography is possible under amazingly weak assumptions. Quantum simulators cherish long important promises but the field needs clear short-term objectives. Many quantum systems (QSs) are too complex to calculate their properties. Quantum simulation allows recreation of behavior via systems formally analogous and easy to control in the laboratory.

To calculate the properties of numerous complex QSs, quantum computers (QCs) are required. However, the construction of a functional QC is still far off. An alternative consists in employing quantum simulators: controllable QSs, with a behavior formally analogous of the system that one wants to study. Some problems that would benefit especially from this approach are the study of many-body systems or those with a considerable amount of entanglement (whose actions/states are linked). Provided the great amount of possible simulations, the new field should mark itself some specific goals, for example, to achieve the interactions of a system or check the reliability of a simulation.

In earlier publications, fractal hybrid-orbital analysis,[1,2] resonance,[3] molecular diversity,[4] periodic table of the elements (PTE),[5,6] law, property, information entropy, molecular classification, simulators,[7–11] labor risk prevention, and preventive healthcare at work with nanomaterials[12–14] were reviewed. In the present report, the aim is to understand Einstein–Podolsky–Rosen (EPR) paradox, quantum decoherence (QD), and qubits for quantum simulation.

15.2 EPR PARADOX

QM Copenhagen interpretation (CI, Bohr, 1927) reasons that measuring influences a QS, causing to take features that will be observed later.[15] Light properties (for example, wave particle) know when to appear because observer tells them what they must make. Einstein thought it was absurd. The CI meant QSs were in limbo till observation. Before a measurement tell one in what quantum state (QSt) it is, QS exists in an all QSts mixture. Einstein adduced that quantum superposition (QSu) was unrealistic. A particle exists independently of the fact that one should be there to see it. He thought that all exists by its selfsame right, and uncertainties showed that something was wrong with QM and CI. In order to discover cracks in CI, Einstein, Podolsky, and Rosen (EPR, 1935) proposed a thought experiment (TE, gedanken experiment): EPR paradox. Imagine a particle, for example, atomic nucleus, which disintegrates in two smaller ones. After conservation rules, if mother particle was stationary, daughters must present equal and opposed linear and angular momenta. Arising particles go out quickly and rotate in opposed directions. Some other pair QPs are related. If an observer measures one particle spin direction, he instantly knows other's QSt: it must present the opposite spin to adapt to quantum rules (QRs). While neither interacts with others, which would ruin signal, the fact keeps certain independently of how far particles be between themselves or much time pass. In CI, daughters exist at first in an all-result QSu: mixture of all different speeds and rotating directions that they could present. When an observer measures one, wave function (WF) probabilities for both collapse to consolidate result. EPR said this had no sense. Einstein knew nothing moves at a speed higher than light. How could an instantaneous signal be transmitted to a particle that could be far, for example, the other end of the universe? The CI must be wrong. Schrödinger used entanglement to describe estrange action at a distance.

15.2.1   ENTANGLEMENT

Einstein believed in local reality: all exists independently of people and signals carry information at a speed not higher than light. Both TE particles knew in what QSt each was when they came away. They carry knowledge with them, instead of simultaneously changing QSt at remote distances. However, he was wrong. His idea seems reasonable and fit for daily experience. Notwithstanding, quantum experiments (QEs) showed it false. Spooky action at a distance occurs and matched particles instantly talk to each other via space. Physicists entangled QPs of more than two particles and saw how they exchange QSts at kilometers. Quantum signals (QSis) emission at a distance opens applications for new remote communication forms, for example, instantaneous messages transmission via enormous space extensions. It raises possibility of QCs, capable of executing many calculations at the same time via all machine memory. Quantum information (QI) units are quantum binary digits (bits) (qubits). Similar to normal computers that employ binary code (BC) to describe messages as large 0/1 sentences, qubits take either QSt. Nevertheless, they could exist in a QSts mixture so that they would achieve calculations one can only dream. However, uncertainty that their power lends to QSis emission means that one cannot transmit a complete information set from one place to another. Heinsenberg's uncertainty principle means that a gap exists in what one can know. Human (science fiction) teletransportation (TT) is impossible.

15.2.2 ACTION AT A DISTANCE

While atom TT never occurs, to move information via space is possible via quantum TT. If two persons (Alice, Bob) hold a pair of entangled particles (EPs) via measurement, they can transmit qubits. Alice and Bob acquire their pair of coupled particles, for example, two photons, each taking one. Alice's qubit is in some QSt that she wants to send Bob. Even if she does not know what QSt it is, she can influence Bob's photon in order that it transmits him such message. Measuring her photon, Alice destroys it. However, Bob's photon takes the relay. Bob can make his measurement to extract information. As nothing travels nowhere, no matter TT exists. Apart from the first particle exchange, no communication exists between messengers. Alice's original message is destroyed in transmission and its content is recreated in other place. The EPs are used to transmit coded messages, so that only receptors to which they are destined can read them. Any furtive listener would break entanglement with which he would ruin message. Einstein's entanglement discomfort is understandable: It is difficult to imagine universe as a quantum net (QN), with an unknown number of particles that talk to their distant couples. Notwithstanding, it is a QS.

15.3 QUANTUM DECOHERENCE

In the quantum world (QW), all is uncertain. Particles and waves cannot be distinguished. The WFs collapse when one establishes something via measurement. In the classical world, all seems solider. A speck of soot is day after day. Where does split between classical and QW appear? De Broglie assigned a wavelength (WL) to all objects in universe. Big objects, for example, footballs, present a short WL, so that their behavior is particle-like. Small ones, for example, electrons (e⁻), show a WL closer to their size, so their wave-type properties are clear. In QM CI, Bohr proposed that WFs collapse whenever a measurement is performed. Part of their intrinsic probability gets lost when one recognizes a feature with certainty. It is irreversible. However, what does it happen when a WF collapses or one executes a measure? How do fuzzy uncertainties convert to a solid result? Everett (1957) overcame question proposing many-worlds. He treated universe like presenting an only WF, which evolves but never collapses. A measure is an entanglement between QSs, which produces universe segregation. He could not explain point in which it occurs. In later pilot-wave quantum theories, for example, de Broglie–Bohm, which tried describing wave/particle duality (WPD) in terms of a particle in a quantum potential, measures distort quantum field particle movement. It is like bringing near one mass to another in general theory of relativity (GTR): space/time changes to harmonize gravitational influences. No collapse of particle WF exists, which changes only its form.

The best explanation for substituting certainty for possibility is QD (Zeh, 1970). When two WFs face each other, for example, a measuring device approaches a quantum entity, the way as they interact depends on relative phases. Similar to crossing light or water waves that are amplified/eliminated when interfering, WFs rise/erase when mixing. The more quantum interactions (QInters) a WF face, the more disorganized it turns. It gets QD and loses its wavy aspect. The QD is much more important for large objects: they lose more rapidly quantum cohesion. Small ones, for example, e⁻, conserve quantum integrity (QInt) during more time. Schrödinger's cat, for example, would soon recover its shape although it was not observed, because its WF would demean itself almost instantaneously. It is comforting. It places people's familiar macroscopic world on a firmer base. However, unknowns remain. Why does QD act so uniformly on a quantum giant, for example, cat? Could not half cat stay in quantum shortage and half become real? Could it be half living and half dead? What does it restrict WF result that demeans itself to appropriate observables? Why does a photon appear when it is needed or light wave, when an aperture is placed in its way? The QD tells people little about WPD.

15.3.1   BIG QSs

A way to learn is to design and study a quantum behavior (QB), macroscopic phenomenon, or object. Brune, Haroche, and Raimond groups (1996–98) manipulated electromagnetic fields (EMFs) to produce QSts QSu via Rb and saw QInt decomposed. Others constructed hypotheses, for example, Schrödinger's cat, but great and better. Big molecule QB is another route. Zeilinger's group (1999) observed C_{60} diffraction. The QE was like pitching a football to a goal and seeing the ball interfered and behaved like a wave. The WL was 1/400 C_{60} size. Another big QS is a superconducting (SC) magnet, which frequently shows a supercooled metallic ring shape of centimeters of diameter. The SCs present an unlimited conductivity: e^- lay via material without hindrances. Ring of SC takes concrete energy levels or QSts. To see how they interfere is possible if observer puts one close to other, for example, with currents that flow in opposed directions (counter/clockwise). Any number of studies showed the greater QS, the more rapidly it gets QD.

15.3.2   QUANTUM LOSES

The QD is imagined like QI loss to environment via many small QInters. It does not cause that WFs collapse but result is similar as QS components easily uncouple. The QD does not solve measurement problem. As measuring devices must be big enough so that one could read them, they are simply complex QSs placed in the way of pristine QS that one tries observing. Each particle that constitutes detector interacts with its prey in complex ways. Multiple entangled QSts gradually get QD till one gets an isolated QSts mess. Quantum sandpile becomes final measurement result, from which original QS estrange information was extracted. The QInters entangled net scene shows that realism died. Similar to localism, signals transmission via communication limited by speed of light, realism (particle exists like separated entity), is a riddle. World apparent reality is a mask that is put to hide circumstance that it is made from quantum ashes.

15.4   QUBITS

Tiny QSs dimensions and capability of existing in different QSts raise possibility of building computer types. Instead of electronic devices to store and process digital information, atoms become core of a QC, which was proposed in 1980s and developed rapidly but far from reality. Physicists connected only 12 atoms to perform calculations because isolating atoms (constituents) are difficult, so that their QSts could be read but stay immune to perturbations. Conventional computers function decomposing numbers and instructions into a BC: a series of 0/1. While people count in multiples of 10, computers think in factors of 2: numbers 2 and 6 express as 10 (a 2 and zero 1 s) and 110 (a 4, a 2, and zero 1 s). Each bit can be 0/1. A computer translates BC into physical states (for example, disconnected/connected) in its equipment. Any distinction (either this or that) will function as a means of storing bits. Bit strings are manipulated via logic gates banks connected in Si chips.

15.4.1   QUANTUM BITS

The QCs are qualitatively different. They are based on disconnected/connected QSts (qubits) but with a variant. Similar to binary signals, qubits can take two QSts. However, unlike bits, they exist in a QSts mixture. An only qubit represents a QSu of two QSts (0/1). A pair of qubit superposes four QSts and three qubits, eight QSts. Each time a qubit is added, number of mixed QSts is doubled. In contrast, a traditional computer would meet at a certain moment in one of such states. Rapid connections duplication between qubits lends power to QC. Another QW benefit that could be mastered for computation is entanglement. The QB of qubits separated from each other is linked by QRs. To bring about that one jump to a certain QSt makes that, simultaneously, of the other change, which brings speed and versatility to mechanisms to solve mathematical problems. The QCs present potential of being much more rapid than conventional ones to perform some types of calculations. The QNs are efficient and adequate to solve problems that require a rapid change of scale or connected communication complex nets. Field received an impulse when Shor (1994) developed an efficient algorithm to factorize large integers in a QC. Different groups started Shor's procedure via many qubits. Although it is about a great technical landmark, results are humdrum ($15 = 3 \times 5$, $21 = 3 \times 7$). However, when one has big QCs, Shor's program will release all its power. It could be used to decode all internet cryptographic codes, which would force to prepare different ways to assure online information.

15.4.2   BEING COHERENT

How can one build a QC? One needs qubits, which one can reunite from any QS with two different QSts. Photons are the simplest, for example, via two different polarization directions (vertical/horizontal). Atoms or ions were tested with different e^- dispositions, and SCs, with e^- currents that flow counter/clockwise. As Schrödinger's cat is living and dead while it is hidden in its box, qubits superpose results till their final QSt is discovered with a measure. Similar to the cat, qubit WFs are susceptible to a partial collapse via many tiny QInters with environment objects. To limit QD is a main challenge. Keeping qubits isolated inside device is important, so that WFs do not alter. Qubits must be susceptible to manipulation. Individual qubits (for example, atoms and ions) are incrusted in tiny cells. A case of Cu and glass protects them from free EMFs and allows electrodes connection. Atoms must be kept in vacuum in order to avoid QInters with each other. One can use light amplifications by stimulated emission of radiation (lasers) and other optical devices to alter qubits quantum energies and QSts (for example, e^- levels, spin). Small quantum recorders prototypes were built from 12 connected qubits. Difficulties exist. To build a qubit and maintain it isolated is complicated. To maintain it stable during long periods without losing quantum coherence is difficult, like making sure it produce precise and reproducible results: every time that one multiply 3 by 5, he wants adequate response. To join, qubits raise complexity. As qubits set rises, difficulty of controlling all sets rises. It raises the possibility of being QInters that get out of hand and affect precision.

15.4.3   FUTURE COMPUTERS

As traditional computers Si-chip technology reaches its limit, one contemplates quantum techniques that provide all a new power level. A QC could simulate almost anything and be key to create a machine that was artificially intelligent. Simultaneously performing so many calculations, QCs make mathematics in many parallel universes, more than parallel machines. Similar to Shor's function, algorithms types will be needed to exploit power. However, a QC strength origin is its weakness. As they are so sensitive to environment, they are fragile.

15.5   QUANTUM SIMULATIONS

Simulation is a crucial tool in the study of many complex problems. It imitates the behavior of the system that one wants to study via other means, in order to be capable of predicting its behavior. The physics of quantum many-body systems raises a great many questions, which exact solutions people do not know or cannot calculate, but which repercussions would include from the most fundamental theoretical level to the technological applications. Here the interest in developing techniques that allow stimulating the systems. Such simulations can be classical, that is, carried out via conventional computers. One of the characteristics of the QSts, entanglement, results a fundamental ingredient to take into account for the success of such simulations. However, provided the complexity of QSs, some problems that are of interest for people will be simulated only by other QSs, that is, the starting point of the field of quantum simulation, which, thanks to the present technological advances that allow the precise manipulation of QSs in the laboratory, turns into a possibility every time closer.

15.6   GOALS AND OPPORTUNITIES IN QUANTUM SIMULATION

Cirac and Zoller proposed hypothesis (Hs), question (Q), and fact (F) on quantum simulation.[16]

H1. (Feynman, 1959). There is plenty of room at the bottom.[17]
H2. (Feynman, 1959). As one goes down and fiddles around with atoms, one is working with different laws and expects to do different things.

H3. *Superposition principle:* For all linear systems, net response at a given place/time caused by two/more stimuli is the sum of responses which would have been caused by each stimulus individually.

Q1. Is it possible to build on experimental advances device performing tasks that classical sets cannot?

H4. (Feynman, 1981). To simulate QSs via classic computers is difficult.[18]

H5. (Feynman, 1981). To overcome such problems, one should use quantum simulators (*cf.* Fig. 15.1.).

H6. (Feynman, 1981). To discretize both space and time.

F1. (Lloyd, 1996). Evolving in small time steps allows efficiently simulating quantum many-body Hamiltonians containing few-particle interactions.[19]

H7. To approximate every time step by sequence of simpler operations after Trotter decomposition.[20]

H8. (Feynman, 1981). A quantum simulator imitates any QS, for example, the physical world.

H9. Main quantum simulators goal is to solve problems unapproachable with classical computers.

H10. A quantum simulator is more robust versus decoherence than a QC.

H11. *Area law:* In thermal equilibrium, the entanglement cannot be arbitrarily high.

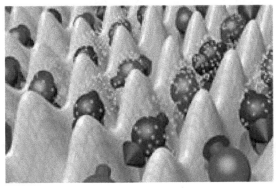

FIGURE 15.1   A quantum simulator: optical network.

They proposed questions and hypothesis on high-temperature (HT) superconductivity.

Q2.   What basic interaction between the electrons is responsible for the superconducting behavior?

Q3.   What minimum Hamiltonian does it describe the phenomenon of HT superconductivity?

H12. A quantum simulator checks the various candidate Hamiltonians for relevant phases.

They proposed an additional question.

Q4.   When will such a system thermalize?

They proposed quantum simulator requisites.[21]

H13. Quantum simulator requisites: (1) QS; (2) initialization; (3) Hamiltonian engineering; (4) detection; (5) verification.

They proposed additional questions, facts, answers, and hypotheses.

Q5.   Can one make a more rigorous statement on quantum simulators' robustness versus decoherence?

F2.   (Lloyd, 1996). QS efficiently simulates another's dynamics by stroboscopic change.

Q6.   However, how is this prone to errors?

Q7.   How to reach the ground or a thermal state of the problem Hamiltonian?

A7.   For the former, one can use adiabatic protocols.

Q8.   How to ensure adiabaticity?

Q9.   How to identify adiabaticity?

Q10. How can one determine for what kind of Hamiltonians the ground state is found efficiently?

H14. To find systems fulfilling the criteria laid out above.

H15. To show in laboratory simulation of a quantum many-body system involving large-scale entanglement that could not be represented classically.

15.7   DISCUSSION

Entanglement constitutes a fundamental quantum phenomenon that does not adapt to the notion of reality to which people is used. Entangled quantum objects contradict the idea of local realism; before a measurement, their properties are not defined in a univocal way; later, they stay strongly correlated. Classically, this would be explainable from only some type of interaction between such objects. Promising future technical developments will be based on quantum entanglement, for example, cryptography, communication, and quantum computation. QM was historically presented as a theory of limits, which imposes an uncertainty inherent in people's observations. Such prejudices find their origin in philosophical doctrines, for example, logical positivism, in fashion during the age in which QM was conceived. In fact, quantum theory does not impose strict limits. Its richness is such that it allows developing new techniques and acquiring new knowledge. The interpretation of quantum theory carries on starting debates. A recent proposal, quantum Bayesianism, combines QM with Bayesian approach to probability theory. Quantum Bayesianism replays one of the fundamental objects of quantum theory: the WF. This mathematical entity allows calculating the probability of obtaining one result or another in an experiment. The new proposal holds that the WF is associated with no objective reality. Instead, it would reflect the subjective mental state of the observer or their expectations of the world. QM seems to insinuate a discrete version of the world. However, its fundamental equations are written in terms of continuous quantities. Discrete properties appear only as an emergent property of such equations. Some experts think that if it were scrutinized in full detail, that appearance of continuity would reveal a discrete subjacent structure. However, this seems to contradict, at least, a fundamental aspect of nature: the chirality of the standard model (SM).

All information is stored and manipulated via physical devices. Quantum information theory investigates the possibilities that arise when such devices are ruled by the laws of QM. Superposition and entanglement, quantum phenomena without classic analogue, offer methods to store, process, and transmit the information much more efficiently than any classical protocol. Such methods should avoid that quantum information filter into the environment, a process known as decoherence. A number of techniques developed in the last years achieved promising advances in this direction. Present cryptographic methods are not intrinsically secure. Their security is based on the long computational time that the present technology would take to decode the cryptographic codes. Quantum laws allow improvement of coding algorithms. However, till not long ago, it was thought that their security would be vulnerable to malicious manipulations of the devices. A number of advances showed that privacy can be guaranteed even without knowing the internal operation of the coding apparatuses. The key consists in the way in which quantum laws treat information. Describing the state of a quantum many-body system, for example, a solid, requires handling huge amounts of information. Calculation of its properties is impracticable even with the best supercomputers of the world. An alternative way to study such systems consists in simulating their behavior via a reduced number of controllable quantum objects, for example, ultracold atoms trapped in optical nets. Thanks to quantum simulation techniques, physicists can study in controlled conditions all types of phenomena (for example, quantum phase transitions, electronic properties of exotic materials).

QM was traditionally considered the theory of the microscopic world: the physics of molecules, atoms, and subatomic particles. However, it is thought that its applicability is universal. The reason by which its strange properties vanish in great-sized systems would not obey a simple question of scale. During years, experiments showed the appearance of quantum effects in an increasingly greater number of macroscopic systems. The quantum effect par excellence, entanglement, can take place at both high temperatures and great-sized systems, for example, living beings. Schrödinger's cat, an apparent paradox conceived in the 1930s, occupied for decades physicists and philosophers with the following questions: can an unobserved macroscopic object be in a QSu of states? Can a cat be alive and dead at the same time? Under this question, the problem of measurement underlies. On carrying out a measurement on a QS described by a superposition of states, the WF collapses to a unique among all possible results. What principles do they rule that interaction between the quantum and the macroscopic? During years, notable advances were achieved in the experimental race to observe quantum effects in physical systems of great dimensions. The answers that this research field provide will affect in a fundamental way of people's conception of physical reality. In the 1970s, Stephen Hawking discovered that black holes (BHs) radiate particles, so that they would finish vanishing. That implied that they would destroy information, which is forbidden by QM. Some ideas from string theory seemed to point to a solution of the problem. According to them, the process of a BH vanishing would respect quantum laws and would not eliminate information. In order to preserve the information, a BH must be enclosed by a wall of high-energy particles (firewall). That undermines one of the basic predictions of GTR. According to GTR, matter and energy change the geometry of the space. A 100 years after Einstein formulated his theory, physicists continue searching for a quantum description of the space and time. QM and GTR predict two phenomena that seem to allow the instantaneous transmission of information: quantum entanglement and wormholes. Einstein studied both in 1935. A number of reports showed that such phenomena are related: entanglement can originate a geometric connection between distant regions of space. It suggests a new principle of quantum gravity. Since 90 years, the predictions of quantum physics were confirmed in no end of experiments. Most researchers opine that nothing exists that quantum formalism cannot explain. Quantum theory is also extraordinarily robust: since now, all attempts to modify it worked out theories that violate some basic principle, for example, the impossibility of transmitting information in an instantaneous way. A new research program, known as reconstruction of quantum theory, tries to determine to what point quantum is the only law compatible with a series of essential physical requisites. A number of recent studies suggest that it is possible to conceive generalized probabilistic theories wider than quantum physics but violate no fundamental principles. Such theories seem to bear an intriguing relationship with the macroscopic formulation of gravity.

15.8 CONCLUDING REMARKS

From the present discussion the following concluding remarks can be drawn:

1. Einstein's discomfort with entanglement is understandable: it is difficult to imagine the universe as a quantum connections net, with an unknown number of particles that talk to their distant couples. The universe is an enormous QS.
2. The panorama of quantum interactions entangled net shows that realism died. Similar to localism, signals transmission via communication limited by the speed of light, realism, that a particle exists

like a separated entity, is a riddle. World apparent reality is a mask that is put to hide the circumstance that it is really made from quantum ashes.

3. On carrying out so many calculations simultaneously, QCs make, in fact, mathematics in many parallel universes, more than parallel machines. Similar to Shor's function, new algorithms types will be needed to exploit the power. However, a QC strength origin is its weakness. As they are so sensitive to the environment, they are essentially fragile.

4. The advent of quantum information processing, as an abstract concept, gave birth to a great deal of new thinking, of a concrete form, about how to create physical computing devices that operate in the hitherto unexplored quantum mechanical regime.

5. The interdisciplinary spirit, which was fostered as a result of quantum computing, is one of the most pleasant and remarkable features of the field. The excitement and freshness that was produced bodes well for the prospect for discovery, invention, and innovation in the endeavor.

6. Feynman was correct that QCs could provide efficient simulation of other QS.

7. Two interesting directions closely related to quantum simulation should be mentioned. One is the study of entanglement in many-body systems and its relation with quantum phase transitions, the other is the development of classical numerical algorithms, inspired by the methods in quantum information and computation, for the simulation of quantum many-body systems.

8. Quantum simulation constitutes an exciting field that contains great promises for the future. However, short-term goals should be clearly defined, for example, to find systems that satisfy the above-exposed criteria and, in particular, to demonstrate in the laboratory the simulation of a quantum many-body system, in which a great-scale entanglement (already shown) take part, which could not be represented with classic means.

15.9 ACKNOWLEDGMENTS

Francisco Torrens belongs to the Institut Universitari de Ciència Molecular, Universitat de València. Gloria Castellano belongs to the Departamento de Ciencias Experimentales y Matemáticas, Facultad de Veterinaria y Ciencias Experimentales, Universidad Católica de Valencia *San Vicente Mártir*. The authors thank support from Generalitat Valenciana (Project No. PROMETEO/2016/094) and Universidad Católica de *Valencia San Vicente Mártir* (Project No. PRUCV/2015/617).

KEYWORDS

- **quantum information**
- **entanglement**
- **quantum computer**
- **quantum mechanics**
- **quantum theory**
- **general theory of relativity**

REFERENCES

1. Torrens, F. Fractals for Hybrid Orbitals in Protein Models. *Complexity Int.* **2001,** *8*, 1.
2. Torrens, F. Fractal Hybrid-Orbital Analysis of the Protein Tertiary Structure. *Complexity Int.* (submitted for publication).
3. Torrens, F.; Castellano, G. Resonance in Interacting Induced-Dipole Polarizing Force Fields: Application to Force-Field Derivatives. *Algorithms* **2009,** *2*, 437–447.
4. Torrens, F.; Castellano, G. Molecular Diversity Classification via Information Theory: A Review. *Trans. Complex Syst.* **2012,** *12*, 10–12, e4–1–8.
5. Torrens, F.; Castellano, G. Reflections on the Nature of the Periodic Table of the Elements: Implications in Chemical Education. In *Synthetic Organic Chemistry*; Seijas, J. A.; Vázquez Tato, M. P.; Lin, S. K.; Eds. MDPI: Basel, Switzerland, 2015,Vol. 18; pp 1–15.
6. Putz, M. V., Ed., *The Explicative Dictionary of Nanochemistry;* Apple Academic–CRC: Waretown, NJ, in press.
7. Torrens, F.; Castellano, G. Reflections on the Cultural History of Nanominiaturization and Quantum Simulators (Computers). In *Sensors and Molecular Recognition*, Laguarda Miró, N., Masot Peris, R., Brun Sánchez, E., Eds.; Universidad Politécnica de Valencia: València, Spain, 2015; Vol. 9, pp 1–7.
8. Torrens, F.; Castellano, G. Ideas in the History of Nano/Miniaturization and (Quantum) Simulators: Feynman, Education and Research Reorientation in Translational Science. In *Synthetic Organic Chemistry*, Seijas, J. A., Vázquez Tato, M. P., Lin, S. K., Eds.; MDPI: Basel, Switzerland, 2016; Vol. 19, pp 1–16.

9. Torrens, F.; Castellano, G. Nanominiaturization and Quantum Computing. In *Sensors and Molecular Recognition,* Costero Nieto, A. M., Parra Álvarez, M., Gaviña Costero, P., Gil Grau, S., Eds.; Universitat de València: València, Spain, 2016; Vol. 10, pp 31–1–5.

10. Torrens, F.; Castellano, G. Nanominiaturization, Classical/Quantum Computers/ Simulators, Superconductivity and Universe. In *Methodologies and Applications for Analytical and Physical Chemistry,* Haghi, A. K., Thomas, S., Palit, S., Main, P., Eds.; Apple Academic–CRC: Waretown, NJ; in press.

11. Torrens, F.; Castellano, G. Superconductors, Superconductivity, BCS Theory and Entagled Photons for Quantum Computing. In *Innovations in Physical Chemistry,* A. K. Haghi, Ed.; Apple Academic–CRC: Waretown, NJ; Vol. 4, in press.

12. Torrens, F.; Castellano, G. *Book of Abstracts.* Certamen Integral de la Prevención y el Bienestar Laboral, València, Spain, September 28–29, 2016; Generalitat Valenciana– INVASSAT: València, Spain, 2016; p 3.

13. Torrens, F.; Castellano, G. Nanoscience: From a Two-Dimensional to a Three-Dimensional Periodic Table of the Elements. In *Methodologies and Applications for Analytical and Physical Chemistry,* Haghi, A. K., Thomas, S., Palit, S., Main, P., Eds.; Apple Academic–CRC: Waretown, NJ; in press.

14. Torrens, F.; Castellano, G. *Book of Abstracts.* Congreso Internacional de Tecnología, Ciencia y Sociedad, València, Spain, October 19–20, 2017; Universidad Cardenal Herrera CEU: València, Spain, 2017; p 1.

15. Baker, J. 50 *Quantum Physics Ideas You Really Need to Know*; Quercus: London, UK, 2013.

16. Cirac, J. I.; Zoller, P. Goals and Opportunities in Quantum Simulation. *Nat. Phys.* **2012,** *8,* 264–266.

17. Feynman, R. P. There is Plenty of Room at The Bottom. *Caltech Eng. Sci.* **1960,** *23,* 22–36.

18. Feynman, R. P. Simulating Physics with Computers. *Int. J. Theor. Phys.* **1982,** *21,* 467–488.

19. Lloyd, S. Universal Quantum Simulators. *Science* **1996,** *273,* 1073–1078.

20. Buluta, I.; Nori, F. Quantum Simulators. *Science* **2009,** *326,* 108–111.

21. DiVincenzo, D. P. The Physical Implementation of Quantum Computation. *Fortschr. Phys.* **2000,** *48,* 771–783.

CHAPTER 16

NOVEL BEAM SHAPING

P. SURESH*

Department of ECE, Veltech Dr. RR, Dr. SR University, Avadi, Chennai, Tamil Nadu 600062, India

Corresponding author. E-mail: P.SURESH@vel-tech.org

CONTENTS

ABSTRACT

Beam shaping is generally defined as a process to rearrange the intensity and phase of an optical light beam. One of the simplest examples of beam shaping is probably that a plane wave is focused into a spot by a convex lens. The term "beam shape" stands for the intensity profile. The phase profile determines how the intensity profile evolves during propagation.

A general beam shaping problem is to find an optical system that operates the incident beam to generate the desired intensity distribution, such as a uniform distribution at a certain area on the target plane (focal region).

16.1   INTRODUCTION

Laser light has a high degree of coherence, good directionality, and a high intensity, which exhibits various properties like reflection, refraction, diffraction, polarization, dispersion, and absorption among others. Some of these properties have been used in the field of near-field optics which is suitable for the optical trapping and other optical manipulation applications of focused optical beams. The trapping of nano- and microparticles by using the radiation forces produced by highly focused optical beams (so-called optical tweezers) has become very widely used in the past two decades in physical, chemical, and biological experiments where precise manipulation of microscopic objects is required.

16.2   FUNDAMENTAL THEORY OF TIGHT FOCUSING

Focusing with high apertures is important to all disciplines requiring highly localized fields of light. It is not only vital to optical microscopy, but also to optical data storage and optical micromanipulation applications. In particular, the detection of single molecules on surfaces, and in solution where there is a high aperture focusing helps to provide high sensitivity and spatial localization. Optical trapping also relies on high aperture focusing, because tight focusing leads to a large field intensity gradient, which is necessary for trapping microscopic particles.

The scattering and gradient optical forces exerted on the trapped objects depend on the intensity and phase distributions in a trapping beam. For this reason, optical trapping has been studied for different types of optical beams, for example, Gaussian, Laguerre–Gaussian and Bessel Gaussian.[11] The optical manipulation using basic Gaussian beams has resulted in many applications, the scope for innovation expands dramatically with the addition of novel optical beam shapes: beams that are not only able to confine objects, but rotate them, beams with unusual transverse intensity profiles that are capable of optically sorting objects[55] and even beams that do not propagate in a straight line,[43,1] which increases the interest, application and turns the world around it.

16.3   VECTORIAL DEBYE THEORY

The paraxial approximation is applicable to focusing systems when the lenses involved are weakly convergent, that is for low-numerical aperture (NA) systems (-NA<0.4). As such, the optical fields can be described as scalar waves in this low-NA limit and they retain their initial polarization structure at the focal plane of the lens. However, there is a polarization scattering effect imparted by lenses such that for higher NA's (-NA>0.4) the polarization state at the focus of the lens is three-dimensional.[55] In this situation, the vector nature of the light must be considered to describe the focusing action of the lens. The method of Richards and Wolf is useful for describing this vector diffraction problem and is detailed below.

16.3.1   ANGULAR SPECTRUM REPRESENTATION

In essence, Richards and Wolf diffraction involves formulating the angular spectrum representation of a plane wave focused by an aplanatic lens.[43] The angular spectrum representation is a method for determining the propagated, electric field distribution at some distance z from the field distribution at z=0. In particular, the far-field distribution is completely defined by the Fourier spectrum of the source field.[43]

$$E(x,y,z) = \frac{ire^{-ikr}}{2\pi} \int_{-\infty}^{\infty}\int_{-\infty}^{\infty} \frac{\tilde{E}_0(k_x,k_y)}{k_z} e^{i(k_x x + k_y y \pm k_z z)} dk_x dk_y \qquad (16.1)$$

Where, $r = \sqrt{x^2 + y^2 + z^2}$ is the distance from the origin and $k_z = \sqrt{k^2 - (k_x^2 + k_y^2)}$, $\tilde{E}_0(k_x,k_y)$ is the Fourier spectrum of $E(x,y,z)$, and K_x and k_y are the special frequency components.[61] The limits of (2.1) are taken such that only rays propagating into the far-field are considered. The rays which obey $k^2 > (kx^2 + ky^2)$ are evanescent, do not propagate to the far-field and are thus not considered in the far-field angular spectrum representation.

Hence, a quantitative investigation of the focal field of high aperture lenses is of paramount importance. The performance of an optical system can be typically characterized by the optical transfer function (OTF). The topic of electromagnetic (EM) wave focusing has been studied by many authors.[43,56,48] However, the Richards and Wolf who established the theory, in which the focused EM field is given as a superposition of plane waves, whose propagation vectors all fall inside the geometrical light cone.[43] The high NA focusing of EM waves in a single homogeneous material was earlier presented in 1959 by E. Wolf.[55] Later, Wolf and Li[56] showed that the approach based on the Debye integral[5] is valid for systems that satisfy the high aperture condition. Later, the problem was thoroughly investigated by Stamnes.[48] It is now understood that, while at small semi aperture angles, a scalar wave theory satisfactorily describes the focusing process, at higher angles (when the NA of lens is larger than 0.7), where the vectorial properties of light plays an important role, the vectorial Debye theory is necessary to represent the field distribution in the focal region of an objective.

16.4   EFFECT ON LIGHT BEAMS OF DIFFERENT POLARIZATION AND AMPLITUDE PROFILES

The basic principle behind optical tweezers is photon momentum transfer during the light reflection and refraction. The particular interest in this discussion of near-field optics is a Gaussian beam. A promising type of beam for optical trapping is Bessel–Gaussian vector beam, which is the solution of the vector wave equation in the paraxial limit.[19,14]

The polarization of light is classified into two types. They are spatially homogeneous and spatially inhomogeneous distribution. The distribution in terms of the state of polarization (SOP) for the light beam is known as spatially homogeneous distribution and its types of optical community are linear, circular, and elliptical polarization shown in Figure 16.1.

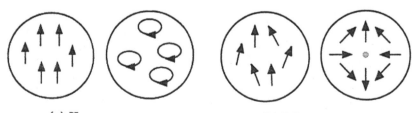

(a) Homogeneous   (b) Inhomogeneous

FIGURE 16.1   Polarization types.

The spatial variant SOP is called as spatially inhomogeneous distribution. Such kind of light beam is expected to lead to new effects and phenomena in optical systems, which increases much interest among researchers and is shown in Figure 16.1b. An example of such spatially inhomogeneous SOP with cylindrical symmetry is called as cylindrical vector (CV) beams.[7]

$$\vec{E}(r,\varphi,z) = E_r \vec{e_r} + E_\varphi \vec{e_\varphi} + E_z \vec{e_z} \qquad (16.2)$$

Where $\vec{e_r}$, $\vec{e_\varphi}$, and $\vec{e_z}$ are the unit vectors in the radial, azimuthal, and z directions, respectively. The amplitudes of the three orthogonal components are given by

$$E_r(r,\varphi,z) = A\cos\phi \int_0^\alpha \sqrt{\cos\theta} P(\theta)\sin\theta \cos\theta J_1(kr\sin\theta) e^{ikz\cos\theta} d\theta$$

$$E_z(r,\varphi,z) = iA\cos\phi \int_0^\alpha \sqrt{\cos\theta} P(\theta)\sin^2\theta J_0(kr\sin\theta) e^{ikz\cos\theta} d\theta \qquad (16.3)$$

$$E_r(r,\varphi,z) = A\sin\phi \int_0^\alpha \sqrt{\cos\theta} P(\theta)\sin\theta J_1(kr\sin\theta) e^{ikz\cos\theta} d\theta$$

Where, $P(\theta)$ is the pupil apodization function, k is the wave number and J_n is the Bessel function of the first kind with order n, A is the amplitude of the field, which is defined by the beam power P. The beam has a polarization rotated by ϕ_0 from its radial direction.

The CV beams are vector beam solutions of Maxwell's equations that obey axial symmetry in both amplitude and phase[14] CV beams can be divided into radial polarization, azimuthal polarization, and generalized cylindrical polarization, according to the actual polarization pattern (Fig. 16.2c). Figure 16.2c shows the polarization pattern of a generalized cylindrical vector beam. Instead of radial polarization or azimuthal polarization, each point of the beam has a polarization rotated by ϕ_0 from its radial direction. The electrical field of this beam can be expressed in a cylindrical coordinate system as

$$\vec{E}(r,\varphi) = P\left[\cos\phi_0\,\vec{e}_r + \sin\phi_0\,\vec{e}_\varphi\right] \tag{16.4}$$

Where, e_r is the unit vector in the radial direction, and e_φ is the unit vector in the azimuthal direction. P is the pupil apodization function denoting the relative amplitude of the field, which only depends on radial position. Thus, a generalized cylindrical vector beam is just a linear superposition of a cylindrically symmetric radial polarization and a cylindrically symmetric azimuthal polarization. The radially polarized or azimuthally polarized light beams can be converted into a generalized CV beam conveniently, or vice versa[64] using two cascaded half-wave plates.

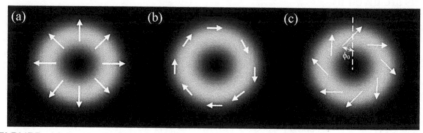

FIGURE 16.2 (a) Radial polarization, (b) azimuthal polarization, (c) generalized cylindrical polarization.

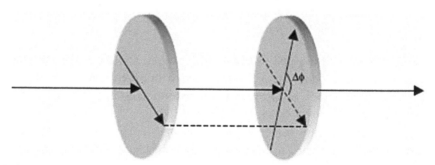

FIGURE 16.3 Polarization rotator.

The polarization rotator consisting of two half-wave plates is shown in Figure 16.3. To make use of the CV beams in different applications, devices that can perform basic manipulations such as reflection, polarization rotation, and retardation are necessary. The key to these operations is to maintain the polarization symmetry. A polarization rotator using two cascaded $\lambda/2$ plates has been designed and demonstrated[65] to maintain polarization symmetry by tuning the angle of two half-wave plates. The angle between the fast axes of the two cascaded $\lambda/2$ plates is $\Delta\phi$. The Jones matrix of this polarization rotator can be written as

$$T = \begin{bmatrix} \cos(2\Delta\phi) & -\sin(2\Delta\phi) \\ \sin(2\Delta\phi) & \cos(2\Delta\phi) \end{bmatrix} = R(-2\Delta\phi) \qquad (16.5)$$

Initially, polarization is independent of rotation of cascaded polarization rotator of two half-wave plates. The angle of rotation between two half-wave plates determined by angle $\Delta\phi$. The generalized cylindrical vector can be obtained when $\Delta\phi = \phi_0/2$ as shown in Figure 16.2.

Nowadays, researchers have much interest in these beams, because of its novel focusing properties under the high-NA lens. Researchers have reported many techniques to generate radially polarized beams or azimuthally polarized beams by inserting a specially designed optical element into laser resonators.[32,51] The elements such as conical elements,[26,46,21] complex Brewster-type windows,[51] polarization selective mirrors,[32,29] c-cut Nd:YVO4 crystals,[57] liquid crystal gels,[42] or phase elements which allow for significant mode discrimination.[36] In order to generate CV beams, some of the other methods are metal strip subwavelength grating,[4] space-variant inhomogeneous media,[38] or diffractive optical element (DOE) interferometer.[50] However, the cylindrical vector beams (CVB) found wide applications in the optical field because of its unique properties, such as optical trapping and manipulation,[24,8,62,61,66] scanning optical microscopy,[59] lithography,[15] laser cutting,[33,31] particle acceleration,[52,13] and single molecule imaging.[47,34] Among these applications, particular interest has been given to the high NA focusing property of these beams and their application as a high-resolution probe. Due to the cylindrical symmetry of the polarization, the electric field at the focus of a cylindrical vector beam has unique polarization properties. For example, it has been shown that the longitudinal component of the focus from such a cylindrical beam is much stronger than the transversal component, and the size of the longitudinal focus is much smaller than the transversal focus.[38,39] This property could find applications in high-resolution microscopy, microlithography, metrology, and nonlinear optics, and so forth. There is continued interest among researchers and scientist of spatially inhomogeneous polarization beams because of propagation and focusing properties.

The total electric field light intensity distribution near the focus depends on the numerical aperture of the focusing objective. This leads to change in the trapping properties of the input beam at the focus by changing NA. Especially, this should be important for the radial illumination of the input beam consists of two orthogonal components namely, transversal (Er) and longitudinal (Ez) component. The Ez-component decreases when NA increases, while the Er does not change essentially. When focused with a high-NA objective, radially polarized light leads to strong longitudinal electric field component in the vicinity of the focus. The low-NA objective produces a doughnut shape of the total intensity distribution; however, the high-NA objective produces a peak at the focus. The radial gradient force traps the high-index particle. The axial gradient force permits to achieve a stable trapping of high-index particles for any value of NA. For low-index particles, the scattering force together with the gradient force may provide the stable axial trapping. In particular, a radially polarized CVB focused by a high-NA objective has a peak at the focus, and an azimuthally polarized incident beam has a null in the center.[58] Switching between radial and azimuthal polarizations can be done by using two half-wave plates. The basic focusing property of highly focused polarized beams can be analyzed with the Richards and Wolf vectorial diffraction method.[55,43] This method has been extensively used to study cases in which the illumination of the pupil has no spatial variation in polarization.[1] This method has also been used to calculate the electric fields in the vicinity of the focal spot for radial and azimuthal polarization.[58,2] This may provide a convenient means of polarization manipulation. However, careful control is necessary due to the sensitivity and increase in the application.

It has been found, that the condition for tighter focusing of CV beam is complicated in fact for above application and degrades in performance and resolution. On the other hand, focal depth is also a very important parameter in many optical systems and can be used to enhance the performance.[18,35,28,44,27] For some applications, a beam with very narrow diffraction pattern with a tunable axial extent is necessary. For example, in optical data storage, one would expect that the focal point possesses a long focal depth but a small transverse dimension;[12] this leads to a larger data density as well as a better tolerance for beam focusing. In biomedical imaging, temporal resolution is strongly enhanced using beams with a long depth of focus in two-photon laser scanning microscopy[7] or plane illumination microscopy.[37] Some other applications requiring high-resolution are second-harmonic generation[3] and material ablation.[16]

In order to generate a high-resolution beam with the reduced focal spot, several methods scheme has been proposed based on far-field apodization technique and handling of evanescent waves with near-field diffraction structure.[15,58,30,54] The binary phase filter has been widely studied and the structured illumination has been applied to optical lithography and confocal microscopy.[30] However, as the key property of optical beam, the polarization state of incident light should be considered.[63,15,58,54,6] Therefore, based on the polarization of light, a variety of filter (Amplitude filter, binary phase filter, and complex filter were proposed to improve focusing characteristics.[45,6,49] Recently, the high-resolution intensity profile of tightly focused incident beam can only be considered in the focal region. For example, the sharper focal spot was achieved by higher-order radially polarized Laguerre–Gaussian (LG) beam and Bessel–Gaussian beam.[49,22,53,23,17] Wang et al. generated a longitudinally polarized beam over a full width at half maximum (FWHM) of long focal depth 4 λ with spot size FWHM 0.43 λ without divergence of incident radially polarized Bessel–Gaussian beam tightly focused through the high-NA lens in combination with the binary optical element.[54] Kitamura et al. produced spot size approximately 0.4 λ FWHM with a depth of focus of greater than 4 λ in the focal region by tight focusing a finite annulus of light with a high-NA lens.[20] Rajesh et al. generated a subwavelength (0.395 λ) longitudinally polarized beam with the large uniform depth of focus (~6 λ) for a radially polarized Bessel–Gaussian input field of focal field of high-NA lens axicon with a binary phase optical component.[40] Yuan et al. generated nondiffracting transversally polarized beam by means of transmitting an azimuthally polarized beam through a multibelt spiral phase hologram focused by a high-NA lens of focal depth ~4.84 λ of the electric field with only radial and azimuthal components is achieved.[60] Rajesh et al. generated a longitudinally polarized beam with focal depth of 8 λ and a transverse FWHM of 0.45 λ of by tightly focused double ring radially polarized beam in the focal region of high-NA lens axicon.[41]

16.5   BESSEL BEAMS

The idea of the Bessel beam first arose in 1987 when Durnin spotted the Bessel solution to the Helmholtz equation. The first experimental realization of the equivalent optical beam soon followed. The electric field, $E(r,\varphi,z)$ of a theoretical Bessel beam, is given by[31]

$$E_z\left(r,\varphi,z\right)=E_0\exp\left(ik_z z\right)J_m\left(k_r r\right)\exp\left(\pm n\varphi\right) \qquad (16.6)$$

where E_0 is the field amplitude, k_z and k_r are wave vectors $\left(k=\sqrt{k_z^2+k_r^2}\right)$, J_m is the Bessel function of mth order, and r, φ, and z are cylindrical coordinates. A zero-order Bessel beam has a transverse intensity profile with a bright central spot surrounded by concentric rings. The transverse intensity profiles of Bessel beams with different m values are shown in Figure 16.4.

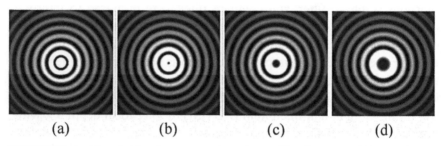

(a)   (b)   (c)   (d)

FIGURE 16.4   The simulated transverse intensity profiles for a Bessel beam with (a) m=0, (b) m=1, (c) m=2, (d) m=3 are shown.

In theory, the intensity profile of a zero-order Bessel beam can propagate for an infinite distance without spreading. In practice, the beam can propagate "diffraction-free" for only a finite distance. This is because an infinite "diffraction-free" propagation distance would require the Bessel beam to have an infinite number of intensity rings and therefore infinite energy. However, an approximation to the ideal Bessel beam, which has a finite "diffraction-free" propagation distance and finite energy.

16.6   LAGUERRE–GAUSSIAN (LG) BEAM

The LG beams are also known as the doughnut beams. This is due to their characteristic intensity distribution of a dark spot in the middle surrounded by a bright ring, because of carrying orbital angular momentum has been exclusively employed in many novel optical trapping and optical manipulation applications. The focusing properties of an LG beam with a high-NA objective have also attracted lots of research interests[51,9] Recently, the successful near-field trapping using a focused evanescent LG beam has been demonstrated.[10] For illumination by a Laguerre–Gaussian beam TEMple* beam with its waist in the pupil, this function is given by[57]

$$A(\theta) = \beta^2 \frac{\sin\theta}{\sin^2\theta} \exp\left[-\left(\beta\frac{\sin\theta}{\sin\alpha}\right)^2\right] L_p^l\left[2\left(\beta\frac{\sin\theta}{\sin\alpha}\right)^2\right] \quad (16.7)$$

Where, β is the parameter that denoted the ratio of pupil diameter to the beam diameter and L_p^1 is the generalized Laguerre polynomial.

16.7 HOLLOW GAUSSIAN BEAM (HGB)

In the cylindrical coordinate system $E\ (r,\ \varphi,\ z)$ are the field distribution of hollow Gaussian beam (HGB) at its waist plane ($z = 0$) and can be written as,

$$E(r,\varphi,0) = E_0(r,\varphi,0)n_r \quad (16.8)$$

Where, n_r is the radial unit vector of HGM in the polarized direction. The optical field value distribution can be written as,

$$E(r,\varphi,0) = D\left(\frac{r^2}{\omega_0^2}\right)^n \exp\left(-\frac{r^2}{\omega_0^2}\right)\exp(i\phi) \quad (16.9)$$

$$E(r,\varphi,0) = D\left(\frac{\sin^2(\theta)}{\omega^2 NA^2}\right)^n \exp\left(-\frac{\sin^2(\theta)}{\omega^2 NA^2}\right)\exp(in\phi) \quad (16.10)$$

Where, n=0, 1, 2 ....

The optical intensity in focal region is proportional to the modulus square of Eq. 16.10. Where $\omega = \omega_0/r_0$ is called relative waist width and ϕ is the phase distribution.

KEYWORDS

- **beam shaping**
- **plane wave**
- **intensity distribution**
- **uniform distribution**
- **optical forces**

REFERENCE

1. Advanced Optical Imaging Theory. Gu, M.; Ed.; Springer-Verlag: New York, 1999; p 75.
2. Biss, D. P.; Brown, T. G. Cylindrical Vector Beam Focusing through a Dielectric Interface. *Opt. Express.* **2001,** *9,* 490–497.
3. Biss, D. P.; Brown, T. G. Polarization-Vortex-Driven Second-harmonic Generation. *Opt. Lett.* **2003,** *28,* 923–925.
4. Bomzon, Z.; Biener, G.; Kleiner, V.; Hasman, E. Radially and Azimuthally Polarized Beams Generated by Space-Variant Dielectric Subwavelength Gratings. *Opt. Lett.* **2002,** *27,* 285–287.
5. Debye, P. Das verhalten von lichtwellen in der nahe eines brennpunktes oder einer brennlinie. *Ann. Phys.* **1909,** *30,* 755.
6. Dorn, R.; Quabis,S.; Leuchs, G. Sharper Focus for a Radially Polarized Light Beam. *Phys. Rev. Lett.* **2003,** *91,* 233901 1–4.
7. Dufour, P.; Piché, M,; De Koninck, Y.; McCarthy, N. Two-Photon Excitation Fluorescence Microscopy with a High Depth of Field Using un Axicon. *Appl. Opt.* **2006,** *45,* 9246–9252.
8. Gahagan, K. T.; Swartzlander, G. A. Simultaneous Trapping of Low-Index and High-Index Micro Particles Observed with an Optical-Vortex Trap. *J. Opt. Soc. Am. B.* **1999,** *16,* 533–537.
9. Ganic, D.; Gan, X.; Gu, M. Focusing of Doughnut Laser Beams by a High Numerical-Aperture Objective in Free Space. *Opt. Express.* **2003,** *11,* 2747.
10. Ganic, D.; Gan, X.; Gu, M. Trapping Force and Optical Lifting under Focused Evanescent Wave Illumination. *Opt. Express.* **2004,** *12,* 5533.
11. Grier, D. G. A Revolution in Optical Manipulation. *Nature.* **2003,** *424,* 810–816.
12. Grosjean, T.; Courjon, D.; Bainier, C. Smallest Lithographic Marks Generated by Optical Focusing Systems. *Opt. Lett.* **2007,** *32,* 976–978.
13. Hafizi, B.; Esarey, E.; Sprangle, P. Laser-Driven Acceleration with Bessel Beams. *Phys. Rev. E.* **1997,** *55,* 3539–3545.
14. Hall, D. G. Vector-Beam Solutions of Maxwell Wave Equation. *Optics Lett.* **1996,** *21,* 9–11.

15. Helseth, L. E. Roles of Polarization, Phase and Amplitude in Solid Immersion Lens Systems. *Opt. Commun.* **2001,** *191,* 161–172.

16. Hnatovsky, C.; Shvedov, V.; Krolikowski, W.; Rode, A. Revealing Local Field Structure of Focused Ultrashort Pulses. *Phys. Rev. Lett.* **2011,** *106,* 123901.

17. Huang, K.; Shi, P.; Cao, G. W.; Li, K.; Zhang, X. B.; Li, Y. P. Vector-Vortex Bessel-Gauss Beams and their Tightly Focusing Properties. *Opt. Lett.* **2011,** *36,* 888–890.

18. Indebetouwg, G.; Bai, H. Imaging with Fresnel Zone Pupil Masks: Extended Depth of Field. *Appl. Opt.* **1984,** *23*(23), 4299–4302.

19. Jordan, R. H.; Hall, D. G. Free-Space Azimuthal Paraxial Wave Equation: The Azimuthal Bessel Gauss Beam Solution. *Optics Lett.* **1994,** *19,*.427–429.

20. Kitamura, K.; Sakai, K.; Noda, S. Sub-wavelength Focal Spot with Long Depth of Focus Generated by Radially Polarized, Narrow-Width Annular Beam. *Opt. Express.* **2010,** *18,* 4518–4525.

21. Kozawa, Y.; Sato, S. Generation of A Radially Polarized Laser Beam by Use of a Conical Brewster Prism. *Opt. Lett.* **2005,** *30,* 3063–3065.

22. Kozawa, Y.; Sato, S. Sharper Focal Spot formed by Higher-Order Radially Polarized Laser Beams. *J. Opt. Soc. Am.* **2007,** *A24,* 1793–1798.

23. Kozawa, Y.; Sato, S. Focusing of Higher-Order Radially Polarized Laguerre-Gaussian Beam. *J. Opt. Soc. Am.* **2012,** *A29,* 2439–2443.

24. Kuga, T.; Torii, Y.; Shiokawa, N.; Hirano, T.; Shimizu, Y.; Sasada, H. Novel Optical Trap of Atoms with a Doughnut Beam. *Phys. Rev. Lett.* **1997,** *78,* 4713–4716.

25. Lerman, G. M.; Levy, U. Effect of Radial Polarization and Apodization on Spot Size under Tight Focusing Conditions. *Opt. Express.* **2008,** *16,* 4567–4581.

26. Li, J.; Ueda, K.; Musha, M. Generation of Radially Polarized Mode in Yb Fiber Laser by Using a Dual Conical Prism. *Opt. Lett.* **2006,** *31,* 2969–2971.

27. Lin, J.; Yin, K.; Li, Y.; Tan, J. Achievement of Longitudinally Polarized Focusing with Long Focal Depth by Amplitude Modulation. *Opt. Lett.* **2011,** *36*(7), 1185–1187.

28. Mikuła, G.; Jaroszewicz, Z.; Kolodziejczyk, A.; Petelczyc, K.; Sypek, M. Imaging with Extended Focal Depth by Means of Lenses with Radial and Angular Modulation. *Opt. Express.* **2007,** *15*(15), 9184–9193.

29. Moser, T.; Balmer, J.; Delbeke, D.; et al. Intracavity Generation of Radially Polarized CO_2 Laser Beams-Based on A Simple Binary Dielectric Diffraction Grating. *Appl. Opt.* **2006,** *45,* 8517–8522.

30. Neil, M. A. A.; Juskaitis, R.; Wilson, T. Method of Obtaining Optical Sectioning by Using Structured Light in a Conventional Microscope. *Opt. Lett.* **1997,** *22,* 1905–1907.

31. Nesterov, A. V.; Niziev, V. G. Laser Beams with Axially Symmetric Polarization. *J. Phys. D.* **2000,** *33,* 1817–1822.

32. Nesterov, A. V.; Niziev, V. G.; Yakunin, V. P. Generation of High-Power Radially Polarized Beam. *J. Phys. D: Appl. Phys.* **1999,** *32,* 2871–2875.

33. Niziev, V. G.; Nesterov, A. V. Influence of Beam Polarization on Laser Cutting Efficiency. *J. Phys. D.* **1999,** *32,* 1455–1461.

34. Novotny, L.; Beversluis, M. R.; Youngworth, K. S.; Brown, T. G. Longitudinal Field Modes Probed by Single Molecules. *Phys. Rev. Lett.* **2001,** *86,* 5251–5254.

35. Ojeda-Castaneda, J.; Landgrave, J. E. A.; Escamilla, H. M. Annular Phase-Only Mask for High Focal Depth. *Opt. Lett.* **2005,** *30*(13),1647–1649.
36. Oron, R.; Blit, S.; Davidson, N. The Formation of Laser Beams with Pure Azimuthal or Radial Polarization. *Appl. Phys. Lett.* **2000,** *77*, 3322–3324.
37. Planchon, T. A.; Gao, L.; Milkie, D. E.; Davidson, M. W.; Galbraith, J. A.; Galbraith, C. G.; Betzig, E. Rapid Three-Dimensional Isotropic Imaging of Living Cells using Bessel Beam Plane Illumination. *Nat. Methods.* **2011,** *8*, 417–423.
38. Quabis, S.; Dorn, R.; Eberler, M.; Glockl, O.; Leuchs, G. Focusing Light to a Tighter Spot. *Opt. Commun.* **2000,** *179*, 1–7.
39. Quabis, S.; Dorn, R.; Eberler, M.; Glöckl, O.; Leuchs, G. The Focus of Light-Theoretical Calculation and Experimental Tomographic Reconstruction. *Appl. Phys. B.* **2001,** *72*, 109–113.
40. Rajesh, K. B.; Jaroszewicz, Z.; Anbarasan, P. M. Improvement of Lens Axicon's Performance for Longitudinally Polarized Beam Generation by Adding a Dedicated Phase Transmittance. *Opt. Express.* **2010,** *18*(26), 26799–26805.
41. Rajesh, K. B.; Veerabagu Suresh, N.; Anbarasan, P. M., Gokulakrishnan, K.; Mahadevan, G. Tight Focusing of Double Ring Shaped Radially Polarized Beam with High NA Lens Axicon. *Opt. Laser Technol.* **2011,** *43*, 1037–1040.
42. Ren, H.; Lin, Y.; Wu, S. Linear to Axial or Radial Polarization Conversion using a Liquid Crystal Gel. *Appl. Phys. Lett.* **2006,** *89*, 051115.
43. Richards, B.; Wolf, E. Electromagnetic Diffraction in Optical Systems II. Structure of the Image Field in an Aplanatic System. *Proc. R. Soc. London Ser. A.* **1959,** *253*, 358–379.
44. Sauceda, A.; Ojeda-Castañeda, J. High Focal Depth with Fractional-Power Wave Fronts. *Opt. Lett.* **2004,** *29*(6), 560–562.
45. Sheppard, C. J. R.; Choudhury, A. Annular Pupils, Radial Polarization, and Super-resolution. *Appl. Opt.* **2004,** *43*, 4322–4327.
46. Shoham, A.; Vander, R.; Lipson, S. G. Production of Radially and Azimuthally Polarized Polychromatic Beams. *Opt. Lett.* **2006,** *31*, 3405–3407.
47. Sick, B.; Hecht, B.; Novotny, L. Orientational Imaging of Single Molecules by Annular Illumination. *Phys. Rev. Lett.* **2000,** *85*, 4482–4485.
48. Stamnes, J. J. *Waves in Focal Regions*; Adam Hilgar: Bristol, UK, 1986.
49. Tan, Q. F.; Cheng, K.; Zhou, Z. H.; Jin, G. F. Diffractive Superresolution Elements for Radially Polarized Light. *J. Opt. Soc. Am.* **2010,** *A27*, 1355–1360.
50. Toussaint, K. C, Park, S.; Jureller, J. E.; Schere, N. F. Generation of Optical Vector Beams with a Diffractive Optical Element Interferometer. *Opt. Lett.* **2005,** *30*, 2846–2848
51. Tovar, A. A. Production and Propagation of Cylindrically Polarized Laguerre–Gaussian Laser Beams. *J. Opt. Soc. Am. A.* **1998,** *15*, 2705–2711.
52. Varin, C.; Piche, M. Acceleration of Ultra-Relativistic Electrons Using High Intensity TM01 Laser Beams. *Appl. Phys. B.* **2002,** *74*, S 83–S88.
53. Vyas, S.; Niwa, M.; Kozawa, Y.; Sato, S. Diffractive Properties of Obstructed Vector Laguerre-Gaussian Beam under Tight Focusing Condition. *J. Opt. Soc. Am.* **2011,** *A28,*1387–1394.

54. Wang, H.; Shi, L.; Lukyanchuk, B.; Sheppard, C.; Chong, C. T. Creation of a Needle of Longitudinally Polarized Light in Vacuum using Binary Optics. *Nat. Photonics* **2008**, *2*, 501–505.

55. Wolf, E. Electromagnetic Diffraction in Optical sSystems I. An Integral Representation of The Image Field. *Proc. R. Soc. Ser. A.* **1959**, *253*, 349–357.

56. Wolf, E.; Li, Y. Conditions for The Validity of The Debye Integral Representation of Focused Fields. *Opt. Commun.* **1981**, *39*, 205.

57. Yonezawa, K.; Kozawa, Y.; Sato, S.Generation of Radially Polarized Laser Beam by Use of the Birefringence of A C-Cut Nd:YVO4 Crystal. *Opt. Lett.* **2006**, *31*, 2151–2153.

58. Youngworth, K. S.; Brown, T. G.; Focusing of High Numerical Aperture Cylindrical-Vector Beams. *Opt. Express.* **2000a**, *7*(2), 77–87.

59. Youngworth, K. S.; Brown, T. G.; Inhomogeneous Polarization in Scanning Optical Microscopy. *Proc. SPIE.* **2000b**, *3919*, 75–85.

60. Yuan, G. H.; Wei, S. B.; Yuan, X. C. Nondiffracting Transversally Polarized Beam. Opt. Lett. **2011**, *36* (17), 3479–3481.

61. Zhan, Q. Radiation Forces on A Dielectric Sphere Produced by Highly Focused Cylindrical Vector Beams. *J. Opt. A. Pure Appl. Opt.* **2003**, *5*, 229–232.

62. Zhan, Q. Trapping Metallic Rayleigh Particles with Radial Polarization. *Opt. Exp.* **2004**, *12*, 3377–3382.

63. Zhan, Q. Cylindrical Vector Beams: From Mathematical Concepts to Applications. *Adv. Opt. Photonics* **2009**, *1*, 1–57.

64. Zhan, Q.; Leger, J. R. Focus Shaping Using Cylindrical Vector Beams. *Opt. Express.* **2002a**, *10*, 324–331.

65. Zhan, Q.; Leger, J. R. Microellipsometer with Radial Symmetry. *Appl. Opt.* **2002b**, *41*, 4630–4637.

66. Zhao, Y, Q.; Zhan, Q.; Zhang, Y. L. Li, Y. Creation of A Three-Dimensional Optical Chain for Controllable Particle Delivery. *Opt. Lett.* **2005**, *30*, 848–850.

CHAPTER 17

FLUID CATALYTIC CRACKING UNIT IN PETROLEUM REFINING AND OPTIMIZATION SCIENCE: SCIENTIFIC VISION AND THE ROAD TO SCIENTIFIC WISDOM

SUKANCHAN PALIT*

Assistant Professor (Senior Scale), Department of Chemical Engineering, University of Petroleum and Energy Studies, Post Office-Bidholi via Premnagar, Dehradun, Uttarakhand 248007, India

43, Judges Bagan, Post-Office- Haridevpur, Kolkata 700082, India

Corresponding author. E-mail: sukanchan68@gmail.com, sukanchan92@gmail.com

CONTENTS

ABSTRACT

Science and technology are witnessing drastic and dramatic challenges today. Engineering science is moving from one paradigm toward another. Technology of petroleum refining stands between deep scientific introspection and deep scientific vision. The depletion of fossil fuel sources has challenged the visionary world of petroleum engineering and chemical process engineering. In this treatise, the author rigorously points out the application of optimization science and multi-objective optimization in designing fluidized catalytic cracking unit, a component in petroleum refining. In the beginning of the treatise, the author deals with fluidized catalytic cracking in particular and then delves deep into the science of multi-objective optimization. Optimization science has changed the scientific landscape. Technological vision, scientific motivation, and deep scientific vision are the pillars of scientific endeavor in optimization science and the vast domain of modeling and simulation of petroleum refining unit. The crux of this treatise is to pinpoint the difficulties and the intricacies of modeling, simulation, optimization, and control of fluid catalytic cracking unit (FCCU) with overall objective of furtherance of science and engineering. Scientific cognizance, scientific sagacity, and deep scientific understanding are of utmost need in the pursuit of scientific research today. This paper goes beyond wide scientific imagination and opens up newer avenues of scientific research pursuit in decades to come. Modeling and simulation are the heart of a chemical engineering endeavor today. The science of optimization needs to be reframed and reenvisioned with the progress of scientific and academic rigor in design of a FCCU today. The paper comprehensively reviews the recent status and future research trends in the field of modeling and simulation of petroleum refining units.

17.1   INTRODUCTION

The world of petroleum refining is witnessing immense scientific challenges, barriers, and hindrances. Depletion of fossil fuel resources is of immense concern to the progress of human civilization today. Scientific vision, scientific fortitude, and deep scientific profundity are of utmost importance in the progress of science of modeling, simulation, and optimization of a fluid catalytic cracking unit (FCCU). Fluid catalytic cracking unit plays a pivotal role in the scientific and academic rigor of petroleum refining as a whole. Optimization science, particularly multi-objective optimization is changing the wide and visionary scientific horizon. Multi-objective optimization science is robust and highly effective in the design of petroleum refining unit. Chemical process engineering and technology are today entering a newer visionary eon. This treatise unfolds the immense technological vision and the scientific profundity behind modeling and simulation of a petroleum refining unit. Mankind's immense scientific prowess, futuristic vision, and scientific determination will go a long and visionary way in the true realization of environmental and energy sustainability today. Petroleum refining and energy sustainability are two opposite sides of the visionary coin. Sustainable development as defined by Dr

Gro Harlem Brundtland targets the development that meets the needs of the present without compromising the ability of future generations to meet their own needs. The vision and the challenges of science are immense and far-reaching today with the progress of human civilization. The author deeply comprehends the scientific hindrances and the intricacies in the design of a particular unit such as the fluid catalytical unit in a petroleum refinery. Today, the immense scientific rigor in design of a petroleum refining unit is replete with scientific vision and deep scientific understanding. This treatise pointedly focuses on the modeling, simulation, and optimization of a FCCU with the application of multi-objective optimization as the sole aim and vision.[12,13]

17.2   THE VISION AND AIM OF THE STUDY

The vision and the challenges of science today are wide and far-reaching. Scientific validation and technological vision are the veritable forerunners toward a greater scientific understanding and deep scientific contemplation. The author in this treatise pointedly focuses on the immense scientific vision and scientific potential in the application of multi-objective optimization in the design of a FCCU in a petroleum refinery. Science and technology today are huge colossi with a vast vision of their own. This treatise is a wide eye-opener toward the success of FCCU in petroleum refining with the sole objective and aim toward the furtherance of science and engineering. Scientific cognizance, scientific discernment, and scientific fortitude are the challenging avenues of science and engineering today. Fluid catalytic cracking process is of vital scientific understanding in the pursuit of engineering science. The depletion of fossil fuel resources and the burgeoning cause of energy sustainability have urged the scientific domain to target new modeling tools and mathematical techniques. The vision and aim of this study targets this area of scientific endeavor, particularly the mathematical and modeling tools to the design of a FCCU.[12,13]

17.3   THE NEED AND THE RATIONALE OF THE STUDY

Scientific vision, scientific profundity, and the world of technology are undergoing drastic challenges. The depletion of fossil fuel resources has urged the scientific domain and the scientific generation to move toward newer innovation and newer avenues in mathematical techniques. The needs and the rationale of this study have surpassed scientific imagination and are replete with deep scientific contemplation. Petroleum refining technology is highly advanced today and is widely replete with scientific vision and fortitude. Petroleum refining technology needs to be reenvisioned and revamped with the passage of scientific history, scientific contemplation, and time. The efficiency of the fluid catalytic cracking process with more regeneration of catalysts is of immense concern toward the progress of scientific rigor. The vision of scientific research pursuit, the futuristic vision of petroleum refining, and the wide scientific introspection will all lead a long way in the true realization of chemical reaction engineering of petroleum refining. Today, the chemical process engineering and petroleum engineering science are two opposite sides of the visionary coin. The tenets of chemical engineering are immensely advanced today, surpassing visionary frontiers. Fluid catalytic cracking is an immense necessity with the progress of petroleum refining and petroleum engineering science. The need and rationale of this study of design of fluid catalytic cracking goes beyond scientific imagination and fortitude. In this treatise, the author repeatedly stresses on the immense success of science of modeling and simulation in designing chemical engineering and petroleum engineering systems. Today, science and engineering are huge colossi with definite and positive vision of their own. This is the age of nuclear science, nuclear engineering, atomic physics, and space technology. The success of science of petroleum refining and the vast design aspects of refining units are veritably opening up new avenues of innovation and scientific instincts in decades to come.[12,13]

17.4   WHAT DO YOU MEAN BY FLUID CATALYTIC CRACKING?

Fluid catalytic cracking is one of the most important conversion processes used in petroleum refineries. It is vastly used to convert the high-boiling, high molecular weight hydrocarbon fractions of petroleum crude oils into more valuable gasoline, olefinic gases and other products. Cracking of petroleum hydrocarbons was originally done by thermal cracking, which has been almost completely replaced by catalytic cracking, because it produces more gasoline with a higher octane rating. It also produces by-product gases that have more carbon–carbon double bonds (i.e., more olefins), and, hence of more economic value, than those produced by thermal cracking. Technological and scientific candor and motivation are today gaining immense heights as science and engineering moves into a newer scientific era. Fluid catalytic cracking and petroleum refining are moving into a challenging era and need to be redefined and restructured as technology advances forward. [12,13]

Fluid catalytic cracking unit (FCCU) plays a vital role in the economy of a modern refinery as it is widely used for value addition to the refinery products. Crude oil, as produced from the ground, contains hydrocarbons ranging from light gases, and liquefied petroleum gas (LPG) to residues boiling above 343°C.[12,13] The products of various boiling ranges can be obtained by distillation. Technology of petroleum refining is highly advanced today, and needs to be equally reenvisioned and restructured with the passage of scientific history, scientific vision, and time. Compared to the products' demand, crude oil is short of lighter material in the boiling range of the transportation fuel (gasoline and diesel) and rich in heavier materials. Fluid catalytic cracking units (FCCU) convert a portion of this heavy material into lighter products, chiefly gasoline, and middle distillates. Scientific vision, rejuvenation, and comprehension are of utmost importance in the path toward emancipation of petroleum engineering science today.

The FCCU comprises three stages: a riser reactor, a catalyst stripper, and a regenerator (along with other accessories). From the modeling point of view, the riser reactor is of immense and vital importance amongst these stages.[12,13] Detailed modeling and simulation of the riser reactor is an immense challenging task for theoretical and experimental investigators not only due to complex hydrodynamics, and the fact that there are thousands of unknown hydrocarbons in the FCC feed, but also because of the involvement of different types of reactions taking place simultaneously.[12,13]

The traditional and global approach of cracking kinetics is lumping. Mathematical models dealing with riser kinetics can be categorized into two main types. In one category, the lumps are made on the basis of boiling range of feed stocks, and corresponding products in the reaction system. Cracking kinetics and scientific validation of fluid catalytic cracking are of utmost importance in the furtherance of science and engineering of petroleum refining. This is the heart of the petroleum refining process. This kind of model has an increasing trend in the number of lumps of the cracked gas components. The other approach is that in which the lumps are made on the basis of molecular structure characteristics of hydrocarbon group composition in the reaction system.[12,13]

More recently, models based upon "single events" cracking, structure-oriented lumping, and reactions in continuous mixture were proposed by different investigators. Scientific vision, scientific contemplation, and a deep scientific forbearance are the pivots and pillars toward a newer visionary era in the field of mathematical modeling and multi-objective optimization. The science and engineering of sustainability science are entering into a newer era of scientific genre. Fluid catalytic cracking is a primary reaction in the petroleum refining process. Engineering science of petroleum refining needs to be refurbished with the progress of scientific and academic rigor.[12,13]

17.5 PETROLEUM REFINING, ENERGY SUSTAINABILITY, AND THE VISION FOR THE FUTURE

Energy sustainability and petroleum refining are today connected by an unsevered umbilical cord. The futuristic vision of sustainable development is opening up new avenues of scientific discernment in the field of petroleum refining. The modeling, simulation, and optimization of an FCCU today stand in the midst of immense scientific vision and scientific forbearance. In this treatise, the author pointedly focuses on the immense scientific success, its potential, and the wide scientific vision of mathematical modeling and design of an FCCU with the sole and veritable purpose of furtherance of science and engineering. Energy sustainability is the utmost need of the hour. The vision of sustainable development, the futuristic vision of science of petroleum refining, and the wide scientific rigor will all lead a long and visionary way in the true emancipation, realization of energy, and environmental sustainability today. Technological revamping and scientific profundity are the pillars of scientific success today. The world is today moving toward renewable energy paradigm. The vision of scientific advancements today wholly depends upon energy and environmental sustainability. Scientific cognizance, scientific candor and deep scientific contemplation are the necessities of science today. The depletion of fossil fuel resources are challenging the wide scientific landscape, and in a similar manner opening wide avenues of scientific profundity, and scientific brilliance in decades to come.[12,13]

17.6   SCIENTIFIC DOCTRINE IN THE FIELD OF PETROLEUM ENGINEERING SCIENCE

Scientific doctrine and scientific sagacity are the pillars of petroleum engineering science today. Modeling, simulation, and optimization of petroleum refining units are the futuristic visions of scientific endeavor today. Technological challenges, scientific motivation, and scientific forbearance are the pillars of scientific research pursuit in today's present day human civilization. The world of petroleum engineering, energy engineering, and chemical process engineering today stand in the midst of deep crisis. Petroleum engineering science today is in the midst of a deep crisis and immense pessimism as depletion of fossil fuel sources aggravates bringing in scientific derision.

Petroleum engineering science and chemical process engineering are moving from one visionary scientific paradigm toward another. Energy sustainability and holistic sustainable development are the pillars toward a newer scientific genre and scientific advancement. Mankind today stands in the midst of a deep scientific comprehension and pessimism. Technological vision, scientific advancements, and a deep scientific introspection are the forerunners toward a newer era of petroleum engineering, sustainability science, and scientific paradigm. Alternate energy sources and renewable energy technology today are in the path of immense scientific regeneration. Today, renewable energy technology is changing the wide scientific frontier. Alternate energy resources, holistic sustainable development, and energy sustainability are the veritable pillars toward a newer visionary future.[12,13]

17.7   WHAT DO YOU MEAN BY OPTIMIZATION SCIENCE?

Optimization science and mathematical modeling today stands in the midst of immense scientific discernment and scientific fortitude. Multi-objective optimization is a robust procedure in modeling, simulation, and optimization of the FCCU in a petroleum refinery. Scientific validation and technological objectives are the vital pillars of the scientific forays in chemical process engineering and petroleum engineering science. The scientific success of human civilization and the wide world of scientific rigor are opening new challenges in the progress of petroleum engineering. This is the age of nuclear engineering and space technology. Every nation is faced with the vexing issue of loss of fossil fuel resources. In such a crucial juncture of scientific history, scientific vision and time, the optimization of science garners immense importance.[12,13]

In mathematics, computer science, and operation research, mathematical optimization is the selection of the best element (with regard to some criterion) for some sets of available decisions and availabilities.[12,13] In the simplest meaning, optimization problem refers to the maximization and minimization of a real function by systematically choosing input values from within an allowed set and computing the function.[12,13]

17.8   WHAT DO YOU MEAN BY MULTI-OBJECTIVE OPTIMIZATION?

Nowadays, multi-objective optimization is utilized in the process of immense scientific regeneration and scientific girth. The vision and the challenges of science are embarking on a new scientific history. Technological validation needs to be reenvisioned and redefined as petroleum engineering and refining ushers in a new eon in the field of science and engineering. Mankind today stands in the midst of deep scientific knowledge and wide applications of applied science. Multi-objective optimization today has an unsevered umbilical cord with modeling and simulation. The science of modeling and simulation is entering into a new phase of scientific validation and technological vision. Scientific potential and success are gaining immense heights as petroleum engineering science faces immense barriers and hindrances. Petroleum refining is an avenue of science which needs immense scientific enrichment and scientific reenvisioning. Efficiency and effectivity of the petroleum refining procedure are the important cornerstones of recent research trends, and the futuristic vision.

Multi-objective optimization (also known as multi-objective programming) is an area of multi-criteria decision-making that is concerned with mathematical optimization problems involving more than one objective function to be optimized simultaneously. Multi-objective optimization has been widely applied in many fields of science including engineering, economics, and logistics where optimal decisions need to be taken in the presence of trade-offs between two or more conflicting objectives. Minimizing cost while maximizing comfort while buying a car, and maximizing performance whilst minimizing fuel composition and emission of pollutants of a vehicle are examples of multi-objective optimization problems involving two or three objectives, respectively. In practice, there can be more than three objectives.[12,13]

For a nontrivial multi-objective optimization problem, no single solution exists that simultaneously optimizes each objective. In that case, the objective functions are said to be conflicting and there exists a (possibly infinite) number of Pareto optimal solutions.[12,13]

17.9   SCIENTIFIC DOCTRINE OF MULTI-OBJECTIVE OPTIMIZATION AND VISIONARY SCIENTIFIC ENDEAVOR

Scientific doctrine of multi-objective optimization is today entering into a newer eon of vision and forbearance. Science and engineering today are subjects with a wide and vast vision of their own. Applied mathematics and chemical process engineering are linked by an unsevered umbilical cord. Science and technology are highly advanced today, crossing vast and versatile scientific boundaries. Multi-objective optimization and mathematical modeling need to be reenvisioned and restructured with the progress of scientific and academic rigor. Technology of multi-objective optimization and the scientific profundity of applied mathematics are ushering in a new age in science and technology.

Zitzler[14] redefined and revisited evolutionary algorithms for multi-objective optimization. Multiple, often conflicting objectives arise naturally in most real-world optimization paradigms. Technological splendor and profundity are the forerunners of vision and forbearance today. Human civilization and human scientific endeavor are today in the path of immense scientific rejuvenation.[14] Multi-objective optimization stands today in the midst of scientific quagmire and scientific regeneration. The vision and the challenges are immense and surpassing visionary boundaries. Evolutionary multi-objective optimization is transforming the world of mathematical modeling and applied mathematics as a whole. As evolutionary algorithms possess several characteristics due to which they are well suited to this type of problem, evolution-based methods have been widely used for many years till now. In this paper, the author rigorously points out the basic principles of evolutionary multi-objective optimization with the pivotal aim toward furtherance of science and engineering.[14] The more focused issues in this paper are: fitness assignment, diversity preservation, and elitism in general rather than on particular algorithms. [14] Scientific vision, scientific fortitude, and technological validation are the pillars and the foundations of evolutionary multi-objective optimization today. This treatise rigorously points out the immense scientific vision, the scientific stature, and the vast scientific introspection in application of multi-objective optimization.[14,12,13]

Garg et al.[5] lucidly discussed optimization by genetic algorithm. Genetic algorithm and multi-objective optimization are today the two opposite sides of the visionary coin. The genetic algorithm is a search and optimization technique that generates solutions to optimization problems using techniques inspired by natural evolution. The frontiers of science are slowly evolving into newer knowledge dimensions and futuristic scientific vision. Optimization is central to any problem involving vision whether it is engineering or economics. This paper presents the experimental results of the most important benchmark function, that is, Dejong function by genetic algorithm.[5] These results show that genetic algorithm provides more optimal solution. This visionary paper unfolds the basic theory of genetic algorithm and will open the wide windows of innovation in optimization science in years to come. Genetic algorithms are search and optimization algorithms based on the principles of natural evolution, which were first introduced by Dr. Holland in 1970.[5] The course of scientific research needs to be reenvisioned and redefined in the field of genetic algorithm in decades to come.[5]

Harik et al.[6] lucidly discussed and with cogent insight the compact genetic algorithm. This paper introduces the compact genetic algorithm (GA) which represents the population as a probability distribution over the set of solutions and is operationally equivalent to the order-one behavior of the simple GA with uniform crossover.[6] This treatise is well researched and brings to the forefront the scientific hindrances and the intricacies in the application of genetic algorithm in design of chemical and petroleum engineering systems. This work raises vital and intricate questions about the use of information in a genetic algorithm, and its vast ramifications show us a fixed direction that can lead to the more efficient design of GAs. Genetic algorithm today stands in the midst of immense scientific vision and deep scientific introspection.[6] Technological validation and scientific forbearance are in a state of immense restructuring in chemical and petroleum engineering systems. The success of scientific endeavor is in the midst of deep crisis as petroleum engineering is on the brink of an impending disaster, that is, the depletion of fossil fuel resources.[6] There is a wide tendency in the community of evolutionary computation to treat the population with some mystical reverence and certainly the population deserves great reverence as it is the source of all that goes right (or wrong) in a GA with respect to function evaluation, schema evaluation, and partition identification.[6] In this paper, the authors discuss a minimalist approach for the population and create a GA that mimics the order-one behavior of a simple GA using finite memory bit by bit. Technological understanding and scientific divinity are of utmost importance in the path of scientific vision today. Genetic algorithm is slowly gaining importance in this decade and the present century. Research work is far-reaching and crossing wide boundaries. This treatise is a phenomenal work of immense vision and fortitude and will surely open a new chapter in optimization science.[6,2,3]

17.10   SCIENTIFIC VISION, SCIENTIFIC FORTITUDE, AND THE SUCCESS OF MULTI-OBJECTIVE OPTIMIZATION

The scientific success and potential of multi-objective optimization is moving forwards by leaps and bounds. Human scientific endeavor in applied mathematics is in the path of new scientific regeneration. Optimization science is ushering in a newer era and a newer vision in the field of chemical process engineering and petroleum engineering science. Chemical process engineering and sustainability science today stand in the midst of immense scientific forbearance and deep scientific profundity. Scientific vision, scientific fortitude, and the success of multi-objective optimization are revamping the entire world of applied mathematics and petroleum refining in particular.[2,3]

17.11   SCIENTIFIC DOCTRINE, SCIENTIFIC UNDERSTANDING IN PROCESS DESIGN, AND THE VISION FOR THE FUTURE

Scientific understanding in the field of chemical process design is veritably opening up a new chapter in the field of chemical process engineering and petroleum engineering science. Today, science and engineering should be more inclined toward the success of environmental and energy sustainability.

Energy sustainability is the cornerstone of all future research endeavors. Energy engineering science and petroleum engineering science today stands in the midst of immense scientific rejuvenation. Chemical process design and chemical process technology are delving deep into the murky depths of human scientific genre. Scientific predilection toward energy engineering and environmental engineering science are opening up new chapters in the field of holistic science and engineering. Technology and engineering science are moving leaps and bounds in this visionary century. The vision for the future needs to be revamped and restructured with the passage of scientific history, the futuristic vision, and the time frame. The depletion of fossil fuel resources is a positive warning to human civilization and human scientific research pursuit. Today, energy and environmental sustainability are the cornerstones of scientific endeavor. The success of human civilization, the immense scientific genre, and the wide futuristic vision will all lead a long way in the true emancipation of petroleum engineering science and petroleum refining today. Human scientific forays and wide scientific endeavors are the pillars of scientific regeneration today.[12,13]

17.12 MODELING, SIMULATION, AND OPTIMIZATION OF CHEMICAL PROCESSES

Modeling, simulation, and optimization of chemical processes are the challenges of today and tomorrow. The heart of chemical process design lies in the world of modeling, simulation, and applied mathematics. Technology is highly advanced today. The technological motivation and scientific might are in the path of newer scientific regeneration. Chemical process engineering and petroleum engineering science are in the avenues of immense scientific rejuvenation and visionary regeneration. Petroleum refining and refining units are poised today for wide and vast scientific revamping. Vision of science, mankind's immense scientific girth, and the grave concerns for energy sustainability will all lead a long and visionary way in the true realization of science of optimization. Modeling and simulation of chemical engineering processes are in the heart of scientific research pursuit in applied science. In this treatise, the author repeatedly points out to the veritable success and scientific potential in the application of multi-objective optimization in designing chemical engineering and petroleum engineering systems.

17.13   MODELING, SIMULATION, OPTIMIZATION, AND CONTROL OF FLUID CATALYTIC CRACKING UNIT IN PETROLEUM REFINING

The modeling, simulation, optimization, and control of FCCU are the heart of chemical process technology and petroleum refining. Fluid catalytic cracking and petroleum engineering science are the scientific success of today. Fluid catalytic cracking unit is the heart of a petroleum refinery. In this treatise, the author points out to the deep scientific vision and the scientific discernment in the field of design of petroleum refining units. Technology is highly advanced today and crossing visionary boundaries. This scientific endeavor deeply comprehends the vast scientific potential, the scientific determination, and the technological vision behind the operation of the FCCU, its modeling and simulation.[12,13]

Today, the modeling and simulation of a FCCU stands in the juncture of deep scientific understanding and vision. Different research work tends to rely upon evolutionary mathematical computation in the design of chemical and petroleum engineering systems. Technology has changed drastically as petroleum refining trudges a weary and difficult path of scientific forbearance and scientific fortitude. Genetic algorithm and multi-objective optimization has revolutionized the deep visionary scientific genre.[12,13]

Elnashaie et al.[4] lucidly discussed with deep insight the modeling, simulation, and optimization of industrial fixed bed catalytic reactors. Technology and engineering science of fixed bed and fluid bed catalytic reactors are drastically changing today. Human scientific vision, scientific profundity, and technological prowess in the domain of modeling, simulation and optimization are today challenging the scientific landscape. The authors with deep scientific vision elucidated the systems theory and principles for developing mathematical models of industrial fixed bed reactors.[4] Today, the challenge of science and technology has changed the vast scientific genre of optimization and mathematical modeling. This treatise also gives a wide and sharp glimpse of chemisorption and catalysis, intrinsic kinetics of gas-solid catalytic reactions, and practical relevance of bifurcation, instability, and chaos in catalytic reactors. The authors also discussed the effect of diffusional resistances and the single pellet problem. Elnashaie et al.[4] also described the overall reactor models and the catalyst deactivation problem. This book primarily deals with the mathematical modeling of industrial fixed bed catalytic reactors which are extremely important to the petrochemical and petroleum refining industries. For example, the ammonia production line consists of about seven fixed bed gas-solid catalytic reactors. It will not be an overestimation to say that more than 90–95 % of gas-solid catalytic reactors operating industrially are of the fixed bed type. This treatise delves deep into the murky depths of scientific intricacies and scientific hindrances in the design of fixed bed reactors. The modeling of catalytic processes combines knowledge from many disciplines in applied chemistry and chemical process engineering. It involves the following aspects:

- Surface phenomenon involved in catalytic activity and the wide vision of chemical kinetics.[4]
- Modeling of intrinsic catalytic reaction rates.[4]
- Thermodynamic equilibrium of the reaction mixture.
- External mass and heat transfer resistances between the gas and solid phase which are again function of the fluid flow conditions.
- Intraparticle mass diffusion and heat conduction.
- Pressure drop associated with the fluid flow.
- Heat evolution (for exothermic reactions) or heat absorption (for endothermic reactions).[4]
- Integration of all the above procedures.[4]

Technological profundity is gaining immense and vibrant heights in today's world of scientific research pursuit. Mathematical modeling of diffusion and reaction in petrochemical and petroleum refining systems is a strong and effective tool in petrochemical and petroleum refining systems. The science of optimization and genetic algorithm is applied in the design of petroleum refining units today. The immense success, the wide scientific potential, and the futuristic targets are the veritable forerunners toward a newer visionary petroleum engineering paradigm today.

17.14 SCIENTIFIC RESEARCH PURSUIT IN MODELING AND SIMULATION OF PETROLEUM REFINING UNITS

Scientific research pursuit in modeling and simulation of petroleum refining units are the pivots and pillars of science of petroleum refining. The challenge of science, the futuristic vision, and the vast scientific rejuvenation are the veritable forerunners toward a visionary era in the field of petroleum refining today. In this treatise, the author repeatedly focuses on the intricacies and scientific hindrances in the field of design of petroleum refining unit. Technology and engineering are highly challenged today. The immense scientific vision, girth, and profundity are the challenging parameters toward greater emancipation of petroleum engineering science today. [12,13]

Pinheiro et al.[10] discussed with deep and cogent insight the process modeling, simulation, and control in the FCC process. The authors focused on the FCC process and reviews on recent developments in its modeling, monitoring, control, and optimization. Vision of science and technological prowess are today gaining immense heights as petroleum engineering science moves from one visionary paradigm over another. This challenging process investigates complex behavior requiring detailed models to elucidate nonlinear effects and extensive interactions between input and control variables that are observed in industrial paradigm. Scientific vision, forbearance, and sagacity are today changing the scientific panorama. The FCC models currently available differ widely in terms of their scope, level of detail, modeling hypothesis, and solution approaches used. Transformation of knowledge dimensions are of utmost need today in the world of scientific validation. Petroleum engineering science and energy sustainability are regaining new heights as science and civilization marches forward.[10] This review describes and compares the different mathematical frameworks that have been applied in the modeling, simulation, control, and optimization of this key downstream unit. Success of technology and engineering are today crossing visionary boundaries. This paper also highlights the importance of understanding the nonlinear behavior of the FCC process. Fluidized catalytic cracking veritably opens up new knowledge dimensions in the avenues of petroleum engineering. FCC remains a key and pivotal unit in many refineries; it consists of a three step process: reaction, product separation, and regeneration. Technological boundaries in the chemistry of catalytic cracking are widely surpassed. In this cyclic process of FCC, gas oils from vacuum distillation towers and residues from atmospheric distillation towers are converted into lighter and more valuable products. One of the most desired products is cracked naphtha, which stands as a major component. Operating conditions comprise of high reaction temperatures in the range of 750–800 K and pressure close to atmospheric conditions.[10] Sagacity of science remains a major pillar of scientific pursuit today. Like all industrial processes involving heterogeneous catalysis, the FCC process also encompasses catalytic deactivation. Actually, a significant fraction of the FCC feedstock is converted into a mixture of compounds (called coke) that are entrenched in the catalyst structure after stripping. The authors deeply comprehended mathematical modeling of cracking kinetics, deactivation, riser models, stripper/disengager models, regenerator models, and finally the dynamic models. The authors also touched upon steady state multiplicities in FCCUs, control and optimization of fluid catalytic cracking units.[10]

Sadeghbeigi[11] discussed with immense insight FCC chemistry. The author delineated in details the design, operation, and troubleshooting of FCC facilities. Technology of FCC is highly advanced today. Vision of science, technological prowess, and the futuristic academic rigor of engineering science will go a long and visionary way in the true emancipation of petroleum engineering science and energy sustainability today. FCC chemistry is a veritable pillar toward the progress of scientific and academic rigor in chemical process engineering and petroleum engineering. The author delineated process description in FCC, FCC feed characterization, chemistry of FCC reactions, unit monitoring and control, products and economics, project management and hardware design, debottlenecking and optimization, and emerging trends in FCC.[11] It continues to play a pivotal role in an integrated refinery as the primary conversion process. For many refiners, the cat cracker is the key to profitability, in which the successful operation of the FCC unit determines whether or not the refiner can remain competitive in today's vast market. Scientific candor, scientific profundity, and the wide technological vision are of vast importance in the avenues of academic and scientific rigor today. This treatise rigorously points out the deep scientific understanding and wide scientific vision in the research pursuit of FCC unit. Approximately 350 cat crackers are operating worldwide, with a total processing capacity of over 12.7 million barrels per day. Energy sustainability today is in the path of immense scientific regeneration and deep scientific rejuvenation.[11] Since the start-up of the first commercial FCC unit in 1942, many improvements have been envisioned.[11] These improvements have enhanced the unit's mechanical reliability and its vast ability to crack heavier, lower value feedstocks.[11] Technological revamping is of utmost importance in our present day-to-day scientific endeavor. The FCC unit uses a microspheroidal catalyst, which behaves like a liquid when properly aerated by gas. Technological and scientific validation will be the future forerunners of emancipation of petroleum engineering science. The main purpose of the FCC unit is to convert high-boiling fractions called gas oil to high-value, high octane gasoline and heating oil.[11]

A petroleum refinery is composed of several processing units that convert raw crude oil into usable products such as gasoline, diesel, and jet fuel. The crude unit is the first unit in the refining process. Here, the raw crude oil is distilled into several intermediate products: naphtha, kerosene, diesel, and gas oil. Scientific vision and technological prowess are of profound and vital importance in the progress of human endeavor. Sadeghbeigi[11] discussed with deep scientific profundity the wide scientific prowess and the vision behind future research trends in the field of petroleum refining and FCC, in particular. The heaviest portion of the crude oil which cannot be distilled in the atmospheric tower is heated and sent to the vacuum tower where it is spilt into gas oil and tar. Technological and scientific challenges are immensely high in today's human civilization. Such is the vision of separation phenomenon in petroleum refining. The tar from the vacuum tower is sent to be further processed in a delayed coker, deasphalting unit, or visbreaker or is sold as fuel oil or road asphalt. The gas oil feed for the conventional cat cracker comes primarily from the atmospheric column, the vacuum tower, and the delayed coker. The FCC process is very complex and robust. For clarity and vision, the FCC process has been broken down into the following classification:

- Feed preheat
- Riser-reactor-stripper
- Regenerator—heat/catalyst recovery
- Main fractionators
- Gas plant
- Treating facilities

Hudec[8] deeply discussed FCC catalyst as a key element in refining technology. A short history of FCC development is presented, dealing with the history of technology of catalytic cracking on one side and with the development of catalyst composition on the other side. Today science is ushering in a new era in petrochemistry and mathematical modeling. The author deeply comprehends the scientific success, potential and vision in the field of FCC catalyst technology.[8] The paper mainly focuses on the role of catalysts used for catalytic cracking from the first fixed bed cracking reactors to the modern FCC technologies and wide innovations. A special and instinctive approach is presented toward the immense scientific potential of zeolites.[8] The author deeply discussed the short history of crude oil, kerosene, and gasoline, history of thermal cracking, history of catalytic cracking, development of FCC technology, development of FCC catalysts, and lastly the immense scientific vision behind application of zeolites. At the heart of FCC units are the catalysts themselves. The development of stable FCC catalysts went parallel with the FCC development. Technology and engineering science are veritably changing the wide scientific horizon. In the 1940s, silica–alumina catalysts were created and greatly improved over the natural clay catalysts. It was Houdry, who for the first time used acid-activated bentonite as active-acid catalyst for catalytic cracking. It was a veritable challenge in those years to delve deep into the murky depths of science. In 1962, a catalyst known as Zeolite-Y was added to the active alumina catalyst.[8] The challenge, the vision, and the success of scientific endeavor were then slowly emerging. That vision and that technological prowess and splendor changed the catalyst development scenario. Zeolites as acid component of FCC catalysts were known from 1765.[8] Zeolites reframed and redefined the status of chemical reaction engineering scenario after technological reframing in 1950. Generally, the philosophy of FCC catalyst preparation is to have weak acid centers in the macroporous part of catalyst particles to ensure pre-cracking the great molecules of residue to smaller molecules which could enter into the mesopores with stronger acidity. The author in this paper revisits and elucidates on the success of catalyst chemistry in the wider furtherance of petroleum science and engineering.[8]

Ahmed et al.[1] delineated with deep and cogent insight modeling and simulation of FCCU. Today, technology and engineering science are vastly sharpened with the passage of scientific history, scientific contemplation, and time. This study investigates the dynamic model for an industrial Universal Oil Products (UOP) fluid catalytic cracking unit on the basis of mass and energy balance and the transfer functions used.[1] The riser and regenerator are simulated by using Matlab/Simulink software.[1] The vastly robust dynamic behavior of the process is carried out by measuring the temperature response of the riser and regenerator to stepwise change in gas oil flow rate, gas oil temperature, catalyst flow rate, air flow rate, and air temperature. The challenge of solving optimization problems are slowly evolving with vision and scientific forbearance. Universal Oil Products is a premier research organization which envisions and envisages FCC technology.[1] Science of catalytic cracking is highly advanced today. Fluid catalytic cracking is also surpassing wide and vast visionary frontiers. FCCU is the essential transformation unit in numerous refineries and one of the most important and complex processes in the petroleum refining industry. It converts heavy material feeds consisting of high boiling points like gas oil into lighter and more valuable products like gasoline, LPG, and olefins by using a zeolite catalyst and it helps to produce about half of the total gasoline output in a refinery.[1] The FCC process vaporizes and breaks the long chain molecules of the high boiling hydrocarbon liquids into much shorter molecules by contacting the feedstock at high temperature and moderate pressure with a fluidized powdered catalyst. Mathematical modeling stands as a vexing issue in the furtherance of science and engineering of petroleum refining. There are many mathematical models for the FCC in the literature, some of them use a very simplified cracking process description, and very few of them present integration between regenerator and riser. The FCC unit consists of the riser and the regenerator. The cracking reaction is carried out in the riser where desired reactions include cracking of the high boiling gas oil fractions into the lighter hydrocarbons. The undesired reactions include carbon formation reactions and a regenerator where the carbon removal reactions take place. The wide vision of science, the immense technological prowess, and the vast scientific frontiers will today lead a long and effective way in the true realization of energy sustainability and petroleum engineering science. This treatise rigorously points out the scientific vision behind mathematical modeling and the vast domain of multi-objective optimization.

Jimenez-Garcia et al.[9] comprehended in a well-researched review on the topic of the fluidized bed catalytic cracking unit and how it is building its future environment. Fluidized-bed catalytic cracking has been widely considered as one of the largest catalytic processes in the world.[9] Fluidized-bed catalytic cracking is the widely used terminology for a complex process unit that cracks long molecules from gas oils and residuals into added value shorter fuel compounds; additionally, this process can be veritably used to produce important petrochemical precursors such as propylenes. This work is widely devoted to review some propositions about the use of FCC converters and how this vast body of knowledge targets riser reactors, change in methodology to estimate the reaction rates and the overall catalytic activity. Revamping and refurbishing of technology are of utmost need in the pursuit of science today. This paper intricately targets the vast scientific divinity and profundity with the sole aim of furtherance of petroleum engineering science. The authors elucidates environmental concerns, process concerns, the wide domain of FCC operating conditions such as riser pressure, riser outlet temperature, product concerns, and the concerns for alternate feedstocks.[9] In such a critical junction of science and engineering, the author delineates the immense scientific potential, the success, and the knowledge dimensions behind the operation of FCC unit.[9]

Han et al.[7] discussed with deep and cogent insight dynamic modeling, simulation of a fluidized catalytic cracking process, and its process modeling scenario. The aim and objective of this study targets a detailed dynamic model of a typical FCC unit that consists of the reactor, regenerator, and the catalyst transfer lines.[10] A distributed parameter model is presented for the reactor riser to investigate the distributions of the catalyst and the gas-phase velocities, the molar concentrations of 4-lump species and the temperature.[7] Today, technological vision and prowess are the pillars of research pursuit in optimization science and modeling paradigm.[7] Challenges and shackles of science are immense and groundbreaking today. In this paper, an efficient model solver was constructed on the basis of a modular approach in which the model equations are grouped into 12 modules each corresponding to a specific part of the vast unit and type of equations.[7] Scientific profundity, divinity and contemplation are the vast forerunners toward the world of energy sustainability today. The author has discussed and delineated process modeling of the reactor, feed vaporization section, reactor riser, reactor cyclones, regenerator, and finally the overall regenerator. Then, the author has touched upon numerical algorithms, degree of freedom analysis, the model equation solvers, and the immense domain of mathematical modeling as a whole.[7]

The visionary aisles of science and engineering are vast and versatile. Petroleum engineering science is witnessing immense scientific hindrances and deep scientific instinct. Technological and scientific prowess and profundity are the challenging forerunners of vision today. This chapter widely researches the deep insight, the technological hindrances, and shackles in the mathematical modeling of a FCC unit. The vision of science and the vast technological prowess of multi-objective optimization are veritably changing the scientific horizon and the deep knowledge dimension of today. FCC design and multi-objective optimization are today two opposite sides of the visionary coin. Future work and future research trends are vast and far-reaching. Modeling, simulation, and optimization of petroleum refining unit are understandably opening up new frontiers of research endeavor. Scientific vision, clarity, and lucidity are the pillars of endeavor in mathematical modeling today. The author in this treatise pointedly focuses on the immense potential, the technological forbearance, and the scientific instinct in the field of modeling and simulation of petroleum refining unit.

17.15 ENERGY SUSTAINABILITY AND THE FUTURE OF PETROLEUM REFINING

Energy sustainability and sustainable development are the true parameters toward global scientific forays and a nation's growth. This treatise widely focuses on the wide scientific vision, attenuation, and the deep scientific girth in the design of a petroleum refining unit. The application of multi-objective optimization and applied mathematics in the process design of petroleum refining units are ushering in a new era in the field of petroleum refining. The science of sustainability needs to be reenvisioned and revamped with the grave concern of depletion of fossil fuel resources. Scientific vision, scientific, and adjudication are in the path of a new beginning in science and technology. Energy and environmental sustainability are rigorously changing the scientific landscape of the future. In this treatise, the author deeply focuses on the success of scientific girth and determination in solving intricate design issues with the sole objective in the furtherance of science and engineering.

17.16 FUTURE WORK AND FUTURE RESEARCH TRENDS

Science and technology of multi-objective optimization and genetic algorithm are today surpassing vast scientific frontiers. Petroleum and chemical engineering systems are today replete with scientific vision, scientific contemplation, and a deep scientific understanding. The depletion of fossil fuel resources and negative sustainable development are the cause of immense scientific concern today. Technology of petroleum refining has few answers to the numerous research questions of mathematical modeling and simulation. The design of FCC is at a state where there is immense scientific hindrance and vicious barriers. The future of research pursuit needs to be effectively reenvisioned and reenvisaged with the passage of scientific history and time. The research questions of modeling, simulation, and optimization of petroleum refining units need to be veritably pursued with scientific grit. The tenacity and vision of science will then witness a new beginning and open up new chapters in petroleum refining and petroleum engineering science.

17.17   SUMMARY, CONCLUSION, AND FUTURE PERSPECTIVES

Scientific vision and determination are in the path of new beginning of science and technology today. The perspectives of science of petroleum engineering and chemical process engineering are today changing the wide scientific landscape. Today, the world of scientific research pursuit is evolving into a new beginning in nuclear engineering and space technology; today is a visionary era of science and engineering. Technological vision and scientific profundity are the forerunners of the efficiency and effectivity of a petroleum engineering system and the wide path toward future research pursuits. This treatise opens up a new chapter in scientific understanding and deep scientific knowledge in the field of petroleum refining and thoroughly reviews the scientific potential, success, and the deep scientific understanding in the design of petroleum refining units. Multi-objective optimization and mathematical modeling are today in the scientific forefront of design of an FCCU. Knowledge dimensions in petroleum refining are today revamping and revising the wide technology of modeling and simulation. The author in this treatise widely focuses on the immense scientific endeavor, the definite vision, and the fruits of science in petroleum refining with the sole aim and mission in the furtherance of science and engineering.

17.18   ACKNOWLEDGMENT

The author with great respect wishes to acknowledge the contribution of Shri Subimal Palit, the author's late father and an eminent textile engineer from India from whom the author learnt the rudiments of chemical engineering science.

KEYWORDS

- **optimization**
- **catalysis**
- **vision**
- **science**
- **engineering**

REFERENCES

1. Ahmed, D. F.; Ateya, S. K. Modelling and Simulation of Fluid Catalytic Cracking Unit. *J. Chem. Eng. Process Technol.* **2016,** *7*(4), 308. DOI: 10.4172/2157-7048.1000308.
2. Bandyopadhyay, S.; Saha, S.; Maulik, U.; Deb, K. A Simulated Annealing-Based Multiobjective Optimization Algorithm: AMOSA, (2008). *IEEE Trans. Evol. Comput.* **2008,** *12*(3), 269–283.
3. Deb, K. *Multi-objective Optimization Using Evolutionary Algorithms: An introduction, Kanpur Genetic Algorithm;* Report No. 2011003; 2011.
4. Elnashaie, S. S. E. H.; Elshishini, S. S. *Modeling, Simulation and Optimization of Industrial Fixed Bed Reactors;* Gordon and Breach Science Publishers S. A.: Great Britain, 1993.
5. Garg, R.; Mittal, S. Optimization by Genetic Algorithm. *Int. J. Adv. Res. Comput. Sci. Software Eng.* **2014,** *4*(4), 587–589.
6. Harik, G. R.; Lobo, F. G.; Goldberg, D. E. The Compact Genetic Algorithm. *IEEE Trans. Evol. Comput.* **1999,** *3*(4), 287–297.
7. Han, I. S.; Chung, C. B. Dynamic Modeling and Simulation of a Fluidized Catalytic Cracking Process. Part I: Process Modeling. *Chem. Eng. Sci.* **2001,** *56*, 1951–1971.
8. Hudec, P. FCC Catalyst-Key Element in Refinery Technology, 45th International Petroleum Conference, Bratislava, Slovak Republic, 2011.
9. Jimenez-Garcia, G.; Aguilar-Lopez, R.; Maya-Ymeescas, R. The Fluidized-bed Catalytic Cracking Unit Building its Future Environment. *Fuel* **2011,** *90*(12), 3531–3541.
10. Pinheiro, C. I. C.; Fernandes, J. L.; Domingues, L.; Chambel, A. J. S.; Graca, I.; Oliveira, N. M. C.; Cerqueira, H. S.; Ribeiro, F. R. Fluid Catalytic Cracking (FCC) Process Modeling, Simulation, and Control. *Ind. Eng. Chem. Res.* **2012,** *51*, 1–29.
11. Sadeghbeigi, R. *Fluid Catalytic Cracking Handbook,* 2nd Ed.; Gulf Professional Publishing: Houston, USA, 2000.
12. www.google.com.
13. www.wikipedia.com.
14. Zitzler, E. Evolutionary Algorithms for Multiobjective Optimization, (Conference Proceedings), Evolutionary Methods for Design, Optimization and Control, Giannakoglou, K., Tsahalis, D., Periaux, J., Papailiou, K., Fogarty, T., CIMNE: Barcelona, Spain, 2002.

CHAPTER 18

TEXTURAL QUALITY OF READY TO EAT "SHRIMP KURUMA" PROCESSED IN RETORTABLE POUCHES AND ALUMINIUM CANS

C. O. MOHAN[1,*] AND C. N. RAVISHANKAR[2]

[1]Senior Scientist, Fish Processing Division, ICAR Central Institute of Fisheries Technology, CIFT Junction, Matsyapuri P.O., Willingdon Island, Kochi, Kerala 682 029 India

[2]ICAR-Central Institute of Fisheries Technology, CIFT Junction, Matsyapuri P.O., Willingdon Island, Kochi, Kerala 682 029, India

*Corresponding author. E-mail: comohan@gmail.com

CONTENTS

ABSTRACT

Physical properties of food products are influenced by preservation methods and packaging materials. Evaluation of textural properties of food during thermal processing in different containers provides useful information to the industry and consumers. Hence, the present study was conducted to assess the extent of textural changes in ready-to-eat (RTE) shrimp processed in different containers. Shrimp kuruma was prepared from Indian white shrimp (*Penaeus indicus*), packed in conventional 301×206 and 401×411 aluminum cans and in thin profile retort pouch having three-layer configuration of 12.5 μ polyester, 12.5 μ aluminum foil, and 85 μ cast polypropylene of size 16×20 cm and 17×30 cm. The process time and physical properties of shrimps processed in these containers were evaluated. Processing in 16×20 cm and 17×30 cm retortable pouch resulted in 35.67 and 56.56% reduction in process time compared to 301×206 and 401×411 cans, respectively with equal pack weight. Hardness 1 and 2 decreased upon thermal processing in both the containers. However, the extent of texture loss was least in the samples packed and processed in retortable pouches compared to the metal container.

Fish and shellfish are highly nutritious and perishable food items. They have to be preserved properly. The preservation of food was practiced before the beginning of recorded history, and some of the methods adopted by the ancients are still in use in a modified form. The preservation of food is a traditional field for research activities. Fish and shellfish are preserved and processed in many forms like icing, freezing, canning, drying, curing, etc. these methods have their own advantages and disadvantages. Consumers prefer convenient, ready to cook/eat, wholesome, safe, preservative free products, which can be achieved by canning. The food preservation methods are aimed at preventing undesirable changes in the wholesomeness, nutritive value, and sensory quality of food by controlling the growth of microorganisms and obviating contamination by adopting economic methods. Thermal processing is one such method, by which food is given sufficient heat treatment in a hermetically sealed container to destroy pathogenic and/or spoilage-causing microorganisms and their spores, antinutrients, and enzymes that cause degradation in the food. An Italian naturalist Spallanzani concluded from his experiments that organisms causing spoilage in a number of food products were carried in the air and by heating the contaminated infusions in an airtight container, the development of the organism was prevented. Although Spallanzani's work was the key to the preservation of food by heat, little use appears to have been made of it until the early part of the 19th century when Nicolas Appert first succeeded in preserving food in airtight glass containers. So, the Frenchman Nicolas Appert is credited as the inventor of this noble technology.

Packaging materials are an important part of this preservation method. Appert's pioneering work, which established thermal processing as a method of preservation, was conducted using glass jars sealed with a cork. Shortly after this, many workers started to use metal containers for this technique. The metal can, the oldest form of packaging and preserving of foods for long periods has contributed very significantly to the growth of food processing and food packaging technologies. Tinplate cans are one of the most popular and traditional containers for canned products. Packaging plays an important role in the canning technology. The packaging today is viewed as a multifunctional activity. It not only protects or preserves the food but also makes it easy to sell, offering great amounts of convenience to the consumers. India is the largest producer of farm commodities, second largest producer of fruits and vegetables, and ranks seventh in fish production. The Indian packaging industry, growing at an annual rate of more than 15%, is valued at $ 15.6billion (INR 85,000 crore), and it is expected to reach $ 73billion in 2020. In India, presently the tin containers have become a major constraint for the development and expansion of food processing industry due to the spiraling cost as well as diminishing availability. This is mainly attributed to the dependence on imported material for fabricating tin containers. The price of the tin can alone work out to nearly 33% of the cost. When added the cost of labels, cartons, etc this cost shoots up to 50% of the total product cost making it ill affordable to the average Indian consumer and not competitive in most of the overseas markets. Looking at the resource potentials of aluminum ore and the demand for canned fishery products in the country and the world markets, there exists a tremendous potential to develop aluminum packaged canned products. Many researchers have felt that the most attractive and viable alternate material for the development and expansion of thermal processing in India is aluminum and its alloys. Aluminum used for making food cans is often reinforced by alloying with manganese and/or magnesium. Aluminum and its alloys are being widely used in a variety of forms in the field of packaging. The most common ones include meat product cans, fruit juice cans, beverage cans, milk bottle tops, toothpaste tubes, and so forth. Aluminum is an acknowledged material for cans and is fast supplanting tin cans in most countries. The advantages of aluminum cans over the tin cans certainly made the packaging industry offer the largest market for aluminum. Resistance to corrosion, lightweight, pleasing appearance, easy opening properties, high thermal conductivity, better recyclability, and recovery rate make aluminum cans far more superior to tin cans. Aluminum containers were in use for packing meat and fish products as early as 1918. Although aluminum can is a later entrant in the global canned seafood sector, it has picked up very fast. The aluminum, when used to pack sensitive products such as food or pharmaceuticals, should be hygienic, nontoxic, non-tainting, and retain the product's flavor. The aluminum barrier also plays the essential role of keeping the contents fresh and protecting them from external influences, thereby guaranteeing a long shelf life. In recent years, the sanitary cans made of aluminum have moved into a position of commercial importance. The aluminum cans are now extensively used in European countries mainly due to the abundant availability of raw material and their low cost of production.

Although the canning as a method of food preservation was started in glass jars, the rigid metal containers became very popular. Rigid containers have played a very significant role over several years in food processing and built up consumer acceptance as well as confidence in preserved foods including canning. The tin is the most ideal metal for this purpose and has a lion's share as far as the packaging of food products is concerned. But in India, the situation is changing due to the high cost of containers (nearly 33%), use of thicker gauge tin plates which causes difficulties in can opening and poor quality of lacquer. The traditional tin plate cans have progressively been replaced by aluminum cans. The aluminum was first discovered and named in 1809 by an English electrochemist, Sir Humphry Davy.[1] Aluminum containers were used for packing meat and fish products as early as in 1918. In 1930, A/S Norsk Aluminum Co. carried out an extensive investigation on the use of aluminum sheets for making food cans.[13] The standard aluminum of 99.5–99.7% purity is obtained by addition of one or more elements like magnesium, silicon, manganese, zinc, copper, and so forth.[24] Lahiri[17] described the suitability of different aluminum alloys for various food products. He also reported on the corrosion behavior of aluminum cans. Naresh et al.[29] studied the corrosion behavior of aluminum cans by electrochemical studies and found that corrosion reaction is faster in plain aluminum cans as compared to lacquered ones. Griffin, Jr. and Sacharow,[12] suggested a suitable food grade lacquer coating for interior corrosion resistance. Balachandran et al.[3] reported that the best promising alternative to the tin plate was aluminum alloyed with manganese and magnesium. Lopez and Jimenez[22] reviewed the use of aluminum cans for canning fruits and vegetable products. Srivatsa et al.[35]

studied the suitability of indigenously prepared aluminum cans for canning different food products. The advantages and disadvantages of aluminum alloys have been described by Balachandran.[2] Lakhsminarayan[18] who reported that aluminum containers are 100% recyclable and biodegradable. Gargoming and Astier-Dumas[8] studied the canning of vegetables and reported that the acidity of tomatoes resulted in the greater migration of aluminum into the products. Ranau et al.[30] studied the aluminum content in fish and fishery products and concluded that aluminum content of seafood does not present a significant health hazard. He also studied the changes in the aluminum concentration of canned herring fillets in tomato sauce and curry sauce. Although aluminum containers are advantageous over tin containers cost wise, the container strength is one of the important factors, which limits the use of aluminum. Aluminum cannot be substituted for the tin plate on a gauge-for-gauge basis. The pure aluminum is quite weak and can be strengthened by the addition of small quantities of magnesium. With aluminum–magnesium alloys, the gauge must be increased about 35% over that of tin plate to provide equal strength for resistance to paneling, buckling, and denting. Further, soldered side seams are still considered impractical for aluminum cans which hinder the expansion of aluminum containers into some product fields.

In recent years, there has been an increasing interest in the possibility of replacing metal can with a retortable pouch as a cost reduction strategy. A retortable pouch is a flexible laminated pack having sufficient strength, and heat resistance to allow it to be used in place of a can for the heat processing and storage of food products. The early retort pouches varied in their composition. Experience has led to the considerable standardization of retort pouch structures. The retort pouch offers various advantages over conventional metal cans; the foremost among them are their shape, increased surface area to volume ratio, and a thin cross-section, which permits faster heat transfer to the cold point. The cold point may be only 10–20 mm from the surface in a pouch compared to 30–40 mm in a can of equal volume. Thus, processing time is reduced and sterility is achieved without overcooking of the contents and, hence retains the original flavor, color, and texture better than those products packed in metal cans. Other advantages are lightweight, cheap, and easy to open and reheat. A retort pouch is a relatively new type of container for packing foods, which enjoyed rapid growth in demand since its introduction in the late 1950s. The US Army promoted the concept of flexible retortable pouches for use in combat rations in the 1950s, which replaced the metal containers and glass jars. The choice of materials for the manufacture of retort pouches is very important. The package must protect against light, degradation, moisture changes, microbial invasion, oxygen ingress, package interactions, toughness, and puncture resistance. It is very difficult to get a single material with all the desirable properties. Hence, laminates or coextruded films are used[31]. The most common form of pouch consists of three-ply laminated material, with outer polyester, middle aluminum foil, and inner polypropylene. The materials used should be tough with good barrier property and heat sealability. Rubinate[32] and Schulz[33] suggested the material requirements for the retortable pouch. The retortable pouches are usually of three-ply laminated ones, for example, 12 μ polyester, 12 μ aluminum foil, and 75 μ cast polypropylene. The outer polyester layer provides strength, abrasion resistance, atmospheric barrier properties, and carries the label and decorations. The inner cast polypropylene provides a heat-sealing medium and protects the middle aluminum from food contact, and contributes to overall pack strength while the middle aluminum foil provides a barrier to gas, water, and light. Transparent pouches without aluminum foil are also available but give shorter shelf life. The development of the retort pouch has been considered as the most significant advance in food packaging since the metal can and has the potential to become a feasible alternative to the metal cans and glass jars.[26]

One of the early studies on the use of pouch was by Hu et al.[14] He reported the feasibility of using plastic film packages for heat-processed foods. Ishitani et al.[15] reported the effect of light and oxygen on the quality changes of retortable pouch packed foods. Lampi[19] reported the microbiological problems faced in foods packed in retortable pouch. The review on flexible packaging material including the hi story has been documented.[23,20,21,10,11,38,31,9] Mohan et al.[27,28] highlighted the advantage of retortable pouches in terms of savings in process time and better quality. The retortable pouch has been used successfully in Japan but in Western countries such as Europe and the United States, cost of retort pouch is higher than cans where tin and aluminum cans are relatively cheap and available. Also due to less robustness, the retortable pouch is enclosed in overwraps and cartons to provide extra protection which offers little price advantage over cans. While filling the pouches, it is essential that the seal area is kept free from contamination from the product, as this could impair sterility either by spoilage or leakage at the seal. Further, the pouches are sterilized by "overpressure retorting" either by processing underwater in conventional canning retorts or in special steam or air systems. The other reasons for the low acceptance of retortable pouch in some countries are slow filling and heat sealing speeds, and high capital investments required for filling and processing.

Physical changes that result in the decline of freshness are mainly related to texture and color. The texture, appearance, and flavor are the three major components of food acceptability. The texture is one of the most important quality parameters of fish and shellfish for producers, processors, and consumers. Processors want a texture that makes the food easy to process, and which gives high-quality products with high yields. Various researchers have given different definitions to texture.[37,16,25] There is a long history of efforts to measure texture by instrumental methods, going back to the 18th century. Instrumental methods for texture measurement have been divided into three classes[37] such as fundamental tests, empirical tests, and imitative tests, where texture profile analysis (TPA) falls in the imitative test. The major breakthrough in texture profile analysis came with the development of the general foods texturometer.[7,37] According to Sigurgisladottir et al.,[34] the recent trend is away from one-point measurements that reflect either only one parameter or an overall value for a group of parameters, and towards a multiple points or curve method that can give information on several parameters. The most common types of measurements of instrumental methods are based on rheological principles; shear strength, puncture, and compression. Compression tests can include one or two successive compressions. Those with two successive compressions from the TPA result in curves from which several texture parameters can be obtained directly or by calculation. Two compressions are said to be necessary if parameters such as cohesiveness, elasticity, adhesiveness, chewiness, and gumminess are to be measured, but only one compression is needed to evaluate the hardness or firmness, and fracturability of the sample.[7] Compression tests are very sensitive to parameters like measurement location and setting (degree of compression, dimension, speed of probe/plunger, etc.). Charnley[5] and Charnley and Bolton[6] tested the firmness or softness of canned salmon as a measure of its condition. For shrimps hardness, fracturability, adhesiveness, springiness, cohesiveness, chewiness, and resilience are the most commonly used texture parameters. Hardness is the effort required to bite through the sample with front teeth or maximum peak force during first compression cycle (first and second bite). Fracturability is the ease at which the sample fractures, crumbles, crunches or becomes brittle under increasing compression load. Adhesiveness is the degree to which sample sticks to the mouth. Springiness is the height that the food recovers during the time that elapses between the end of the first bite and the start of the second bite. Cohesiveness is the strength of the internal bonds making up the body of the sample before rupture. Gumminess is the product of hardness × cohesiveness; or perception of the dimensions and shape of sample's particles. Chewiness is the product of gumminess × springiness (which equals hardness × cohesiveness × springiness). Resilience is associated with the elastic recovery of a sample in terms of speed and force. Typically, a firm product has moderate resistance to deformation whereas a product with higher hardness indicates it showed substantial resistance to deformation. TA Plus Stable microsystems, Ametek Lloyds, Bestech Australia, TMS Pilot texture instruments, Shimadzu are few leading companies supplying food texture analyzing instruments. Few instruments are shown in Figure 18.1. Depending on the product to be tested, the probes are decided (Fig. 18.2).

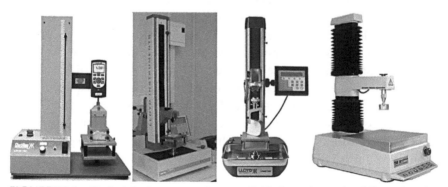

FIGURE 18.1   Typical food texture analyzer available in market under different brands.

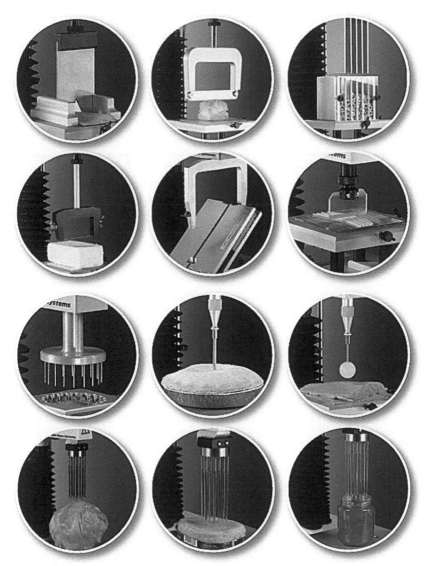

FIGURE 18.2   Different types of probes for assessing various properties of food.

A typical force by time graph obtained during texture profile analysis of food sample is given in Figure 18.3. Single hardness is commonly measured for assessing the texture of fresh, frozen, processed as well as the dried food product. It is the effort required to bite through the sample with front teeth or maximum peak force during first bite (Fig. 18.4).

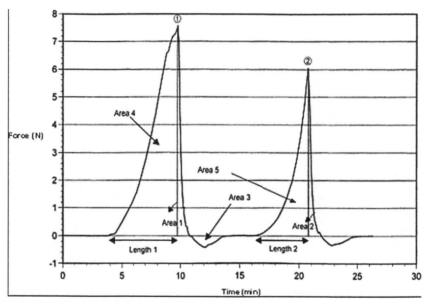

FIGURE 18.3 Typical force by time curve plots to determine texture profile analysis parameters. Peak forces 1 and 2 are hardness 1 and 2; cohesiveness=(Area 2/Area1); springiness=(Length 2/Length1); chewiness=(hardness 1 × springiness × cohesiveness).

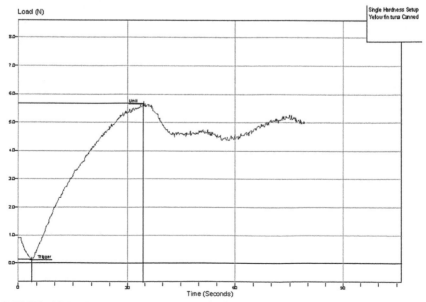

FIGURE 18.4 Single hardness of sample highlighting the maximum force (N) for breaking the product.

The world demand for seafood products is so diverse that the multiplicity in the species makes up in marine landings, and the possibility of processing them into various value-added products could go a long way in satisfying the demands from both domestic and overseas consumers. Appearance, consumer acceptability, packaging, and display are important factors leading to successful marketing of diversified value-added products. Most of the diversified products are either ready-to-serve or ready-to-cook convenient foods. One such ready-to-serve product "Shrimp kuruma" was prepared using the commercially important and most abundantly available species "Indian white shrimp" (*Penaeus indicus*). Relatively few comparative studies on the retortable pouch and metal cans in terms of physical quality of the product have been reported in the seafood area. The present study was, therefore, undertaken with the objectives of comparing the relative processing time required and physical properties of "Shrimp kuruma" packaged and processed in retort pouches and aluminum cans.

The commercially important and most commonly available species, Indian "white shrimp" (*P. indicus*) was used in the present study (Fig. 18.5). The shrimp were collected from Fort Kochi fish market at Cochin. Utmost care was taken to bring the raw material in the freshest form. The standard body length of the shrimps used was in the range of 120–130 mm with the size designation in the range of 8–9 shrimps for 100 g.

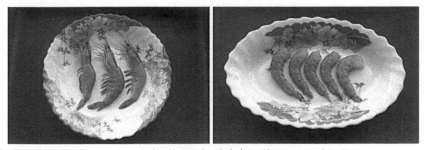

FIGURE 18.5   Raw and peeled and deveined shrimp (*Penaeus indicus*).

A two-piece drawn aluminum can of 8 oz capacity (301 × 206) and A 2 ½ (401 × 411), manufactured by M/s. Klass Engineering Pvt. Ltd., Bangalore, were used in the present study. The cans were internally coated with sulfur resistant lacquer. A flexible pouch of three-ply laminates consisting of outer polyester, middle aluminum foil, and inner cast poly-propylene of size grade 16×20 cm and 17×30 cm, manufactured by M.H. Packaging, Ahmedabad were used for the study. The shrimps (*P. indicus*) were procured from the local market in iced condition. As soon as they were brought to the laboratory, they were washed with chilled water and weight was taken and dressed in peeled-deveined style. Precooking was done for 4 min. About 1282 ± 2 g shrimps were packed along with 68 ± 2 g kuruma into the 301×206 size aluminum cans and 16×20 cm size pouches to maintain a pack weight of about 197 ± 2 g. In case of A 2 ½ size cans (401×411) and 17×30 cm size pouches about 505 ± 2 g shrimps were packed along with 272 ± 2 g kuruma to maintain a pack weight of about 775 ± 2 g. Utmost care was taken to avoid the contamination of seal area in both the containers. An adequate number of cans and pouches were fixed with glands and thermocouples and the tip of the thermocouple were inserted into the meat pieces. Steam exhausting was done for 10 min to remove the air present in the containers. Immediately after, the exhausting cans were closed using the double seaming machine and sealing machine was used to seal the pouches. The thermal processing was carried out for each kind of size of the container separately at 121°C to an F value of 8.0 min. The data was measured using an Ellab CTF 9008 data recorder. The processing was carried out using overpressure autoclave (John Fraser and sons Ltd, UK. Model. no. 5682). After completion of the process, cooling was done rapidly by spraying water under pressure. Then they were wiped to dryness and kept in a dustproof cabinet at ambient temperature. The process data was taken by inserting thermocouple needles into the centre of the cold spot (positioned one-third from the bottom). Thermocouple outputs were measured by using an Ellab CTF 9008 data recorder. The recorded data was analyzed using a computer. The heat penetration data was plotted on a semi logarithm paper with temperature deficit (RT-CT) in logarithmic scale on Y-axis against time in linear scale on X-axis. Lag factor for heating (J_h), lag factor for cooling (J_c), slope of the heating curve (f_h), and time in minutes for sterilization at retort temperature (U) were determined. The process time (B) was calculated by mathematical method.[36] Actual process time (T) was determined by adding process time (B) and the effective heating period during come up time, that is, 58% of the come up time.

Process time $(B) = f_h [\log I \times J_h - \log g]$

Total Process time $(T) = B + 58\%$ of come up time

The texture of the sample was assessed objectively using Universal Testing Machine (Lloyd Instruments LR×plus, Lloyd Instruments Ltd., Hampshire, UK). It imitates the human biting at specified force.[4] A cylindrical probe of 50 mm diameter equipped with 50 N load cell was used in the study to assess the texture profile of uniformly cut samples. Texture measurement consisted of compression of samples two times consecutively to a sample height of 40% to cause deformation of the sample. Force by time data from each test was used to calculate mean values for the TPA parameters. The values for hardness 1 and 2 (the resistance at maximum compression during the 1st and 2nd compression), cohesiveness (the extent to which the sample could be deformed before rupture, that is, the ratio of the positive force area during the 2nd compression to that during the 1st compression {Area 2/Area 1}), springiness (the ability of the sample to recover its original form after the deforming force is removed, that is, the ratio of the time duration of force input during the 2nd compression to that during the 1st compression {length 2/length 1}) and chewiness (the work needed to chew a solid sample to a steady state of swallowing {hardness 1 × cohesiveness × springiness in kg}) were determined as described by Bourne (1978).[4]

The processing was carried out at 121.1°C. In the pouches, the heating lag factor (J_h) was less than that of the cans, whereas the cooling lag factor (J_c) was almost similar in all the containers. The f_h values in the pouches were found to be 19 min and 23.3 min in 16×20 cm and 17×30 cm, respectively, whereas in the cans it was very high, that is, 32 and 62 min in 301×206 and 401×411, respectively. Although the lethality was targeted at around 8.0 min, a slight deviation in the targeted values was observed. The cook value in the case of pouches was less than that of cans. A very high cook value was obtained for 401×411 can. The process time (B) was calculated using formula method[36] and is presented in Table 18.1. It was observed that the pouched products experienced a less process time as compared to canned ones. The 16×20 cm pouches packed with 197±2 g had a process time of 33.79 min as compared to 52.53 min in the case of 301×206 can with equal pack weight. In the case of 17×30 cm pouches, a process time of 38.37×min was obtained as compared to 88.34 min in 401×411 cans packed with 775±2 g. This study pointed out that there is a significant reduction in the thermal processing time required to achieve an equal lethality for retortable pouched products when compared with cans containing equal weights of product. Processing in 16×20 cm retortable pouches resulted in 35.67% reduction in process time for equivalent lethality when compared with 301×206 cans. For 17×30 cm retortable pouches, a reduction of 56.56% process time was obtained than the 401×411 cans.

TABLE 18.1   Thermal Process Parameters for Shrimp Kuruma Processed in Retortable Pouches and Aluminum Cans.

Parameter	Aluminum can		Pouch	
	301×206	401×411	16×20	17×30
Heating rate index f_h (min)	32	62	19	23.3
Heating lag factor (J_h)	1.444	1.445	0.962	0.8735
Cooling lag factor (J_c)	1.09	1.0	0.951	1.064
F_o value (min)	8.43	8.10	8.289	8.199
Temperature deficit (g)	2.382	4.134	1.363	1.712
Cook value (C_g) (min)	104.7	121	86.14	83.19
Process time (B) (min)	52.53	88.34	33.79	38.37
Total process time (T) (min)	53.69	90.08	39.59	43.59

The texture is the combination of the physical structure of the food and the characteristics of the food during various treatments. Texture attributes were analyzed for the raw shrimp, canned and pouched "shrimp kuruma." Various parameters analyzed include hardness I and II, springiness, cohesiveness, chewiness, resilience, and fracture force which are given in Tables 18.2 and 18.3 and Figures 18.6–18.8 for canned and pouched products. The decrease in the hardness upon thermal processing could be attributed to the heat treatment which reduces the water content of meat, thereby affecting the firmness of the meat. The decrease in the hardness 1 and 2 is also attributed to the loss of binding properties of connective tissue due to thermal denaturation of muscle collagen. Processing in both the containers resulted in reduced hardness. However, the extent of decrease was more in metal containers compared to retortable pouches indicating a lesser quality loss in retortable pouches. During the storage period, the hardness 1 and 2 show an increasing trend in both the containers. Cohesiveness and springiness increased upon heat processing as well as during storage period in both the containers. Instrumental hardness, chewiness, and springiness were higher in pouched samples than canned samples. The study indicated that the products processed in retortable pouches resulted in better quality products compared to canned products.

TABLE 18.2 Texture Profile of "Shrimp Kuruma" Processed in Aluminum Container.

Storage period (Days)	Raw shrimp	0	30	60	90	120
Hardness 1 (kgf)	3.88±1.06	1.74±0.85	2.71±0.48	2.99±1.01	2.72±0.33	2.21±0.21
Hardness 2 (N)	30.17±1.06	15.22±1.35	23.11±1.06	23.91±1.29	23.38±1.3	17.79±1.54
Cohesiveness	0.225±0.08	0.436±0.01	0.40±0.02	0.405±0.08	0.415±0.03	0.39±0.01
Springiness (mm)	1.86±0.15	2.59±0.12	2.84±0.34	2.90±0.24	2.92±0.1	2.95±0.22
Chewiness (kgf.mm)	1.53±0.40	2.12±0.14	3.11±0.83	3.50±1.4	3.30±0.48	2.54±0.21
Resilience	0.49±0.05	0.56±0.1	0.60±0.03	0.65±0.08	0.61±0.03	0.60±0.01
Fracture force (kgf)	0.32±0.79	0.051±0.0007	0.0492±0.001	0.049±0.0008	0.05±1.3	0.438±0.67

TABLE 18.3 Texture Profile of "Shrimp Kuruma" Processed in Retortable Pouches.

Storage period (Days)	Raw shrimp	0	30	60	90	120
Hardness 1 (kgf)	3.88±1.06	2.43±0.52	1.99±0.36	2.3±0.56	2.82±0.86	3.16±0.73
Hardness 2 (N)	30.17±1.06	20.72±1.58	14.24±1.34	19.29±1.12	23.38±1.3	26.40±1.54
Cohesiveness	0.225±0.08	0.389±0.01	0.383±0.04	0.40±0.01	0.40±0.03	0.4±0.01
Springiness (mm)	1.86±0.15	2.4±0.17	2.47±0.2	2.82±0.56	3.28±0.57	2.97±0.12
Chewiness (kgf.mm)	1.53±0.40	2.28±0.58	1.76±0.45	2.72±1.19	3.82±1.43	3.84±1.08
Resilience	0.49±0.05	0.610±0.05	0.613±0.08	0.58±0.05	0.653±0.04	0.657±0.02
Fracture force (kgf)	0.32±0.79	0.05±0.0009	0.05±0.97	0.0504±0.002	0.0505±0.001	0.051±0.001

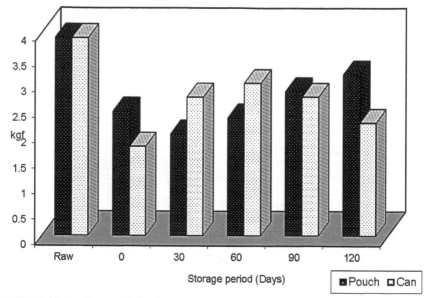

FIGURE 18.6   Changes in hardness I.

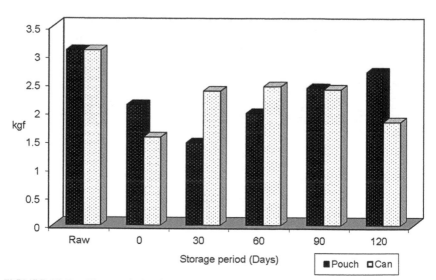

FIGURE 18.7   Changes in hardness II.

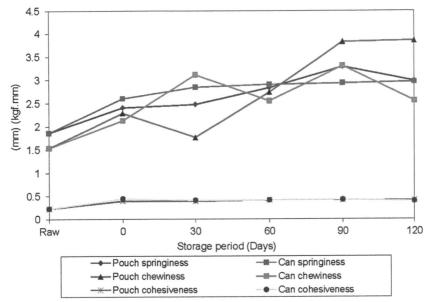

FIGURE 18.8 Changes in the springiness, cohesiveness and chewiness.

KEYWORDS

- **RTE shrimp**
- **retortable pouch**
- **metal can**
- **texture**

REFERENCES

1. Althen, P. C. The Aluminium Can. *Food Technol.* **1965,** *19*(5), 102–106.
2. Balachandran, K. K. Canning. In *Post-harvest Technology of Fish and Fish Products;* Daya Publishing House: New Delhi, **2001,** pp 158–220.
3. Balachandran, K. K.; Gopal, T. K. S.; Vijayan, P. K. Aluminium Container for Fish Canning. In *Aluminium in Packaging;* Cunha, J. F. D., Ed.; Indian Institute of Packaging: Mumbai, 1998; pp 570–576.
4. Bourne, M. C. Texture Profile Analysis. *Food Technol.* **1978,** *22*, 62–66, 72.

5. Charnley, F. Softness of Canned Salmon. In: Progr. Rept. Canned Salmon Inspection Lab. Can. No. 28, 1936, p 14.
6. Charnley, F.; Bolton, R. S. The Measurement of Firmness of Canned Salmon and Other Semi Rigid Bodies by the Dynamic Penetrometer Method 1. Experiments with a Multiple Needle Penetrometer. *J. Fish. Res. Board Can.* **1938,** *4,* 162–173.
7. Friedman, H. H.; Whitney, J. E.; Szczesniak, A. S. The Texturometer—A New Instrument for Objective Texture Measurement. *J. Food Sci.* **1963,** *28,* 390–396.
8. Gargoming, N.; Astier-Dumas, M. Aluminium Content of Foods: Raw Food, Canned Foods in Steel or Aluminium Cans. *Medecine-et-Nutrition* **1995,** *31*(5), 253–256.
9. Gopakumar, K. Retortable Pouch Processing. In *Fish Packaging Technology;* Concept publishing company: New Delhi, 1993; pp 113–131.
10. Gopakumar, K.; Gopal, T. K. S. Retort Pouch Packaging. Packaging India, Apr-June: 1987, 3–4.
11. Griffin, R. C., Jr. Retortable Plastic Packaging. In *Modern Processing, Packaging and Distribution Systems of Food;* Paine, F. A., ed.; AVI Publishing Co. Inc.: West port, Connecticut, New York, 1987; pp 1–19.
12. Griffin, R. C., Jr.; Sacharow, S. Packaging Materials. In *Principle of package development;* AVI Publishing Co. Inc.: West port, Connecticut, New York, 1972; pp 23–58.
13. Howard, A. J. *Canning Technology;* J and A Churchill Ltd.: London, 1949; p. 264.
14. Hu, K. H.; Nelson, A.; Legault, R. R.; Steinberg, M. P. Feasibility of Using Plastic Film Packages for Heat Processed Foods. *Food Technol.* **1955,** *19*(9), 236–240.
15. Ishitani, T.; Hirata, T.; Matsushita, K.; Hirose, K.; Kodani, N.; Ueda, K.; Yanai, S.; Kumura, S. The Effects of Oxygen Permeability of Pouch, Storage Temperature and Light on the Quality Change of a Retortable Pouched Food During Storage. *J. Food Sci. Technol.* **1980,** *27*(3), 118–124.
16. Jowitt, R. The Terminology of Food Texture. *J. Texture Stud.* **1974,** *5,* 351–358.
17. Lahiri, A. Aluminium Rigid Containers for Processed Foods. *Packag. India.* **1992,** *3,* 19–27.
18. Lakhsminarayan, S. Aluminium—The Packaging Tomorrow. *Packag. India.* **1992,** *24*(5), 33–34.
19. Lampi, R. A. Microbial Recontamination in Flexible Films. *Act. Rep. Res. Dev. Assoc. Mil. Food Packag. Sys.* **1967,** *19*(1), 51–58.
20. Lampi, R. A. Flexible Packaging for Thermoprocessed Foods. *Adv. Food Res.* **1977,** *23,* 306–426.
21. Leung, H. K. The Retort Pouch. In *Economics and Management of Food Processing;* Greig, W. S., ed.; AVI Publishing Co. Inc.: Westport, Connecticut, New York, 1984; pp 219–222.
22. Lopez, A.; Jimenez, M. A. Canning Fruits and Vegetable Products in Aluminium Container. *Food Technol.* **1969,** *23*(10), 1200–1206.
23. Mahadeviah, M. Plastic Containers for Processed Food Products. *Indian Food Packer* **1976,** *30*(4), 35–46.
24. Mahadeviah, M.; Gowramma, R. V. Aluminium Container. In *Food packaging materials;* Tata Mc Graw-Hill Publishing Company Ltd.: New Delhi, 1996; pp 73–83.
25. Meilgaard, M. C.; Civille, G. V.; Carr, B. T. Sensory Evaluation Techniques, 3rd ed.; CRC Press Ltd.: Boca Raton, Florida, 1999; p. 416.

26. Mermeistein, N. H. Retort Pouch Earns 1978 IFT Food Technology Industrial Achievement Award. *Food Technol.* **1978**, *32,* 22–23, 26, 30, 32–33.
27. Mohan, C. O.; Ravi Shankar, C. N.; Bindu, J.; Geethalakshmi, V.; Srinivasa Gopal, T. K. Effect of Thermal Processing on Texture and Subjective Sensory Characteristics of Prawn Kuruma in Retortable Pouches and Aluminium Cans. *J. Food Sci.* **2006,** *71*(6), S496–500.
28. Mohan, C.O.; Ravi Shankar, C. N.; Srinivasa Gopal, T. K.; Bindu, J. Thermal Processing of Prawn Kuruma in Retortable Pouches and Aluminium Cans. *Int. J. Food Sci. Technol.* **2008,** *43,* 200–207.
29. Naresh, R.; Mahadeviah, M.; Gowramma, R. V. Electrochemical Studies of Aluminium with Model Solutions and Vegetables. *J. Food. Sci. Technol.* **1988,** *25*(3), 121–124.
30. Ranau, R.; Oehlenschlaeger, J.; Steinhart, H. Aluminium Content of Stored Industrially Manufactured Canned Herring Products. *Archiv-fuer-lebensmittelhygiene.* **2001,** *52*(6), 135–139.
31. Rangarao, G. C. P. Retortable Plastic Packaging for Thermo—Processed Foods. *J. Indian Food Ind.* **1992,** *11*(6), 25–32.
32. Rubinate, F. J. Army's Obstacle Course Yields a New Look in Food Packaging. *Food Technol.* **1964,** *18*(11), 71–74.
33. Schulz, G. L. Test Procedures and Performance Values Required to Assure Reliability. In *Proceeding of the symposium on flexible packaging for heat processed foods.* Nat. Acad. Sci-Natl. Res. Counc. Washington DC, 1973; pp 71–82.
34. Sigurgisladottir, S.; Torrissen, O.; Lie, O.; Thomassen, M.; Hafsteinsson, H. Salmon Quality: Methods to Determine the Quality Parameters. *Rev. Fish. Sci.* **1997,** *5,* 223–252.
35. Srivatsa, A. N.; Ramakrishna, A.; Gopinathan, V. K.; Nataraju, S.; Leela, R. K.; Jayaraman, K. S.; Sankaran, R. Suitability of Indigenously Fabricated Aluminium Cans for Canning of Indian Foods. *J. Food Sci. Technol.* **1993,** *30*(6), 429–434.
36. Stumbo, C. R. *Thermobacteriology in Food Processing,* 2nd ed.; Academic Press. Inc.: New York, 1973; p 329.
37. Szezesniak, A. S. Classification of Textural Characteristics. *J. Food Sci.* **1963,** *28,* 385.
38. Yamaguchi, K. Retortable Packaging. In *Food packaging;* Academic Press, Inc.: New York, 1990; pp 185–211.

CHAPTER 19

WORKING OUT OF AN OPTIMUM CONFIGURATION OF A SCRUBBER FOR THE INTENSIFICATION OF THE PROCESS OF CLEARING OF GAS EMISSIONS

R. R. USMANOVA[1,*] and G. E. ZAIKOV[2]

[1]*Ufa State Technical University of Aviation, Ufa 450000, Bashkortostan, Russia*

[2]*N. M. Emanuel Institute of Biochemical Physics, Russian Academy of Sciences, Moscow 119991, Russia*

[*]Corresponding author. E-mail: Usmanovarr@mail.ru

CONTENTS

ABSTRACT

In this chapter an optimum configuration of a scrubber for the intensification of the process of clearing of industrial gas emissions is reviewed in detail.

19.1 INTRODUCTION

In the modern chemical industry, for conduction of mass transfer processes, various types of devices with multiphase systems and direct contact of phases have found application. The heterogeneous processes proceeding in system "gas–liquid–solid" take a special place among other processes, after all speed of their leakage is defined by regularity of a mass transport and heat between cooperating phases. Various ways of clearing of gas emissions refer to such processes.[2]

One of the most effective methods of realization of mass transfer processes at direct contact of phases is application of the weighed layer. The basic advantages of such hydrodynamic system are noted in works of domestic and foreign scientists.[1]

Despite numerous advantages, apparatuses with the classical weighed layer are characterized by a row of defects: irregularity of a dwell time of a dispersoid and low stability of a layer in a wide range of change of loadings on liquid, firm, and gas phases.

In such devices, the intensification of proceeding processes for the account of simple turbulization of streams is essentially restricted, as it is accompanied by raise of intensity of physical effect on a dispersoid. Besides, the increase in working speed of a gas phase results not only in increase in intensity of work of the weighed layer but also to raise power expenses for functioning of such system. It is necessary to note that increment of intensity of work of the weighed layer is not so intensive, as increment of expenses of energy on dispersoid weighting.

Implementation of new forms of the organization of mutual motion of streams (at conservation of principles of contact of phases in a suspension) would allow to intensify machining of dispersion materials without substantial growth of expenses of energy a perspective heading of development of mass transfer processes in heterogeneous systems.

Now, the use of twirled streams gains the increasing extension in mass transfer processes.[2,4] The twisting of streams allows to raise essentially intensity of their leakage for the account of the presence of velocity gradients, intensive mixing, and enough high extent of a turbulization of streams.

Among variety of ways of an intensification of processes of applied chemistry, the twisting of streams is one of the most simple and widespread ways. It is possible to explain it by the use of twirled streams leading to betterment of efficiency of a mass transfer, and also leveling of temperature drops and stabilization of currents.

In dedusters, the twisting of a stream by means of various devices (air swirlers) affects all characteristics of a field of a current on the large-scale, and consequently, and mass transfer. The characteristic for the twirled streams, three dimensionality of a field of speed, and comparability of tangential and axial blending agents of speed cause formation of a three-dimensional field of pressure with the transverse and the longitudinal gradients. Thanks to presence of the transverse components of full speed—tangential and the radial—the convective carrying over of a pulse, energy, and weight fade-ins and the whirlwind formation of the internal twirled streams changes. Therefore, necessary properties in technical applications of the twirled currents also are connected with it, expressed in their ability to intensify mass transfer processes, to level down local temperature inhomogeneity at the expense of the convective mixing.[2]

Whirlwind apparatuses possess the big specific productivity and smaller gabarits. It is also possible to combine simultaneously some processes in them (for example, clearing and cooling).[5]

For implementation of control mechanisms by a mechanical trajectory and a dispersoid dwell(ing) time in a deduster, it is necessary to study hydrodynamic characteristics of motion of the monophase and two-phase twirled streams in its swept volume. The use of computer modeling at the research of hydrodynamics of vortex flows allows to make selection of an optimum configuration of working space and an air swirler build. Results of modeling allow selecting an optimum build of an air swirler at the initial stage of researches before experiment conducting on the natural sample.[3]

In the conditions of considerable abbreviation of financing of scientific researches and funds of development of manufactures, experimental works on creation of new production engineering are rather inconvenient.

In this connection, the problem of development and perfection of numerical methods of research of hydrodynamics becomes especially actual.

19.2   THEORETICAL BASES OF MODELING

Analytical and numerical methods of calculation can be applied to the description of hydrodynamic characteristics of motion of streams in working space of a deduster.

The description of motion of the twirled stream is based on an analytical method from one of the following approaches:[6]

1. The stream is represented in the form of superposition of a flat current on potential twirl. The design procedure is based on the use of empirical factors, and it provides only water resistance definition.
2. Bernoulli's theorem application: the presence of an extreme as one of the components of speed of the twirled stream at conservation along the radius of working chamber of an angular momentum. An approach defect—a coarse schematization of a current, absence of the account of features of motion of streams in an axial zone of the working chamber.
3. The use of Bernoulli's theorem for the description of motion of a liquid in the chamber of spiral type. This method demands preliminary definition of the characteristics depending on geometry of the working chamber, it does not allow to define all components of full speed.

The specified defects reduce the scope of these methods for the description and calculation of vortex flows.

Separately gate out a method in which the description of axisymmetric motion of a gas stream with twirl is based on the application of system of differential Navier–Stokes equations (Eq. 19.1), mean field on Reynolds, and continuity equations of a stream (Eq. 19.2):[6]

$$\frac{1}{r}\left[\frac{\partial}{\partial r}\left(r\rho v_r v_r\right)+\frac{\partial}{\partial r}\left(r\rho v_r v_z\right)\right]=\frac{1}{r}\left[\frac{\partial}{\partial r}\left(r\mu_T\frac{\partial v_r}{\partial r}\right)+\frac{\partial}{\partial z}\left(r\mu_T\frac{\partial v r}{\partial z}\right)\right]$$

$$-\frac{\partial P}{\partial r}-\mu_T\frac{\rho v_r}{r^2}+\frac{\rho v^2\varphi}{r}$$

$$\frac{1}{r}\left[\frac{\partial}{\partial r}\left(r\rho v_r v_\varphi\right)+\frac{\partial}{\partial z}\left(r\rho v_z v_\varphi\right)\right]=\frac{1}{r}\left[\frac{\partial}{\partial r}\left(r\mu_T\frac{\partial v_\varphi}{\partial r}\right)+\frac{\partial}{\partial z}\left(r\mu_T\frac{\partial v_\varphi}{\partial z}\right)\right] \quad (19.1)$$

$$-\mu_T\frac{\rho v_\varphi}{r^2}-\frac{\rho v_\varphi v_r}{r}$$

$$\frac{1}{r}\left[\frac{\partial}{\partial r}\left(r\rho v_r v_z\right)+\frac{\partial}{\partial z}\left(r\rho v_z v_z\right)\right]=\frac{1}{r}\left[\frac{\partial}{\partial r}\left(r\mu_T\frac{\partial v_z}{\partial r}\right)+\frac{\partial}{\partial z}\left(r\mu_T\frac{\partial v_z}{\partial z}\right)\right]$$

$$-\frac{\partial P}{\partial z}$$

$$dev\ \rho\vec{v}=0 \quad (19.2)$$

where v_z, v_r, v_φ are the components of speed on an axis; P, ρ, μ are pressure, density, and turbulent viscosity of a stream.

For the solution of the equations, the two-parametric model of turbulence κ—ε, for which two additional transport equations were solved, defining κ—turbulent kinetic energy of a gas phase and ε—speed of a dissipation of turbulent energy was used:

$$\frac{\partial\rho_c k_c}{\partial t}\alpha_c+\frac{\partial\rho_c u_c k_c}{\partial x_j}\alpha_c=\tau_{ij}\frac{\partial u_c}{\partial x_j}\alpha_c-\alpha_c\cdot\rho_c\cdot\varepsilon_c$$

$$+\frac{\partial}{\partial x_j}\left[\alpha_c\left(\mu_c+\frac{\mu_c^t}{\sigma_k}\right)\frac{\partial k_c}{\partial x_j}\right]$$

$$\frac{\partial\rho_c\varepsilon_c}{\partial t}\alpha_c+\frac{\partial\rho_c u_c\varepsilon_c}{\partial x_j}\alpha_c=C_{\varepsilon1}\frac{\varepsilon_c}{k_c}\tau_{ij}\frac{\partial u_c}{\partial x_j}-C_{\varepsilon1}\frac{\varepsilon_c^2}{k_c} \quad (19.3)$$

$$+\frac{\partial}{\partial x_j}\left[\alpha_c\left(\mu_c+\frac{\mu_c^t}{\sigma_\varepsilon}\right)\frac{\partial\varepsilon_c}{\partial x_j}\right]$$

$$\mu_c^t=C_\mu\cdot\rho_c\cdot\frac{k_c^2}{\varepsilon}.$$

where σ_κ, σ_ε—a turbulent Prandtl number for the kinetic energy and dissipation equations, accordingly; μ_c and μ^t_c—molecular and turbulent viscosity of gas, accordingly; τ_{ij}—blending agents of tensor the voltage accepted:

$$C_\mu = 0.09; \ C_{\varepsilon 1} = 1.44; \ C_{\varepsilon 2} = 1.92; \ \sigma_k = 1.0; \ \sigma_\varepsilon = 1.3$$

This method allows spending full definition of hydrodynamic characteristics of motion of streams. However, it is mostly applicable for laminar flows.

Generally, the system of Navier–Stokes equations and continuity of a stream have nonlinear character; they have no general analytical solution without introduction of certain simplifications and assumptions.

Modeling of turbulent flows by the quantitative solution of the Navier–Stokes equations, which have been written down for instant speeds, is an indeterminate problem today.

However, for the solution of separate problems, there is possibly an application of this fundamental equation of hydrodynamics at performance with some conditions:

- Work with the values of speeds averaged on a time at modeling of turbulent flows;
- Sampling of the coordinate system, as much as possible fulfilling a case study and facilitating record of the equations.

Definition of the efficiency of separation was made by two methods:

1. As the share of corpuscles that are carried away by a liquid from total of a dust, arriving with gas:

$$\eta = \frac{L \cdot \rho_g \left(C_k - C_n\right)}{G \cdot \rho_1 \cdot C_n} \tag{19.4}$$

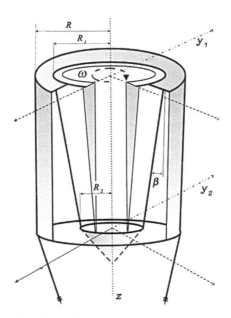

FIGURE 19.1 The analytical model.

The value of an average concentration has been defined from the material balance equation:

$$C_y = C_n + 2\frac{G}{L}\cdot\frac{\rho_1}{\rho_g}\cdot\frac{C_{xn}}{R_2^2 - R_1^2}\int\limits_{R_1/\sin\beta}^{R_2/\sin\beta} y\left(1-e^{-B\cdot b}\right)dy \qquad (19.5)$$

R_1—An element of a conic air swirler;
R_2—An apex of a conic air swirler (Fig. 19.1).

$$\eta_u = \frac{2}{1-m^2}\int\limits_m^1 t_1\left(1-e^{-T}\right)dt,$$

where

$$T = \frac{3}{4}\frac{\rho_g}{\rho_1}\frac{L}{G}\frac{(1-\chi)\varepsilon}{\chi_k}\eta_K\frac{1-m^2}{d_k}\frac{t_1}{t_1^2-m^2}\frac{\sin\beta}{R_2} \qquad (19.6)$$

For modeling conducting to solve the specified equations conveniently numerical methods (discrete element method (DEM)), defining instead of the continuous solution a discrete set of required values in a certain place (a mesh, grid knot) spaces (at a stationary regime of motion of streams).[1] For achievement of the maximum accuracy of the solution, such way of representation of discrete values for this digitization matches to analogues of the algebraic equations is chosen. As a result, the mathematical problem of the solution of system of the differential or integrated equations can be reduced to a problem of the solution of system of the algebraic equations. In practice, various models of the numerical solution of the classical equations of hydrodynamics for turbulent flows with which that or other success are used in various cases, however, have the merits and demerits:[1] direct numerical simulation (DNS), Reynolds-averaged Navier–Stokes (RANS), large eddy simulation (LES).

The further simplification of system of the Equations (19.1–19.3) for modeling of a vortex flow of gas phase in working space of a deduster was possibly at use of such assumptions:

- Presence of a dominating heading of a current along which the axial component of speed of a gas stream everywhere positive and much more exceeds the radial is supposed.
- The component of traverse speed of a gas stream in an axial heading varies much more slowly than in the radial.
- Magnitudes of speeds and pressure in each elementary volume of a gas stream depend only on conditions more low on a stream and do not depend on conditions above on a stream.

These assumptions allow to carry out the analysis of usages of components in the Equations (19.1–19.3) and to bounce those from those which do not render appreciable effect on result of calculation.

19.3   VISUALIZATION OF RESULTS OF CALCULATION

All space of a scrubber has been covered and is final difference grid, according to Figure 19.2. In grid knots, unknown values of speed and pressure were defined. Integration was spent for one mid-flight pass from entrance to target cross section of working space of the apparatus.

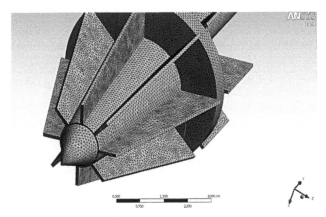

FIGURE 19.2 The settlement grid.

Each knot of a grid is characterized by the heading of a projection of speed of a stream: the radial v_r, tangential v_φ, and axial v_z. Transition between knots is carried out in steps by means of replacement of speeds of a stream or by finding their intermediate value between knots by means of interpolation. Such statement of a regional problem has allowed to implement a sticking condition on each step and, is analogous to a condition for functions ψ and ω, to install it on different boundary lines.

Results of computer modeling of hydrodynamics of a multiphase stream (characteristic pictures of streamlines) in working space of a deduster are presented in Figure 19.3.

The weak twisting $\omega_0 = 15$ c^{-1} (Fig. 19.3(a)) slightly influences character of a current which is close to a usual tangential twisting of a stream; the increase in a twisting to $\omega_0 = 50$ c^{-1} leads to formation of zones of recirculation near to a twirled air swirler, streamlines form a bend. Extent of such zone considerably increases with increase in a Reynolds number and at the further increase in a twisting to $\omega_0 = 100$ c^{-1} (Fig. 19.3(b)) leads to displacement of the center of area of recirculation and an elongation of a zone of a backward flow in axial and radial headings.

The qualitative picture which has been had theoretically will be well coordinated with known experimental data; a divergence, depending on a flow, fluctuates over the range from 4% to 7%. The obtained results are used in the equations of motion of corpuscles for definition of expected efficiency of process of clearing of gas emissions.

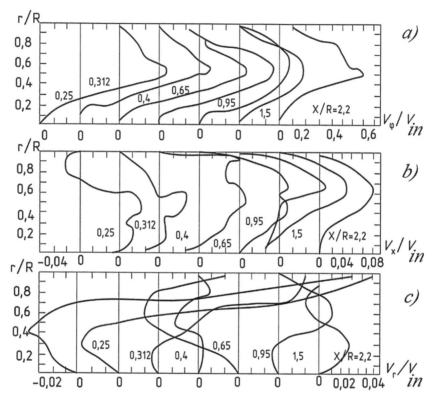

FIGURE 19.3   Streamlines.

It is installed in such a way that in detached flows, considerable pressure decrease both in comparison with a main stream and in a zone of guide vanes of an air swirler is observed. Irregularity of static-making pressures in a scrubber reduces an effect on efficiency of clearing. By comparing empirical data on separation efficiency, it is revealed that decrease in efficiency of separation does not exceed 3%, though on level of irregularity of a pressure pattern a difference is more considerable. It is possible to explain that irregularity of pressure is compensated by positive effect of zones of the breakaway promoting separation of small impurity from main current in a zone of a rarefaction and their removal on a helicoid path from working space, and further on the walls of a conic part of the apparatus in the sludge remover.

The vanes air swirler which has been in the central part of the apparatus considerably complicates a picture of a current of a gas-dispersed stream in a dynamic spray scrubber. It is installed as such that as a result of a turbulent diffusion, dust corpuscles will concentrate at apparatus walls and not on a dense bed, and in the form of the loosened concentrated gas-dispersed ring. On apparatus walls, the showered dust layer is not formed; dust accumulations are localized in a ring wall layer of a certain thickness in the form of braids. The air swirler promotes the formation of spiral dust braids, at dust passage through shovels; there is a concentration of corpuscles on peripheral area of blades. The vanes air swirler divides a homogeneous stream into a row of concurrent flows with an interleaving of the impoverished and enriched concentration of a dust.

In Figure 19.4, visualization of motion of streams is presented at a configuration of working space.

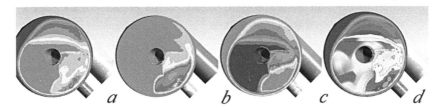

FIGURE 19.4   Pouring of a field of speeds of a gas stream in working space.

At air swirler installation:

$$a - \alpha = 30°, n = 3; b - \alpha = 30°, n = 8; c - \alpha = 60°, n = 3; d - \alpha = 60°, n - 8$$

At air swirler installation, the increase in speed of a gas stream at walls is observed, and in the apparatus center, there are zones of underspeeds. The increase in a slope of blades is accompanied by increase in stagnation zones.

The analysis of results of researches has allowed to define regularity of the effect of a build of an air swirler on distribution of traverse speed of a gas stream.

Air swirler configuration:

- With increase in a slope of blades, the peripheral velocity of a gas stream on cross section of working space decreases.
- With increase in a slope of blades, chaotic eddying of a gas stream at the switching centre is formed.

- With increase in number of blades, there is a nonuniform velocity distribution—speed of a gas stream at an entry is much more than at an exit from the apparatus.
- With increase in a slope of blades, the big areas of stagnation zones of a dust are formed.

Configuration of working space:

- At a configuration of working space in the form of the cylinder irregularity of distribution of a peripheral velocity of a gas stream—speed at an entry is much more than at an exit from the apparatus, and in the center underspeed zones are formed.
- At a configuration of working space in the form of a cone, speed of a gas stream considerably increases in the process of passage of working space of the apparatus.

19.4   CONCLUSIONS

The analytical model of a current of the gas-dispersed stream is devised, allowing to design distributions of all blending agent of speed U'_φ, U'_r, U'_x, and also current functions $\psi\,(r,\,z)$ and to build a characteristic flow pattern of a current in bundled software Ansys CFX.

The analysis of results of researches has allowed to define regularity of the effect of a build of an air swirler on distribution of traverse speed of a gas stream and formation of zones of a return current.

Results of scaling of streamlines and velocity profiles in various cross sections of the apparatus are obtained. Visualization of the results of calculation has allowed to conduct research on motion of gas in a wide range of change of flow parameters and to develop a scrubber build.

Thus, the obtained results of research of hydrodynamics of vortex flows allow to make selection of an optimum configuration of working space, a build of an air swirler and its guide vanes. Necessary efficiency of separation of fine fractions of a dust is thus secured.

KEYWORDS

- **boundary problem**
- **inertial devices**
- **mathematical model**
- **computational grid**
- **twist flow**
- **streamlines**

REFERENCES

1. Artyukhov, A. E. Computer Simulation of Vortex Flow. *Hydrodyn. J. Manuf. Ind. Eng.* **2013**, *12*, 25–29.
2. Kouzov, I. A.; Malgin, V. A.; Skryabin, A. D. Dust Element of Gases and Air in a Chemical Industry. L: Chemistry, 2002.
3. Usmanova, R. R. Dynamic Gas Washer. Patent for the Invention of the Russian Federation, U.S. Patent 2,339,435, Nov 20, 2008; The Bulletin No. 33.
4. Usmanova, R. R.; Zaikov, G. E. Choice of Boundary Conditions to Calculating Parameters Movement of Gas-Dispersion Streams (in Russian), *Enciklopedia Ingenera-Chimika* **2015**, *3*(37), 36–42.
5. Usmanova, R. R.; Zaikov, G. E. The Modern Approach to Modelling and Calculation of Efficiency of Process of a Gas Cleaning (in Canada), *Chem. Eng. Chemoinf.* **2016**, *3*, 36–42.
6. Usmanova, R. R.; Zhernakov, V. S. Simulation and Research of Factors Affecting Aerodynamic Indices of the Gas Purification Process (in Russian), *Vestnik SGAU*, **2014**, *1*(43), 173–180.

INDEX

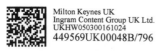

9 781774 630723